Assert

For Churchill Livingstone:

Commissioning Editor Susan Young
Development Editor Catherine Jackson
Project Controller Morven Dean
Designer Judith Wright

Assertive Outreach

A Strengths Approach to Policy and Practice

Peter Ryan DProf MSc CQSW

Professor of Mental Health, Middlesex University
Chair of Mental Health Academic Group
Chair of ENTER Mental Health

Steve Morgan BA BPL DipCOT MA

Independent Mental Health Consultancy, 'Practice-Based Evidence', London

FOREWORD BY
Charles A Rapp PhD

Professor, University of Kansas

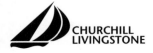
CHURCHILL
LIVINGSTONE

EDINBURGH   LONDON   NEW YORK   OXFORD   PHILADELPHIA   ST LOUIS   SYDNEY   TORONTO   2004

CHURCHILL LIVINGSTONE
An imprint of Elsevier Limited

First published 2004

ISBN 0 443 07375 9

British Library Cataloguing in Publication Data
A catalogue record for this book is available from the British Library

Library of Congress Cataloging in Publication Data
A catalog record for this book is available from the Library of Congress

Notice
Medical knowledge is constantly changing. Standard safety precautions must be followed, but as new research and clinical experience broaden our knowledge, changes in treatment and drug therapy may become necessary or appropriate. Readers are advised to check the most current product information provided by the manufacturer of each drug to be administered to verify the recommended dose, the method and duration of administration, and contraindications. It is the responsibility of the practitioner, relying on experience and knowledge of the patient, to determine dosages and the best treatment for each individual patient. Neither the Publisher nor the authors assume any liability for any injury and/or damage to persons or property arising from this publication.

The Publisher

ELSEVIER SCIENCE your source for books, journals and multimedia in the health sciences

www.elsevierhealth.com

The publisher's policy is to use **paper manufactured from sustainable forests**

Printed in China

Contents

Foreword

This volume is a clarion call for policy and practice to be intelligent and coherent, and anchored by the well-being of the people we are serving. Ryan and Morgan suggest that as long as we stay in the muck and mire of problems, pathology and weakness, assertive outreach cannot help clients achieve. Until we throw off the 'conspiracy of understanding' that centres on deficits, we cannot effectively help.

In the history of mental health, the diagnosis of schizophrenia or other major mental illness was accompanied by a prognosis of life-long disability. For example, in a recent New Zealand study, all the subjects diagnosed with bipolar disorders were told that they would never be well and would always have to rely on medication. In many ways, mental health systems have institutionalized low expectations whereby clients needed to be protected from life and sheltered from stress. Jobs and careers, school and college degrees, apartments and homes were thought to be not only impossible but would lead to acceleration of symptoms.

The last twenty years has produced considerable evidence that major mental illness does not necessarily mean lifelong disability. Three separate bodies of research support the proposition that people with psychiatric disabilities can and often do recover. The first body of research is comprised of seven long-term longitudinal studies in four countries of people with major mental illness. These studies followed clients from 22 to 37 years and found that the average percentage of people who recovered or improved significantly was 55.4 percent. This was true even within systems that were underdeveloped or regressive.

The second body of research is comprised of the thousands of first-person accounts of recovery and ethnographic studies of people's lived experience. These accounts compellingly document the ability of people with psychiatric disabilities to overcome the despair, withdrawal, and alienation caused by this mean-spirited condition and (too often) the services that we have created 'to help'. These are stories of people who have achieved a place they call home, a job that brings satisfaction and income, rich social networks, and opportunities to contribute to others. The third body of research is the intervention research. Through well-controlled experiments, practices are being identified that are successful in helping users avoid psychiatric hospitalization, become employed, reduce dependence on substances, and achieve stable housing.

Despite this corpus of evidence, the policy and resultant practice of the UK, like many countries, continues to focus on 'protection and safety' with its preoccupation with monitoring, resource management and review of needs. Ryan and Morgan argue that (paradoxically) the best route to safety may be the one that seeks to empower users, not control them, which seeks to help them create a better and more fulfilling life.

Their model of practice combines a set of values with evidence-based practices. While the centrepiece of their approach is a strengths model of care, they employ features more commonly associated with assertive community treatment, and skillfully integrate motivational interviewing and the stages of change. They also include a wide range of psychosocial interventions that have evidence of effectiveness.

The strengths model is not just being nice to clients or positively reframing their difficulties and deficiencies, foibles and failures. It is, in fact, an approach that requires new skills, new tools and new perspectives. The practice methods described by the authors make it accessible to a wide variety of people and this same clarity helps unmask the complexity of the work.

This book is analytic and practical. The case examples bring life to the methods. The strengths assessment and case planning tools are here for practitioners to adopt. Checklists and specific guidelines are present for supervisor use.

Every once in a while a book comes along that provides a picture of hope and a path to its achievement. A book that acknowledges the struggle of people with psychiatric disabilities and those of the people who seek to help, but depicts a way out of the oppressive day-to-day existence. This volume does it with clarity and sophistication.

Charles A. Rapp, PhD.
Kansas, USA

Acknowledgements

The creation of a text of this nature arises from the passions and dedication of a cast that stretches way beyond its authors. We are indebted to many people, for their imagination, innovation, and practical help and support throughout our personal journeys of the last few years.

In the first instance, we wish to acknowledge Charlie Rapp for his inspirational development of the Strengths Model of Case Management in the USA since 1982, and for his time and interest in introducing the ideas to the Research and Development for Psychiatry (subsequently Sainsbury Centre for Mental Health) case management project from 1991. This work had a seismic influence on the thinking and practice of the authors of this text.

Regarding the continuing development of a strengths approach to policy and practice in the UK, we particularly wish to acknowledge the contributions of Andrew Bleach. A former colleague of ours in the Sainsbury Centre for Mental Health, his humanitarian approach to his work in developing case management practice has influenced us both immensely.

Two teams have provided a strong practical basis for some of the ideas emerging in this book: Kettering Assertive Outreach Team (Northamptonshire) in the statutory sector, and Julian Housing Active Outreach Team (Norwich) in the voluntary sector. The dedication and love for their work across these two teams has offered invaluable insights into the power of a strengths approach in practice. For this we specifically acknowledge Sue Jugon, Diane Cooke, Tony Torok, Sam Smith, Nigel Collins and Viv Robey in Kettering, and Anne McCrudden, Jayne Burchell, Peter McGuiness, Robby Lewry, Carrie Horgan and Adrian Dicks in Norwich. We wish also to thank Debbie Green, now of the Sainsbury Centre and College of Occupational Therapists, for being an inspirational strengths team leader and practitioner.

Several people have also made significant contributions through their reviews of draft chapters of this book. Without exception, we have been fortunate to receive positive and constructive contributions to our work. We specifically wish to thank and acknowledge the following people for their undoubted understanding and connections to the strengths approach:

- Neville Pettitt, Team Leader Daventry Community Mental Health Team (Northamptonshire)
- Sara Tiplady, Joint Team Leader FOCUS Homeless Outreach Team (Camden and Islington Mental Health and Social Care Trust)
- Toby Williamson, Mental Health Foundation
- Kim Woodbridge, Sainsbury Centre for Mental Health
- Perry Marshall, Julian Housing City Team Manager (Norwich).

Introduction

"Ordinary people have suddenly come out with the most amazing statements, when they find the courage"

Zeldin 1998

What gives you the most sense of enjoyment in your life? What do you enjoy most about your work? Do we make real attempts to ask these simple questions, either of the people requiring, or providing, mental health services? Do we ask our practitioners whether the things they are good at in their personal lives can be translated into the tasks of their working lives? Our preoccupation with problems and deficits is very strongly culturally ingrained into society's thinking, particularly in relation to people experiencing severe and enduring mental distress (Rapp 1998). By focusing our attention on helping people to improve on their areas of greatest deficit, we do little more than achieve mediocrity at best (Buckingham and Clifton 2002). For the potential of promoting greater achievement in people, we need to engage with and help develop individual capabilities, rather than inabilities – this is the 'strengths approach'.

We may consider that we acknowledge people's strengths but all too often it is as an aside to the attempted resolution of problems, or simply as an undeveloped observation from previous interactions, or even as a defensive statement when we feel challenged about not doing so. We are frightened that the problem or deficit left unchallenged will result in a catastrophe, with the responsibility laid clearly on us for not having averted the dangers in the first place. This appears to be the culture driven by most of our organizations in response to a wider blame culture in society. Government policy and mental health services place a huge emphasis upon practitioners to eliminate risks by being more cautious and defensive in their approach to their work. We are committed to an approach to assertive outreach emphasizing positive risk taking (see Chapter 11). We hope that such an approach will lead to energized, skilled and motivated practitioners who are less likely to be caught out by the complex, demanding and high-risk circumstances that assertive outreach practitioners typically face.

Many users have disengaged from mental health services, often because of the kind of experiences illustrated above. They feel that their needs are not properly understood or that services are not set up in a way to respond appropriately, particularly seeing them solely as problems without any recognition of them as people with achievements and further potential. For others, there is the reality of being disconnected from their experiences, misinterpreting or denying the nature of difficulties they are experiencing. Consequently, they retreat from services or become hostile to the traditional approaches of service-based appointments, set up to discuss the very things they do not believe in. There is also the risk, arguably as great, of mental health practitioners becoming burnt out and disengaged

---

Example

A practitioner meets her supervisor and enthusiastically explains that one of the people she is working with has just disclosed their achievements in music lessons many years ago, which led onto qualifications at school and a place on a graduate music course, which they were ultimately unable to take up. The person now wishes to reconnect with this part of their life by practising on their clarinet and maybe finding other people to hook up with, practising and jamming.

The supervisor replies that this is interesting but not relevant in terms of the current high-risk circumstances: what about the forthcoming care review meeting? Has a medication review been set up? Is the risk assessment up-to-date, particularly in light of the high assessed suicide risk? Didn't the carer say something about being kept awake at night recently, causing a strain in the relationship? Might not this increased strain add to the suicide risk?

Such an approach, typical of a risk minimization perspective, can have the effect of demotivating and limiting the aspirations both of the service user and the practitioner. A positive risk-taking approach might come to different conclusions. Perhaps the care review meeting would be best used for encouraging the person to hold onto their musical ambitions for a while, until they can establish a consistent pattern and structure to their day by attending the day centre. Focusing on the user's musical aspirations might be a good way to distract the user from the inherent strains of her relationship with her mother, decrease contact time with her and help with building her esteem – and thereby also decrease suicide risk.

from services, and who also feel that their needs are not met and that they are not listened to by the services that employ them.

**RATIONALE AND
PURPOSE OF
THE BOOK**

We hope that a strengths approach to assertive outreach will prove an enhancing approach to care for service users and practitioners alike. 'Assertive Outreach' is a rapidly developing form of care in the UK endorsed and financially supported by government policy. It is a controversial form of care, emphasizing the need for service providers to persistently 'reach out' towards the service user. It raises ethical issues as to its best practice, and service users may consequently interpret it in a negative way. *The values and ethical base from which it is carried out therefore seem to us to be crucial.* Assertive Outreach can easily become identified with people considered to have the most difficult and complex of problems, who are the most challenging and risky in their behaviours. Attribution of blame and labels are quickly applied to service users. Far less frequently we consider the role services play themselves in people's decisions to reject those services.

Government policy sees it as a 'safety net' for the community, with the task of engaging these service users in care, to minimize the incidence of self-harm or violence towards others in the community (Ryan 2002). Potentially controversial new legislation could give services such as Assertive Outreach the power to return service users to hospital if the 'risk' in the community is too high and/or they fail to adhere to their treatment in the community.

In Assertive Outreach as in many other areas of mental health care, we can rapidly become bogged down by the language and focus of solving problems for problems' sake, caught up in the seemingly intransigent difficulties of resistant or reluctant people. The motivation of service users to comply, and of service providers to repeatedly offer the same failed interventions can easily become sapped. Zeldin (1998) reminds us "When problems have appeared insoluble ... people have sometimes found a way out by changing the subject of their conversation, or the way they talked." This is reflected in the 'strengths approach', which attempts to develop a collaborative approach to working with the service user, emphasizing the achievement of the service user's own aspirations and building upon the service user's own strengths and resources. Empowering service users can be more easily achieved through a workforce that feels empowered in the first place to work flexibly and creatively. The strengths approach upholds the importance of creating the right conditions and working environment that permits the inherent creative capabilities of practitioners to develop and shine through. This crucial issue of providing an enhancing and strengths-oriented organizational context for Assertive Outreach services is explored further in Part 2 of this book (see Chapter 12).

The intention of this shift of emphasis is further encapsulated by Zeldin's thinking: "When minds meet, they do not just exchange facts; they transform them, reshape them, draw different interpretations from them, engage in new trains of thought. Conversation does not just reshuffle the cards, it creates new cards." In this way, the strengths approach envisages that practitioners can connect with service users in ways that produce new ways of thinking about the role of mental health services. Similarly, when the practitioner meets their supervisor, or colleagues across a team, new thinking should be encouraged, to produce new ideas. It recaptures the humanity of delivering mental health services, which easily becomes lost in a rigid emphasis on research evidence, process and outcomes; this is not to say that the latter do not play their part within this approach.

The purpose of this approach is not to ignore the problems, and the detrimental or devastating consequences of the experiences of severe mental distress – it is to explore radically different ways of connecting with people and connecting them with appropriate services for their needs and wishes. It upholds Assertive Outreach as a proven vehicle for achieving difference but also proposes that the principles and practices outlined throughout this book can and should be applied to practitioners, managers and teams in all other parts of the mental health system.

To return to the initial line of inquiry at the head of this introduction, do we really check that our practitioners have the opportunity to do what they are best at, every day? Do our practitioners routinely ask the service users how they might be helped to do what they are best at, every day? The strong likelihood is that we do not – we are probably too frightened to ask the questions, for fear of the answers. The strengths approach gives us the courage to ask these and many other positive questions.

STRUCTURE OF THE BOOK

The 'strengths approach' primarily applies to working directly and indirectly with service users. However, its application to the different functions of service and practice development make it vital for supporting the daily activity and links between "practitioners–teams–organizations" to differing degrees. The content is simply divided into two parts: 'Policy' and 'Practice', reflecting service development and practice development respectively.

The shorter policy section contains three chapters, broadly setting a context for the strengths approach. Chapter 1 explores some definitions of Assertive Outreach, and arrives at a 'strengths definition'. It also outlines the historical origins and evidence for Assertive Outreach, linking the strengths model to the broader concepts of case management and assertive community treatment. Chapter 2 sets the approach within a contemporary UK policy context, reviewing the emergence and apparent demise of the concept of case management from 1985–91 and 1991–7 respectively, and the emergence of Assertive Outreach since 1997. The potential influences of imminent mental health legislation are briefly considered. Chapter 3 specifically outlines the purpose and principles of a 'strengths approach', building on the ground-breaking work established by Rapp (1998) in the USA.

Part 2 focuses on developing the strengths approach in practice. Chapter 4 examines the ethical dilemmas of an apparently controversial approach to service delivery. Chapter 5 focuses attention on the models of team-working by examining different ways of collaborating to deliver a 'team approach'. Chapters 6 to 11 focus on specific areas of strengths practice: targeting; engagement; assessment; care planning; care co-ordination; working with the service user and broader network; and risk taking. Finally, Chapter 12 explores the issues of implementing good practice through research, training, practice development and reflection.

Where appropriate the book is illustrated with extensive case examples, both of service user situations and from two services closely worked with.

FROM A PROBLEMS-ORIENTED TO A STRENGTHS-ORIENTED APPROACH TO MENTAL HEALTH CARE

We would argue that mental health services are commonly built on a problems-oriented approach to mental health care. Such an approach inherently underpins the clinical process of working with service users from assessment, to care planning, through to the co-ordination and delivery of services. It tends to emphasize, as a point of departure, the psychiatric, relational and social problems, disabilities and difficulties in functioning of the individual service user. Once identified, such dysfunctions are then addressed through a problem-solving process leading, over time, to reducing those disabilities, problems or difficulties.

A strengths approach has a different point of philosophical and epistemological departure. It certainly acknowledges the existence of 'problems and difficulties' *but sees them as barriers and obstacles to be overcome in order that a service user may achieve their wants and aspirations, which they themselves have defined.* A strengths approach is about connecting with service users, and with ourselves as practitioners, in ways that help to unearth our mutual creative potentials and by so doing restoring all that is fun and exciting in our work. An essential part in reconstructing the nature of the task of mental health care is the use of language, and the meanings attached to it.

How we refer to the people who need and use mental health services continues to stimulate debate. Patients, clients, service users and survivors are just some of the terms in frequent use. We are clear that the term 'patients' is the most medical, and applies to the periods of hospital admission in our conceptualization of people in services. Primarily people are 'people', and we will endeavour to use 'people' or 'person' wherever possible. In other instances we will use the term 'service users', acknowledging that it is adopted by many but not all in the service user/survivor movement.

By 'wants' we mean the personally stated aims/ambitions/aspirations expressed by the service user in their own terms and language. By 'problem' we mean a barrier or obstacle (sometimes referred to by services as a dysfunction or disability) which may lie in the service user. However, a 'problem' can equally exist in the service user's social environment or in mental health services itself. Wherever a problem is located, the common outcome is one of rendering it more difficult for the service users to achieve their wants or aspirations.

In the context of Assertive Outreach services, we will use the term 'practitioners' to refer to workers within all parts of the mental health system, largely in relation to the role blurring expected in these progressive teams and services. We accept that workers from all professional backgrounds have the potential to be good strengths practitioners but no single profession lays claim to the exclusive rights in the approach. We are interested in the personal qualities and experience that individuals bring to their work, as much as the professional training and experience.

The term 'community' is widely used in mental health but seems to have little clarity of meaning other than being 'non-hospital'. Changes in society have undermined the formerly strong sense of identity with local community. We will continue to use the phrase 'community mental health' in relation to specific teams and a widely recognized part of the health system, as understood by the predominant readership of this book. However, we are persuaded by the arguments presented by Baldwin (1993) for the closer identity with the term 'neighbourhood' for the majority of service users, and for practitioners when considering their own lives away from the work environment. Neighbourhood is primarily distinguished from community by its smaller size (e.g. 10 000–25 000 as opposed to 100 000–250 000 population) and recognition in relation to local physical and social boundaries and services. The shops, pubs, libraries, post office, primary care practice and housing developments are more clearly related to our concept of neighbourhood. When we consider individuals functioning within their own routines, we need to identify them primarily within a definition of their own neighbourhood. It is the individuals themselves who can best identify their neighbourhood.

'Recovery' is a concept that has been widely accepted in mental health services during recent years but its potential implications are rarely acknowledged. O'Hagan (2002) explains some of the service users' concerns – recovery implying the existence of a mental illness in the first place and that a person accepts that their experiences are something to recover from. We adopt her description of recovery as "... living well in the presence or absence of one's mental illness", developing the concept beyond just the sense of individual process to a wider acceptance of social responsibility, connection to one's own culture, and of hope. (O'Hagan 2002). Smith and Morris (2003) suggest that the holistic approach, a central feature of Assertive Outreach, helps to facilitate a person's progress toward recovery. They argue a belief that personal recovery being possible for all requires sufficient resources and time, in order to challenge the low expectations inherent in, and attributed to, the client group. However, this very stance also seems to embody some of the criticisms of the concept of recovery made by service users such as O'Hagan (2002), that it is largely a service-generated and -owned concept – a play on words to make mental health services appear more user-centred. Through a strengths approach, we believe that the concept of recovery can be more service user led, including engaging, hearing and working with the views of those who feel they have nothing to recover from.

References

Baldwin S 1993 The Myth of Community Care: An alternative neighbourhood model of care. Chapman & Hall, London

Buckingham M, Clifton D O 2002 Now, discover your strengths: how to develop your talents and those of the people you manage. Simon & Schuster, London

O'Hagan M 2002 Living well. Openmind 118: 16–17

Rapp C A 1998 The Strengths Model: Case management with people suffering from severe and persistent mental illness. Oxford University Press, New York

Ryan P 2002 The long arm of outreach. Mental Health Today, December: 20–21

Smith M, Morris M 2003 Recovery teams. Openmind 119: 22–23

Zeldin T 1998 Conversation. Harvill, London

PART 1

A guide to policy

PART CONTENTS

This part of the book focuses on the information necessary for understanding and implementing local policy. It is the area of Assertive Outreach that is primarily concerned with service development issues. For this reason, in the practitioner–team–organization triad, the organizational management is required to exercise a prominent role. However, this is not to say that the contributions of practitioners and teams in relation to policy are any less relevant. The role of organizational management should be to articulate an inspirational 'vision' for the local services, creating the environment for practitioners and teams to feel permitted to explore their creativity in response to the need for a different type of service.

The chapters in this section detail the following aspects of assertive outreach:

- Definitions, historical context and research evidence – identifying a strengths model of case management alongside assertive community treatment as two of the most significant developments from the USA that are influencing service development in the UK.
- Policy background – tracing the development of case management and Assertive Outreach within the context of UK government legislation from 1985 to 2003.
- Purpose and principles – outlining a specific framework for underpinning the strengths approach to practice.

CREATING A DIFFERENCE

A strengths approach to Assertive Outreach emerges as a distinctive style of working, which is very different from the traditional approaches developed in community mental health services. It requires practitioners to adopt attitudes and practices that challenge their more usual ways of thinking and working – to respond to complex needs in more flexible and creative ways. It is not about assuming traditional professional roles under a different team name; neither is it about losing the uniqueness of personal and profession-aligned skills.

Chapter **1**

The origins of and evidence for case management

Peter Ryan

Treat history with respect, soon you will be a part of it

INTRODUCTION

This chapter begins by asking the question: What is Assertive Outreach? We review a variety of definitions and then suggest a 'strengths approach' definition, which we use for the purposes of this book. The chapter then continues with an overview of the origins of case management. Finally, it focuses more specifically on the development and early supporting evidence for two of the most established models: assertive community treatment and the strengths approach. Because much of the later evidence for case management has been with nonspecific models of case management or where the model is not clearly specified, the evidence for case management as a whole is presented in terms of some of its major functions: engagement; assuring safety to self or others; prevention of hospitalization; and social and clinical outcomes.

WHAT IS ASSERTIVE OUTREACH?

One of the difficulties in the literature is that there is enormous variation in how this term is defined. In the UK, the present Labour Government has used the term 'Assertive Outreach' in its White Paper (Department of Health 1998). The National Service Framework for Mental Health (Department of Health 1999) also uses the term and, for the sake of clarity, this is the term that will be used here. However, in the mental health policy and research literature, a number of terms are used almost interchangeably. These include assertive community treatment (ACT), clinical case management and intensive case management.

Definitions

In a useful overview, Onyett (1992) defines Assertive Outreach as "A way of tailoring help to meet individual need through placing the responsibility for assessment and service co-ordination with one individual worker *or* team."

This emphasizes the fact that a central feature of Assertive Outreach is that it both co-ordinates and individualizes care. The care needed by individual clients is carefully and comprehensively assessed, leading to a tailored and unique package of care for each client. This can be done either through one individual being specifically responsible for delivery of the care package *or* for the team as a whole to share responsibility for the effective co-ordination of care.

However, one of the centrally defining aspects of Assertive Outreach is the *context* in which it occurs and the *kind of service user* to whom it is offered. These important aspects of Assertive Outreach are highlighted in the government's own definition in its White Paper on Mental Health Services (Department of Health 1998):

> "Assertive outreach is an active approach to treatment and care for those who are at risk of being readmitted to psychiatric hospital. Such people are typically hard to engage because of their negative experiences of statutory services. Assertive outreach… ensures that treatment is delivered early enough to prevent the patient's condition from worsening."

This definition highlights the proactive nature of Assertive Outreach and that it is designed to operate out of the office base and on the client's own 'territory' in the community – it is not an office-based service. It reaches out to the client rather than expecting the client to reach out to it. Assertive Outreach therefore can be very effective in engaging high-risk clients with complex needs who otherwise might have fallen out of contact with services. Equally, Assertive Outreach is designed to avoid unnecessary hospital admissions, and therefore it helps clients to stay in the community, which is where the great majority of clients wish to stay.

However, the government's own definition leaves out a number of essential features. For example, it talks of 'preventing the patient's condition from deteriorating'. This is very much a minimalist definition of the rehabilitation potential of Assertive Outreach. It misses out the central features: enhancing psychosocial functioning; optimizing quality of life; and assisting in recovery.

In summary, Assertive Outreach is an approach to care that:

- Engages high-risk severely mentally ill service users with complex needs who are resistant to contacting services.
- Proactively reaches out to people in their own 'territory' in the community.
- Assesses need comprehensively, develops individually tailored care packages and effectively co-ordinates care across agencies.
- Optimizes the recovery potential of service users.

> ### A 'strengths–based' definition
>
> Assertive Outreach is a collaborative approach to working with people deemed by services to be high risk, with complex needs, and hard to engage in and/or rejecting those services. It emphasizes flexible and creative ways of responding to complex and longterm needs, in a way that combines a quick and immediate response to needs together with a longterm commitment to care. It seeks to enhance the service users' capacities to define and meet their needs and aspirations within their own local neighbourhoods.

ORIGINS OF CASE MANAGEMENT

The need for such an approach as case management first became apparent in the USA in the 1960s and 1970s as a creative response to the historic trend away from institutionally based hospital services and towards care in the community. This historic shift, which has taken place in all developed countries (Rose 2001), was undoubtedly stimulated by the discovery in the 1950s of a whole new range of psychotropic drugs, which were effective in controlling some of the major acute symptoms of schizophrenia and other major mental disorders. This meant that mental hospitals could manage acute episodes far more rapidly and effectively than before, and that service users could therefore be discharged back into the community at a far earlier stage. At around the same time the publication of highly influential sociological critiques of mental hospitals, such as Goffman's *Asylums* (1961), rapidly convinced policymakers and service planners that mental hospitals were in any case noxious and custodial institutions to which service users should be exposed as little as possible.

This encouraged the rapid but almost random development of a vast array of services in the community for mental health service users. Mental hospitals had become a discredited form of care, yet did offer a kind of seamless, co-ordinated care in a designated geographical location. Community care on the other hand was bewilderingly complex. Where users lived might be many miles away from where they collected their welfare benefit, which again would be a long way from a community mental health centre, which users might need to attend during the day – 'community care' had an inbuilt tendency to become disjointed and fragmentary. The implication of this was that the existence of a service in the community did not necessarily mean that it would be used, particularly by severely disabled clients who often found accessing such diverse and fragmented services more of a challenge than they could manage.

It began to be apparent that severely institutionalized service users, with longterm and severe disabilities, were also substantially disadvantaged in the community. Service users often lived in poverty and severe social isolation and were subject to being stigmatized and rejected by the neighbourhood where they lived. Community services were patchy and poorly integrated, and service users themselves were often at a loss to know how to access them effectively. Also, a board and lodging house in the community was not necessarily more humane or any less restrictive to live in than the discredited 'total institution' environment provided by the hospital (Bachrach 1986). Many community resources were in fact geared to the needs of less disabled clients, who were therefore excluded from access to care by restrictive selection criteria, regulations, policies or procedures. Also, mental health professionals were not necessarily particularly well equipped to work with severely disabled service users who previously had stayed quietly in mental hospitals year after year. Often the sophisticated psychotherapeutic and counselling skills developed by mental health professionals were far more appropriate for use with less severely disabled clients, but were inappropriate or inapplicable to the more disabled clients to whom they now had to offer a service. As a result, many clients were unable to cope with the vicissitudes and complexities of life in the community, and simply rapidly returned to hospital, leading to the 'revolving door' pattern of service use (Talbot 1981).

Case management emerged as a means to combat these difficulties. In essence, the case manager did whatever was necessary, for example advocacy, directly providing services themselves, and co-ordinating services across often chaotic and disorganized organizational systems, in order to ensure that the user's needs were met. Holding one worker responsible for the care of a particular service user, and for ensuring the effective co-ordination of needed services, became an effective mechanism for overcoming the fragmentation, neglect and lack of coherent linkage that typically occurred amongst mental health services in the 1970s and indeed today. "In other words, designating one person as the case manager was an attempt to ensure that there is somebody who is accountable, and who is helping the client hold the service delivery system accountable, someone who cannot 'pass the buck' to another agency or individual, when or if services are not delivered quickly and appropriately" (Miller 1983).

In response to the difficulties outlined above, during the late 1970s the American National Institute of Mental Health decided to generate new solutions to these problems, by evolving a new model of community care, which was evaluated in 19 states. This was called the community support system or CSS (Turner 1977). Case management was specified as one of the ten elements necessary for adequate community support for the severe longterm mentally ill. This model had at its core a local agency that was designated with possessing the power and authority to co-ordinate and integrate services at the local level. This 'core CSS agency' would assess the needs of the severe longterm mentally ill in its catchment area and on that basis negotiate the appropriate set of services for each individual service user. Where there were major identified gaps in the local community support system, it would stimulate the development of appropriate new services. This core CSS agency was essentially case management, the authority for which was sanctioned by service contracts, which bound provider agencies to deliver the specified services. During the same period, the US Congress passed legislation requiring that community mental health centres provide case management for severely mentally ill clients.

In summary, by the late 1970s, case management emerged in the USA as an approach with the following functions:

- Ensure continuity of care across services at any given point or over time.
- Ensure that services are responsive to the full range of the service users' needs.
- Help service users gain access to necessary services, overcoming obstacles to access by widening restrictive eligibility criteria, regulations or policies.
- Ensure that the services provided match user need, are provided in an appropriate timescale and add up to a comprehensive range of provision (Intagliata 1982).

As case management itself began to gain popularity, a number of different approaches to conceptualizing or configuring this important intervention began to come into prominence. Initially, four models came to the fore (Solomon 1992): the brokerage model; the rehabilitation model; the strengths approach; and ACT. The brokerage model has subsequently been found to be ineffective (Franklin et al 1987, Curtis et al 1992, Hornstra et al 1993). The rehabilitation model has only had one evaluation (Goering et al 1988). Amongst these leading models, two in particular began to be much more widely known: strengths case management and ACT. The origins, early development and evidence for these two models are presented below.

The origins of and early evidence for ACT

In 1970, Dr Leonard Stein took up the post of Director of Education and Training at Mendota State Hospital in Madison, Wisconsin. Working together with his longterm colleague Mary Ann Test, Stein began to develop what in the early 1970s was a radical departure in the kind and quality of care in the community for clients with longterm mental illness. "We decided to change the focus of our efforts, from activities in an inpatient setting designed to prepare the patients to live in the community, to activities in an outpatient setting designed to help patients make a sustained adjustment to community life" (Stein 1992).

They developed an intensive community support programme for psychiatric inpatients who had proved difficult to discharge. They called the programme 'Total In-community Treatment'. They had concluded that these patients had several features in common, which were independent of diagnosis: a limited range of instrumental and problem-solving skills; strong dependency needs; and a heightened vulnerability to stress. They hypothesized that the community would be a better location than the hospital for treatment of these problems, because the community was more likely to require and reinforce appropriate behaviour, and to present good role models of individuals coping adequately with living in the community. It would also provide a precise focus for skill training in the particular locations where adaptive behaviour was required.

Stein and Test, after much negotiation, managed to secure the agreement of hospital administrators to redeploy hospital ward staff in the community. Instead of being based on an inpatient ward, the staff were located in an old house in downtown Madison. Staff coverage was available 24 hours per day, seven days per week. An individually tailored treatment programme was devised for every patient, based on an assessment of their deficits in the coping skills necessary for independent living in the community. In essence, staff would do whatever was necessary to keep the patient out of hospital. Most treatment took place in vivo, in patients' homes, neighbourhoods and places of work. The focus was on training patients in the specific skills necessary in their particular living situation to survive adequately in the community. This meant that patients were helped to use the particular gas stove, washing machine or bus route that they needed to manage in order to adjust to their particular 'niche' in the community. In addition, patients were given sustained and intensive assistance in finding a job or sheltered workshop placement. Staff would stay in contact afterwards, in order to help resolve any problems that might emerge once a job had been started. Patients were also assisted in exploring their use of leisure time and their development of effective social skills. They tried to build on the strengths and competencies of clients. They worked with the patient's family; where the ties with the family were pathological, they would encourage 'constructive separation'. They would work with friends and neighbours who might be providing additional support. They engaged in assertive outreach in the sense that, if a patient initially refused to see the case manager, they would persist in their attempts at engagement. They would assess the patient's need for medication and ensure that medication compliance was adhered to. Hospital inpatient facilities were used very much as a last resort.

Stein and Test (1980) published their first groundbreaking evaluation of ACT. The study was carried out in Madison, Wisconsin, USA, and had two major stages. During the first stage, which lasted 14 months, patients were randomly allocated either to ACT community treatment or to a control programme consisting of standard hospital and community care. In the second stage, the ACT intervention was stopped, and the effects of reintegrating the ACT patients into standard community care evaluated. All patients were aged between 18 and 62, and had any diagnosis other than primary alcoholism or severe organic brain syndrome.

Over the first stage of 14 months, when the experimental group were receiving ACT, only 18% were hospitalized, for a mean of 11 days; the readmission rate was under 10%. The results for the control group were strikingly different. Here, 88% were hospitalized, with a readmission rate of 60%. Also, inpatient length of stay was much longer, at an average of 36 days. There were also significant differences in favour of the experimental group in terms of reduction in symptomatology, higher levels of employment, a greater number of social relationships and higher patient satisfaction with quality of life.

Striking as these results are, Olfson (1990) advises interpreting them with caution since a lower proportion of the experimental group were diagnosed with schizophrenia (50% versus 79%), and rather more were suffering from acute illness, thus giving greater potentiality for improvement.

In the second 14-month period, when the experimental group were reintegrated into standard community care, all the gains made began to deteriorate. There was a gradual increase in hospital use, social relationships declined in quality, symptomatology increased, time spent in sheltered employment declined, and overall satisfaction with quality of life decreased, until at the end there was virtually no difference between the groups. Stein himself concluded that Assertive Outreach needed to be provided on an ongoing basis, in perpetuity. Concerning the deterioration in functioning during this second 14-month period, Stein (1992) comments:

"At first blush this deterioration in the second phase was a disappointment. However, on further consideration I believe that this was the most important finding of the study. What this experiment made clear is that we need to move from a time-limited model to a model that provided services indefinitely. In retrospect it seems obvious that when we deal with an illness that we do not know how to prevent or cure – and that is thus chronic in nature – the intervention must likewise be long term in nature."

The bold innovations in treatment developed in the ACT model have led to considerable interest, both in the USA and internationally. The positive results obtained through their rigorously conducted research evaluations enhanced the burgeoning reputation of the approach. Programmes borrowing heavily from the ACT model are now found throughout the USA (Bond et al 1995). The ACT model has received considerable attention overseas. Hoult et al (1983) in North Shore, Sydney, Australia, set up and evaluated an ACT programme. Also, a team based at the Maudsley Hospital, London, developed and evaluated the Daily Living Programme, which again was largely based on the ACT model (Marks et al 1994, Muijen et al 1992b).

The first major international replication of the ACT model came from Dr John Hoult and his colleagues, who were setting up an ACT service in Sydney (Hoult et al 1983). Their target group comprised mixed diagnosis, difficult-to-treat patients who were assigned at inpatient admission either to the experimental Total Community Living Programme or to standard inpatient care. They were very comparable to the patient group treated by Stein and Test (1980). Results at the end of the first year indicated much reduced hospital inpatient care (a mean of 8.4 days versus 53.5 days for the control group). Programme costs were also significantly less. On one outcome measure, the ACT group were less symptomatic than the controls, although on others there were no differences; they were also more satisfied with their care and had higher psychosocial performance. There were no differences in occupational outcome although it should be noted that this was the area that was least comparable to the ACT model. Somewhat disturbingly, 10% of patients in the experimental programme made attempts at suicide, compared to none of the controls.

Both the original research carried out by Stein and Test (1980) and the international replication carried out by Hoult et al (1983) produced a comprehensive array of positive results:

- Length of stay in hospital and the number of hospitalizations were reduced.
- Community tenure was increased, and clients stayed for longer periods of time in their accommodation in the community.
- Symptoms were reduced and overall level of psychosocial functioning increased.
- Clients perceived their quality of life as having improved, and much preferred Assertive Outreach to standard services.

The origins of and early evidence for the strengths model

The origins of strengths case management as a clinical intervention can be traced to 1982 (Rapp 1998) when the University of Kansas School of Social Welfare was awarded, by the State of Kansas, a $10 000 contract to provide case management services for people with severe, longterm mental illness. Rona Chamberlain, a new PhD student, was assigned to Professor Rapp to take this project forward. Together they designed a service model of case management: "Discarding the current approaches, we began identifying the elements of practice that we thought would make sense... The notion of individual and community strengths was central to this initial formulation." They selected four social work students, who were about to start a community placement, carried out a brief case management training programme, then monitored and supervised their clinical work using this new approach.

Modrcin et al (1988) reported on the earliest evaluation of strengths case management. This pilot study evaluated the impact upon client outcomes of the strengths approach to case management. Four social work students in the graduate School of the University of Kansas Social Welfare department were given a five-day training programme in strengths case management. None had had any prior experience of working with the severe longterm mentally ill. Case managers in the control group had had three years' prior experience. A total of 89 clients were randomly assigned either to the strengths case managers or to the control condition. However, the drop-out rate was quite high and only 51 clients finally took part in the experiment. Outcomes were assessed on a variety of measures including quality of life, medication compliance, hospitalization, employment, participation in vocational training, and the acquisition of skills in community living, socialization and inappropriate behaviour. On all but one measure, results favoured the clients receiving strengths case management. These clients demonstrated better adjustment in community living skills, more appropriate behaviour, greater participation in vocational training and higher quality of life. However, strengths case management clients were rated by their own case managers as having more 'mild or minor' problems in socialization.

Four years later, a more ambitious study was published, which reviewed the evidence derived over a six-year period, from implementing the strengths model in 12 different community mental health centres in Kansas. Under close supervision from an experienced social worker in the School's doctorate programme, a team of four masters level or final year degree social work students were placed as project teams, for an eight-month basis. Students worked with a caseload of five to seven clients for the first half of this time two days per week, and for the second half three days per week. Apart from providing ongoing supervision for the students, the university also undertook an intensive training programme for all the students prior to their placement. The project was evaluated by a variety of methods including monitoring frequency of hospitalization, interviewing both the students and the clients, and reviewing the number and kind of goals specified in the care plans. With respect to hospitalization, the rate for case-managed clients was half (15.5%) the state average of 30%. With respect to client goals, the proportion of goals achieved increased from 60% in year one to 82% in year six. This study, whilst a useful pointer towards the face validity and efficacy of the model, must be viewed with some caution. Firstly, no overall outcome data are reported in terms of improvements with respect to symptomatic or social adjustment. Secondly, the gains reported refer to only a very limited period of time: some eight months for each individual project. Thirdly, the study was not a randomized controlled trial and cannot therefore compare results achieved with respect to a control comparison group.

Macias et al (1994) published substantial evidence confirming the efficacy of the strengths approach to case management, when linked into input from an existing psychosocial rehabilitation programme, which offered daily activities, group discussion and recreational outings as well as a luncheon club. The case management intervention consisted of care co-ordination (housing and welfare benefit assistance, linkage with medical services, etc.) and direct assistance such as supportive counselling and help in daily tasks such as shopping, cooking, cleaning, etc. Macias et al randomly allocated a cohort of 42 clients. Half received the psychosocial rehabilitation programme alone, whilst the other half received both strengths case management and the rehabilitation programme. At one year and also at 18 months after commencing treatment, both groups received a comprehensive evaluation. This consisted of the psychosocial evaluation of the users themselves, views of their families, views of the case managers, and an examination of use of hospitalization and crisis services. Macias et al found that the results of their study significantly favoured the experimental group receiving both case management and psychosocial rehabilitation. This group experienced fewer problems with a depressed mood, fewer problems with thinking, better overall physical and mental health, greater competence in daily living skills, and greater psychological well-being. Macias et al (1994) concluded: "Overall, the case management group reported lower psychiatric symptomatology, a greater sense of health and well-being, and a higher level of competence in daily functioning, compared to the control group, even though both groups were equivalent in diagnosis, level of support, and other factors known to be related to impaired functioning." The researchers also evaluated family member ratings of user functioning. These also showed that the case-managed group were significantly less disturbed in terms of expressions of paranoia and in overall level of cognitive functioning. Family members whose users were receiving case management were also less burdened, less depressed and less in need of help and support, than those receiving the rehabilitation programme alone. There were also beneficial effects in terms of hospitalization for the case-managed group. In the 18 months prior to receiving case management, one-third had been hospitalized, compared to no hospitalizations for this group in the 18 months after case management had commenced. In comparison, around one-quarter of the group receiving psychosocial rehabilitation alone continued to be hospitalized throughout this period.

Some years later, Macias et al (1997) evaluated strengths case management with respect to a specialized set of issues related to accessing Medicaid payment. Strengths case management was therefore evaluated with respect to the Medicaid criteria of economic independence and the attendance at psychiatric aftercare facilities where comprehensive assessment and diagnosis could be carried out. Ninety-seven service users were randomly allocated either to the strengths case management programme or to the control condition. Both services made significant improvements with respect to residential autonomy and attendance at therapy. In addition, strengths case management was evaluated with respect to its impact upon income, social support and improvement in physical health. In all three areas the strengths case management group made significantly greater improvements compared to the control group.

A study carried out by Stanard (1999) set out to evaluate the efficacy of a 40-hour training programme in the strengths approach in terms of its effect upon clients. Two community mental health centres in rural southeastern Ohio were selected, and mental health staff in one of them received the training. In the 'experimental site', 29 clients were assessed as to their functioning prior to and after the training, and were compared to the functioning of 15 clients in the control site. It should be noted that there was a high drop-out rate in the experimental site (only 29 out of 60 clients actually agreed to participate). Clients were assessed on quality of life, residential living status, vocational and educational status, symptomatology and hospitalization. The results indicated that the quality of life of the clients receiving strengths case management significantly improved compared to that of the control clients. Furthermore, the vocational and educational outcomes for the strengths case management group were significantly better than those of the control group. However, there was no difference between the groups in hospitalization, symptomatology or residential status.

AN OVERVIEW OF THE GENERIC EVIDENCE FOR ASSERTIVE OUTREACH

Since the early 1980s when these early studies were carried out, numerous evaluations on Assertive Outreach have been undertaken, many of which were not so comprehensively successful. As the numbers of studies evaluating case management continued to grow, a number of attempts were made to pull together all these studies. This enabled a wider overview of the overall efficacy of this approach (Mueser et al 2001,

Philips et al 2001, Ziguras and Stuart 2000, Latimer 1999, Mueser et al 1998, Marshall and Lockwood 1998, Marshall et al 1998). Some systematic reviews have drawn a clear distinction between ACT and case management (Marshall and Lockwood 1998, Marshall et al 1998). Others, however, have lumped the two together in their comparisons (Mueser et al 1998). The main findings (from both ACT studies and intensive case management) from these systematic reviews are summarized below, as are the findings of some recent UK-based studies.

Critical ingredients of Assertive Outreach

There has been much debate as to what constitutes the 'critical ingredients' or essential elements of Assertive Outreach. The two approaches that have been most refined in terms of developing model adherence scales applicable to test the adherence of other ACT programmes, and which have received most dissemination, are those of McGrew and Bond (1995) and Teague et al (1998); see also Bond et al (2001). Both approaches have used the same 'expert panel' approach for their development. A listing of all the critical features of ACT is generated. An expert panel of 20 or so 'experts in the field' is convened and asked to rate the relative importance of the contribution of each critical feature to the ACT model. The responses of the expert panel are analysed, critical features of the model where there are high levels of agreement are retained, and those with lower levels of agreement rejected. Both these approaches have been generated in the USA and therefore reflect American assumptions concerning service structures and systems, and staff groupings and categories, which are current in the USA but not necessarily in the UK. Burns et al (2001) have written a fascinating paper exploring some of the underlying cultural differences in patterns of service delivery not only between the USA and the UK but also teasing out European cultural variations in the delivery of case management.

Fiander et al (2003) compared the model fidelity of one London-based ACT team with four American ACT teams based in New Hampshire. Their treatment fidelity was measured by the Dartmouth Scale (Teague et al 1998). All teams were rated as 'high fidelity', although there were some important differences in emphasis between the American and London teams. American teams saw their clients for longer (about six-and-a-half hours per month versus four-and-a-quarter hours). However, the London team spent far longer in the community working 'in vivo' with its clients (83% versus 53% in the USA). It also spent a proportionately longer time on direct-care activities such as arranging for welfare benefits.

McGrew has carried out two studies, one using an expert panel of raters (McGrew and Bond 1995) and one comparing the perceptions of ACT field workers (McGrew et al 2003). This latter study surveyed 121 ACT teams and asked team members to rate the degree to which 27 ingredients were characteristic of their own teams, on a scale of 1 to 5. Table 1.1 summarizes the overall ranking of critical ingredients as rated in this study. The five 'most characteristic' items were:

- presence of a nurse on the team
- team involvement in hospital admission

Table 1.1 Summary of the overall ranking of critical ingredients in a study of 121 assertive community treatment (ACT) teams, as surveyed by McGrew et al (2003)

Critical ingredient	Ranking (%)
Presence of a full-time nurse	97
Team involvement in hospital admissions	93
Team involvement in hospital discharge	90
Involvement of all team members in treatment planning	90
Total team caseload of under 100 clients	91
Daily team meetings	93
Caseload weighting of under 12:1	91
More than 50% of services provided in home or community	89
Shared caseloads for treatment	88
Team has primary clinical authority	86
Presence of a full-time social worker	87
Psychiatrist involved more than eight hours per week	83
Clearly identified treatment criteria	83
Assertive engagement	79
Team works with a client support system	77
More than two client contacts per week	76
Low staff turnover	79
The team is the primary provider of services	79
One member is the clinical team leader	82
Assertive monitoring	71
Team leader provides direct service	75
Team has 24-hour responsibility for the client	76
Daily team meetings of less than one hour duration	63
Presence of full-time substance misuse specialist	57
Presence of full-time vocational specialist	42
Presence of full-time housing specialist	47
Never discharging clients	23

- team involvement in hospital discharge
- shared caseloads for treatment planning
- small caseloads.

A study comparing the perceptions of expert raters concerning the critical ingredients of ACT and case management (Schaedle et al 2002) found a great deal of overlap between the two sets of rater perceptions, except for the area of the team approach, which was emphasized more in ACT. From a strengths perspective, there are some important findings emerging from the studies of Schaedle et al (2002) and McGrew et al (2003). It is interesting to note that in the Schaedle et al (2002) study, the characteristics rated higher by the case management compared to the ACT experts illustrated an inherent emphasis on the strengths approach:

- building on clients' strengths
- maximizing participation in decision making
- ensuring linkage and co-ordination of needed services
- integrating the client into the community.

In McGrew et al's (2003) study, the lowest rated critical ingredient was 'never closing cases'. This would seem to suggest that ACT field workers did not see continuity of care as an essential ingredient of ACT. The strengths approach emphasizes the contrary: the importance of restoring the user to community niches rather than discharging them to other parts of the mental health service system.

Engagement

The meta-analysis of Marshall and Lockwood (1998) confirmed that clients receiving either intensive case management (ICM) or ACT were more likely to stay in contact with services. Thus, the clear conclusion from international studies is that Assertive Outreach/case management is better at engaging clients with services. The results from UK studies are at some variance from this. Both Burns et al (1999) and Johnson et al (1998) found higher engagement levels in control services compared to the case management service. Ford et al (1995), on the other hand, found significantly greater engagement levels with the experimental teams of 96% ($P < 0.05$). A five-year follow-up to this study (Ford et al 2001) still found very high levels of engagement (96%). However, case management was being delivered to only 36 of the 120 clients traced at five years. It would seem that broadly similar engagement levels at five years were achieved through a variety of service mechanisms.

How can the inconsistencies in the UK findings best be accounted for? Careful scrutiny of the sociodemographic data in the PRiSM study (Thornicroft 1998) suggests that, whilst there were no significant differences between experimental and control groups, the trend was for the experimental group subjects to be more disabled on most of the indicators used. It could be that this slightly greater level of disability made engagement more problematic.

However, the levels of disability of clients in the Sainsbury Centre case management study (Ryan et al 1999) were broadly equivalent, and yet the engagement levels were consistently higher. How can this be? One factor may be that teams in this study received intensive training in the strengths model of case management and, in particular, were trained in strengths assessment. An independent user evaluation of the case management teams in this study revealed that: "Users very much valued the responsiveness of their case managers, and were appreciative of the fact that every effort was made to take their needs on board, and to work with them as partners" (Beeforth et al 1995). It may be that this approach to engagement was particularly effective in overcoming resistance and encouraging users to engage with services (Rapp 1998, Bleach and Ryan 1995).

Ensuring safety to self or others

In terms of National Service Framework requirements, the government has made the policy assumption that Assertive Outreach is likely to be effective in managing and reducing episodes of self-harm or violence to others. Yet so far as UK research is concerned, the evidence does not support this. Burns et al (1999) reported no difference between intensive and standard teams with respect to unnatural deaths. No data from this study have so far been reported with respect to the occurrence of violence. Marks et al (1994) reported that during the first 20 months of the Daily Living Programme (DLP) there were three deaths from self-harm and one manslaughter amongst DLP clients, compared to two deaths through self-harm amongst control group clients. Johnson et al (1998) reported higher frequencies of self-harm or harm to others amongst the case management client group. These findings do give cause for concern. A central feature for the government's rationale for promoting Assertive Outreach is precisely to work effectively with high-risk clients: "If personal and public safety and well-being are to be assured, it is essential that mental health services stay in contact with people with severe mental illness, especially individuals who are assessed as at risk of harm themselves, or of posing a risk to others. Services should provide flexible help and outreach support in response to fluctuating need and risk..." (Johnson et al 1998). The assumption would seem to be that assertive outreach would not only engage with this high-risk user group but also be effective in risk management and presumably risk reduction. Neither of the studies that address this issue in some detail provides reassuring evidence.

There were 11 'unnatural deaths' reported in the PRiSM study (Thornicroft 1998) – five of these were in the ICM group and six in the control group. With respect to the 24 incidents of violence recorded in this study, ICM clients committed 18, and there were six by the standard care clients. Three times as many violent incidents occurred with clients of the ICM team compared to the standard team.

It would therefore seem that the ICM did not in any sense act to prevent or reduce the occurrence of violent behaviour. In addition, there would seem to be no automatic linkage between engagement of a client and prevention of violence. For whatever reasons, more incidents of violence occurred in clients of the intensively case managed team. One of the reasons why the ICM team in this study did not have any effect on the prevention of risk events may be linked to the frequency of visiting; this was around once per week for about 40 minutes. This frequency/intensity of contact has been reported in a number of other UK studies (Burns et al 1999, Ford et al 1995). This amount of contact may simply not be enough, in order to effectively monitor clients at particularly high risk of violence. Visiting on average once per week does not allow the client's condition to be sufficiently closely monitored so as to be able to pick up early signs of violent behaviour. A greater frequency or intensity of contact is almost certainly necessary for these clients.

The authors (Johnson et al 1998) gave additional data on factors associated with the occurrence of violence. None of these reported factors was a new finding or in the slightest surprising. Essentially, they were that incidents of violence were significantly linked to a previous history of violence, forensic history and level of disability.

The authors do not say whether systematic risk assessment was carried out with these specifically high-risk clients but there would appear to be a very good case for doing so in the future. The National Service Framework for Mental Health does specifically endorse 'good risk assessment' for all clients on the Enhanced Care Programme Approach, which would certainly include the majority of Assertive Outreach clients. If risks of violence cannot be prevented they can at least be managed more effectively.

The findings from the DLP give additional cause for reflection. It may be remembered that in this study there was one DLP patient who committed manslaughter (killing a neighbour's baby). This was a very traumatic and emotive incident, which caused a national controversy at the time, and nearly led to the closure of the DLP service itself. However, when the steps taken by the DLP with this client are examined (Marks et al 1994), it is difficult to be sure what more the team could have done. Repeated psychiatric examination on the ward of this client showed no psychotic symptoms. On discharge, the DLP team frequently visited him; he still showed no psychotic signs and was sufficiently well to have found employment. He was visited two days before he killed the child and it was only after this incident that he manifested psychotic ideation. It is of course possible that the psychiatric examination on the ward was seriously remiss, but the fact that repeated examinations were made over a five-day period would appear to argue against this.

An unpalatable truth is that, whilst risk may be reduced, it cannot be eliminated. It would seem that although the DLP team did everything they reasonably could a tragic incident still occurred. One of the real causes of concern that stems from this analysis is that government policy-makers, and local service managers for that matter, may be under an important misapprehension with respect to Assertive Outreach.

The evidence presented here does not seem to suggest that, as currently practised in the UK, Assertive Outreach can prevent or reduce the frequency of occurrence of violent or suicidal behaviour. This is clearly a worrying finding, especially given the fact that government policy explicitly tasks Assertive Outreach with securing good engagement, high-quality risk assessment and the prevention of violence. A strengths approach makes a contribution to this debate by emphasizing the importance of positive risk taking (see Chapter 11). By prioritizing working with the client's own aspirations and preferences in the community, a strengths approach engenders a close, trusting and collaborative relationship. It becomes possible to engage the users themselves in their own perceptions, fears and anxieties about risk. By sharing the agenda on risk with the user, it becomes a mutual arena for both action and prevention.

Prevention of hospitalization

A reasonably clear consensus emerges from the systematic reviews, namely that clients receiving ACT are less likely to be admitted to hospital than those receiving standard care, and are likely to spend less time in hospital. However, with the exception of Marks et al (1994), who found an 80% reduction in bed-days in favour of ACT, the UK studies are at some variance with these findings. No other UK study has found a significant reduction in either frequency of hospitalization or length of stay. Both Ford et al (1995) and Thornicroft (1998) found trends towards reduction in hospitalization, which did not however reach significance. The UK 700 study found different patterns of hospitalization, with the case-managed clients being admitted for shorter and longer periods than were the control group clients; however, average lengths of stay were nearly identical (73 days for each group). Similarly, Minghella et al (2002) found disappointing results with respect to hospitalization with two London-based voluntary sector Assertive Outreach teams, whose clients were tracked over a two-year period, the year preceding and the year subsequent to referral to Assertive Outreach. Significant increases were found in both teams' use of inpatient admission. For Team A the number of bed-days occupied increased by 115% in the year after referral to Assertive Outreach. For Team B the proportional increase was 102%. Jones (2002) has similarly found disappointing results: 55 severely mentally ill service users, all with histories of high use of hospital inpatient care, were referred to an ACT team. He tracked their length of hospital stay for two years before acceptance to the ACT team, and for one year thereafter. The overall length of hospital stay remained unaltered, although there were trends towards reduction in frequency of admission and total number of bed-days.

Why have UK studies had such disappointing outcomes with respect to hospitalization? A host of reasons have been given including poor adherence to the model (Tyrer 2000), inadequate staff training (Gournay 1999), and a good standard of control services due to the implementation of the Care Programme Approach (Burns et al 2000). All these factors may well have been in operation. However, a factor that has been given insufficient attention is control of hospital admission and discharge procedures. In the early classic studies, it is certainly the case that both Stein and Test (1980) and Hoult et al (1983) were psychiatrists who were in a position to control inpatient admission and discharge. The DLP (Marks et al 1994) was in a position to make a 'natural experiment' 31 months into the project, in that control of admission and discharge was switched from the ACT team having control, to control returning to the hospital ward. Average length of stay was increased 300% after control returned to the ward, from 20 days on average to 60 days. Marks himself comments: "The pre-audit bed day reduction was due not to DLP care being home-based, but rather to the DLP team's control of discharge from any admissions." Muijen et al (1992a) make a similar observation: "Good community care requires that responsibility for admission, treatment and discharge remains with the community team if a dynamic, proactive and efficient service is to be achieved."

Stability of community tenure

Mueser et al (1998) found that Assertive Outreach significantly increased housing stability in nine out of 12 studies where this outcome was measured. Marshall and Lockwood (1998) also confirmed that ACT (but not case management) had superior outcomes compared to standard services with respect to community tenure. One of the essential features of the strengths approach is the emphasis on regarding the community as 'an oasis of naturally occurring resources', and the notion of developing an individually tailored niche for the user concerned. Inherent in the strengths model therefore is a commitment towards the user living in the community on a longterm basis, supported by the development of a unique support system tailored to the user's own needs and circumstances.

Social and clinical outcomes

On reflection, it would seem that the first two classic studies on ACT (Stein and Test 1980, Hoult et al 1983) gave a somewhat misleading picture of the capacity of ACT to significantly reduce symptomatology and enhance social functioning. The success of these early studies in these areas of functioning has not readily been duplicated in the literature. Mueser et al (1998) found in their systematic review only moderate support for ACT having an effect in terms of reducing symptomatology. Effects were even more restricted when impact on social functioning was considered. Only three out of 14 studies could demonstrate a significant impact in this area. Marshall and Lockwood's (1998) systematic review came to similar conclusions. Of the ten studies Marshall used to analyse psychosocial functioning, there were no clear differences between ACT and standard community care. In this context, results from the UK studies with respect to psychosocial functioning are perhaps not too surprising. Two studies (Thornicroft 1998, Burns et al 1999) showed no differences with respect to psychosocial functioning. Marks et al (1994) found modest and limited improvements in favour of the experimental group clients. Ford and Ryan (1997) found within-group improvements on two sites and no difference on the third. It would seem therefore that symptomatic and social adjustment does not necessarily improve with case management.

A strengths approach would emphasize that, for the user, improvements in psychosocial adjustment are not necessarily the highest priority outcomes they are looking for. A recent user evaluation of Assertive Outreach (Graley-Wetherell and Morgan 2001) found that, from a user perspective, improvements in quality of life were of more relevance to them than improvements in symptomatology or social adjustment. The evaluation found that:

> "There had been improvements in various areas of peoples' lives, but nobody reported improvements in all parts of their lives. The greatest improvements had been in their living situation – many users had previously experienced problems with their tenancies, or had been in supported accommodation. Most were now living in their own flats, and were coping quite well… Relationships with families varied from having no contact to having improved relationships… The assertive outreach team had also helped to find voluntary work for service users who had previously been quite isolated. Others were part of a social group that went bowling, swimming or on trips to various places… One person had just spent several days in a religious retreat, and had enjoyed it so much she was keen to go again."

Users are often far more interested in the fact that a strengths approach emphasizes a collaborative relationship with the case manager, which seeks to achieve their own aspirations.

User satisfaction

Mueser et al (1998) found that six out of seven studies that have evaluated this factor were able to report significantly higher levels of client satisfaction with Assertive Outreach services compared to standard service provision. One UK study (Ryan et al 1999) carried out an independent user-led evaluation. The interview schedules were designed, carried out and analysed by the users themselves. The central message of this user-controlled research was that:

> "In summary, the interviews and discussions elicited an overwhelmingly positive response... it was seen as qualitatively different from other services and as a vast improvement. The central relationship between the service user and the assertive outreach worker, as the means of negotiating a better life in the community, was understood and appreciated. It did not always work perfectly, and could not compensate for service gaps and failures, but it was better than what went before, and its loss was feared" (Beeforth et al 1995).

Of UK studies, Thornicroft (1998) also reports higher levels of client satisfaction. McGrew et al (2002) asked 182 service users in the USA what they thought were the best and worst features of ACT. Nearly half the group (44%) thought there was actually nothing wrong with it as an approach. However, the three features that were most unpopular with service users were the intrusive nature of persistent home visits, the confining nature of the programme and the overemphasis on the use of medication. Unsurprisingly, they also found that the teams with the best implementation (i.e. with highest fidelity to the model) were also the most popular with the service users.

CONCLUSIONS

Over the past 30 years, case management has become a major 'connective tissue' for the systems of community care in most Western democracies. Inevitably, the particular format in which it has developed has taken on the social and cultural characteristics of the society in which it is being implemented. Thus in the UK, and in the UK alone, the term used is Assertive Outreach. Inevitably, case management is expressed within the particular organizational systems favoured by a given society and the levels of financial resourcing available. Also, case management is staffed by the kinds and categories of staff present in each particular society. Thus in the UK nurses and social workers form the backbone of many teams. Psychiatrists, on the other hand, because of their overall scarcity in the UK, are not typically available as a full-time resource for case management teams. In the USA, on the other hand, where psychiatrists are far more commonly available, ACT teams usually do have a full-time psychiatrist.

The two major approaches or models that have emerged over this period of time are assertive community treatment (ACT) and the strengths approach. There is strong supporting research evidence in the international literature to suggest that case management is effective in achieving high levels of engagement with severely mentally ill clients, that community tenure can be increased, and that the impact of hospitalization can be reduced. Depending on the study concerned, this is either by reducing frequency of admission and/or by reducing length of stay. Unfortunately, the UK research literature is less reassuring in these respects. Only one study (Ryan et al 1999) confirms that case management is effective in achieving higher levels of engagement, whilst two do not (Burns et al 1999, Thornicroft 1998). Evidence from three studies suggests that case management as implemented in the UK is no more effective than control services in reducing the occurrence of violence (Johnson et al 1998, Burns et al 1999, Marks et al 1994). Similarly, only one UK study shows good evidence that case management is effective in reducing hospitalization (Marks et al 1994), whilst four do not (Ford and Ryan 1997, Burns et al 1999, Harrison-Read et al 2002, Thornicroft 1998).

There is a strange paradox that at precisely the time (1998–2000) that evidence was accumulating in the UK that there is no demonstrated additional benefit from case management over and above standard services, the Department of Health was launching a major mental health initiative in which case management, relaunched as Assertive Outreach, was playing a leading role. Well over 200 Assertive Outreach teams have now been implemented nationally, and Assertive Outreach plays a crucial role in local mental health services as the treatment of choice for severely mentally ill clients at high risk of self-harm or harm towards others. Whilst the supporting research evidence for Assertive Outreach is equivocal, especially in the UK, clinically there appears little alternative to it as a treatment approach for its target group.

References

Bachrach L L 1986 The challenge of service planning for chronic mental patients. Community Mental Health Journal 22: 170–174

Beeforth M, Conlan E, Graley R 1995 Have We Got Views for You. Sainsbury Centre for Mental Health, London

Bleach A, Ryan P 1995 Intensive Community Support for Mental Health. Sainsbury Centre for Mental Health/Pavilion Publishing, Brighton

Bond G R, McGrew J H, Fekete D 1995 Assertive Outreach for frequent users of psychiatric hospitals: a meta-analysis. Journal of Mental Health Administration 22: 4–16

Bond G, Drake R, Mueser K et al 2001 Assertive community treatment for people with severe mental illness: critical ingredients and impact on patients. Disease Management and Health Outcomes 9: 141–159

Burns T, Creed F, Fahy T et al 1999 Intensive versus standard case management for severe psychotic illness: a randomised trial. The Lancet 353: 2185–2189

Burns T, Fiander M, Kent A et al 2000 Effects of caseload size upon the process of care of patients with severe psychotic illness. Report from the UK700 trial. British Journal of Psychiatry 177: 427–433

Burns T, Fioritti A, Holloway F et al 2001 Case management and Assertive Outreach treatment in Europe. Psychiatric Services 52 (5): 631–636

Curtis J, Millman E, Struening E 1992 Effect of case management on rehospitalisation and utilisation of ambulatory care services. Hospital and Community Psychiatry 43: 895–899

Department of Health 1998 Modernising Mental Health Services: Safe Sound Supportive. HMSO, London

Department of Health 1999 National Service Framework for Mental Health: Modern Standards and Service Models. HMSO, London

Fiander M, Burns T, McHugo G et al 2003 Assertive community treatment across the Atlantic: comparison of model fidelity in the UK and USA. British Journal of Psychiatry 182: 248–254

Ford R, Ryan P 1997 Labour intensive: how effective is intensive community support for people with long-standing mental illness? Health Services Journal 23: 26–29

Ford R, Beadsmoore A, Ryan P 1995 Providing the safety net: case management for people with a serious mental illness. Journal of Mental Health 1: 91–97

Ford R, Barnes A, Davies R et al 2001 Maintaining contact with people with severe mental illness: a five-year follow-up of assertive outreach. Social Psychiatry Psychiatrica Epidemiologica 36: 444–447

Franklin J, Solovitz B, Mason M et al 1987 An evaluation of case management. American Journal of Public Health 77: 674

Goering P, Wasylenki D, Farkas M et al 1988 What difference does case management make? Hospital & Community Psychiatry 39: 272–276

Goffman E 1961 Asylums: Essays on the Social Situation of Mental Patients and Other Inmates. Doubleday, New York

Gournay K 1999 Assertive community treatment – why isn't it working? Journal of Mental Health 8 (5): 427–429

Graley-Wetherell R, Morgan S 2001 Active Outreach – An independent user evaluation of a model of assertive outreach practice. Sainsbury Centre for Mental Health, London

Harrison-Read P, Lucas B, Tyrer P et al 2002 Heavy users of acute psychiatric beds: randomised controlled trial of enhanced community management in an outer London borough. Psychological Medicine 32: 403–416

Hornstra R, Bruce-Wolf V, Sagduyo K et al 1993 The effect of intensive case management on hospitalisation of patients with schizophrenia. Journal of Hospital and Community Psychiatry 44 (9): 844–853

Hoult J, Reynolds I, Charbonneau-Powis M et al 1983 Hospital versus community treatment: the results of a randomised controlled trial. Australian and New Zealand Journal of Psychiatry 17: 160–167

Intagliata J 1982 Improving the quality of care for the chronically mentally disabled: the role of case management. Schizophrenia Bulletin 8 (4): 655–674

Johnson S, Leese M, Brooks L et al 1998 Frequency and predictors of adverse events. PRiSM Psychosis Study 3. British Journal of Psychiatry 173: 376–384

Jones A 2002 Assertive community treatment: development of the team, selection of clients, and impact on length of stay. Journal of Psychiatric and Mental Health Nursing 9: 261–270

Latimer E 1999 Economic aspects of assertive community treatment: a review of the literature. Canadian Journal of Psychiatry 44: 443–454

Macias C, Kinney R, Farley W et al 1994 The role of case management within a community support system: partnership with psycho-social rehabilitation. Community Mental Health Journal 30: 323–339

Macias C, Farley W, Jackson R et al 1997 Case management in the context of capitation financing: an evaluation of the strengths model. Administration & Policy in Mental Health 24 (6): 535–543

Marks I, Connolly J, Muijen M et al 1994 Home-based versus hospital-based care for people with serious mental illness. British Journal of Psychiatry 165: 179–194

Marshall M, Lockwood A 1998 Assertive Community Treatment for People with Severe Mental Disorders (Cochrane Review). Issue 4. Oxford Update Software

Marshall M, Lockwood A, Gray A et al 1998 Case Management with People with Severe Mental Disorders (Cochrane Review). Issue 4. Oxford Update Software

McGrew J, Bond G 1995 Critical ingredients of assertive outreach: judgement of the experts. Journal of Mental Health Administration 22 (2): 113–125

McGrew J, Wilson R, Bond G 2002 An exploratory study of what clients like least about assertive community treatment. Psychiatric Services 53 (6): 761–763

McGrew J, Pescosolido P, Wright E 2003 Case managers' perspectives on critical ingredients of assertive community treatment and on its implementation. Psychiatric Services 54 (3): 370–376

Miller G 1983 Case management: the essential services. In: Sanborn C J (ed) Case Management in Mental Health Services. Haworth Press, New York, p 3–16

Minghella E, Gauntlett N, Ford R 2002 Assertive Outreach: does it reach expectations? Journal of Mental Health 11 (1): 27–42

Modrcin M, Rapp C, Poetner J 1988 The evaluation of case management services with the chronically mentally ill. Journal of Evaluation and Program Planning 11 (4): 307–314

Mueser K T, Bond G R, Drake R E et al 1998 Models of community care for severe mental illness: a review of research on case management. Schizophrenia Bulletin 24 (1): 37–73

Mueser K T, Bond G R, Drake R E 2001 Community-Based Treatment of Schizophrenia and Other Severe Mental Disorders: Treatment Outcomes? http://psychiatry/medscape.com

Muijen M, Cooney M, Strathdee G 1992a Community psychiatric nurse teams: intensive support versus generic care. British Journal of Psychiatry 165: 211–217

Muijen M, Marks I, Connolly J et al 1992b Home-based care and standard hospital care for patients with severe mental illness: a randomised controlled study. British Medical Journal 304: 211–217

Olfson M 1990 Assertive community treatment: an evaluation of the experimental evidence. Hospital and Community Psychiatry 41: 634–641

Onyett S 1992 Case Management in Mental Health. Chapman & Hall, London

Philips S, Burns B, Edgar E et al 2001 Moving assertive community treatment into the community. Psychiatric Services 52 (6): 771–779

Rapp C 1998 The Strengths Model: Case Management with People Suffering from Severe and Persistent Mental Illness. Oxford University Press, New York

Rose N 2001 Historical changes in mental health practice. In: Thornicroft G, Szmukler G (eds) Textbook of Community Psychiatry. Oxford University Press, Oxford

Ryan P, Ford R, Beadsmoore A et al 1999 The enduring relevance of case management. British Journal of Social Work 29: 97–125

Schaedle R, McGrew J, Bond G et al 2002 A comparison of experts' perspectives on assertive community treatment and intensive case management. Psychiatric Services 53 (2): 207–210

Solomon P 1992 The efficacy of case management services for severely mentally disabled clients. Community Mental Health Journal 28: 163–180

Stanard R P 1999 The effect of training in a strengths model of case management on client outcomes in a community mental health center. Community Mental Health Journal 35 (2): 169–179

Stein L 1992 Innovating against the current. New Directions in Mental Health 56: 5–40

Stein L, Test A 1980 Alternatives to mental hospital treatment: conceptual model, treatment program and clinical evaluation. Archives of General Psychiatry 37: 392–397

Talbot J 1981 The Chronic Mentally Ill: Treatment, Programs, Systems. Human Sciences, New York

Teague G, Bond G, Drake R 1998 Program fidelity in assertive community treatment: development and use of a measure. American Journal of Orthopsychiatry 68: 218–232

Thornicroft G 1998 The PRiSM psychosis study articles 1–10. British Journal of Psychiatry 173: 363–431

Turner J C 1977 Comprehensive community support systems for severely disabled adults. Psychosocial Rehabilitation Journal 1 (1): 39–47

Tyrer P 2000 Are small caseloads beautiful in severe mental illness? British Journal of Psychiatry 177: 386–387

Ziguras J, Stuart G 2000 A meta-analysis of the effectiveness of mental health case management over 20 years. Psychiatric Services 51: 1410–1421

Chapter 2

The transformation of case management into Assertive Outreach: the policy context 1985–2003

Peter Ryan

INTRODUCTION

There is an important sense in which over the past 15 years, and under both Conservative and Labour governments, the history and development of community care has been inextricably intertwined with case management. During this period, the term 'case management' has received favourable mention in government White Papers, has been abolished, misinterpreted and latterly, under the Labour Government, reinvented as 'Assertive Outreach'. This chapter provides an overview as to the various ways in which, throughout the last decade, case management/Assertive Outreach has influenced both government social policy and local delivery of mental health services. This is achieved by dividing this period into three broad phases: the emergence of case management 1985–1991; the demise of case management 1991–1997; and the arrival of Assertive Outreach 1997–2002.

1985–1991: THE EMERGENCE OF CASE MANAGEMENT

The development of case management in the UK commenced in the early 1980s through the pioneering work of Bleddyn Davies, David Challis and others at the Personal Social Services Research Unit at the University of Kent, UK. Their work focused on the application of case management to the care of the elderly. The cost-efficiency and -effectiveness of case management was demonstrated in a number of ground-breaking studies (Challis and Davies 1986, Davies et al 1990). Through their work, it became apparent that case management could provide a cost-efficient remedy for the fragmentation and inefficiency that characterized the care in the community for this and many other care groups. At the heart of their approach was an individual case manager who would engage with and assess the needs of the client, and co-ordinate the care needed, using a devolved budget set at two-thirds of the average cost of a residential care placement. The approach offered the promise of personalized care tailored to individualized needs, and at a cost-effective price. The research undertaken to evaluate this approach confirmed that case management was cost-effective and did deliver individually tailored care. The approach became widely known and attracted great interest from the Conservative government which set case management as a central component of its intended community care reforms, laid out in the 1989 White Paper (Department of Health 1989).

The 1989 Conservative White Paper on the future direction of community care endorsed case management, and saw it as an important vehicle for service delivery. "Where an individual's needs are complex, or significant levels of resources are involved, the government sees considerable merit in nominating a 'case manager' to take responsibility for ensuring that individual needs are regularly reviewed, resources are managed effectively, and that each service user has a single point of contact." The White Paper went on to encourage the widest application of the key principles of case management, which it articulated as follows:

1. Identification of people in need, including systems of referral.
2. Assessment of care needs.
3. Planning and securing the delivery of care.
4. Monitoring the quality of care provided.
5. Review of client needs.

In April 1991, the Conservative government launched the Care Programme Approach (CPA). The CPA came as a great shock to supporters of case management: no new money was offered and there were to be no new case management teams as such with devolved budgets, to personalize care at an individual level to individual clients. Instead, a system of administrative monitoring was to be introduced. The accompanying circular HC (90) 23 (Department of Health 1990) stated its operational principles as follows:

"Once an assessment has been made of the continuing health and social care needs to be met if a patient is to be treated in the community... it is necessary to have effective arrangements both for monitoring that the agreed services are, indeed, being provided, and for keeping in contact with the patient and drawing attention to changes in his or her condition... the ideal is for one named person to be appointed as key worker to keep in close contact with the patient and to monitor that the agreed health and social care has been given."

The CPA was designed to ensure that the care in the community of all clients leaving mental hospital would be effectively co-ordinated by ensuring multidisciplinary discharge planning and by appointing a nominated key worker to co-ordinate each client's care package. In 1993, the plans that the Conservative government had been laying to restructure Social Services in terms of the purchaser–provider split came into effect. Care management was strategically important to the government, since it enabled them to cap the community care budget, and at the same time it gave much greater scope to the voluntary and private sectors as providers of social care. Care management was designed to ensure that Social Services targeted care at the most vulnerable and severely disabled clients, assessed need on an individually tailored basis, and monitored the delivery of an appropriate care package on a cost basis. These reforms were undertaken with a view to enhancing the co-ordination and efficiency of care in the community. Both Health and Social Services were given a fixed annual budget within which to operate. There were to be no central government 'bail outs' if this budget was overspent. The requirements of efficiency, bringing with it the pressure to control and reduce costs, had somehow to be reconciled with other policy requirements.

1991–1997: THE DEMISE OF CASE MANAGEMENT

The net effect of the Conservative government's community care reforms was to provide, particularly through Social Services care management, the administrative machinery necessary to cap costs and budgets available for all care groups in the community including the mentally ill. The principles of case management were turned into administrative systems to monitor and control expenditure, and to track the care offered through a system of monitoring by allocating key workers. Case management itself had been offered up on the altar of cost-efficiency and its heart removed. One of the essential principles underlying case management is low caseloads which enable the tailored individualized care to develop between case manager and client. As, in the 1990s, key workers continued to work with high caseloads, there was no real possibility to offer increased quality of care to individual clients, or in any meaningful sense to offer personalized tailored care to individual clients.

At this stage of the early 1990s the term 'case management' was dropped from the official government lexicon. This was because it was thought that it would cause confusion to simultaneously use the term 'case and care management'. Naturally, the government preferred its own invention (care management) and so from this point onwards 'case management' simply disappeared from public usage. Did this matter? If the term that survived (care management) had been functionally equivalent in terms of service delivery to the term it replaced then arguably it would not have mattered in the slightest. However, in fact, the terms referred to profoundly different processes of care.

Care management was essentially a mechanism of financial broker-age, designed to purchase and monitor, within an annually capped budget, cost-effective packages of social care, purchased mainly from the ideologically acceptable private and voluntary sectors. In this sense, Social Services care management is a manifestation of Conservative ide-ological principles, applied to the design and delivery of social care. Essentially, it is an administrative system designed to produce value for money social care packages. The priority of the Conservative govern-ment was to cap the rising tide of social care expenditure that had been causing such concern, and in care management the government had developed an effective mechanism to achieve that.

There was however, a major consequence. By developing both care management and the CPA, these reforms had the paradoxical effect of developing two separate and functionally autonomous systems of administrative care co-ordination in the community. One, the CPA, was administered through health authorities, whilst the other (care manage-ment) was administered through Social Services. Which of these two sys-tems of co-ordination took priority? How did they link in to each other? In this sense, arguably, these reforms created as much confusion and possibilities of duplication as they resolved. In a way, the 1990s can be seen as a forced experiment with administrative brokerage – the antithe-sis of case management. The Conservative government's rationale dur-ing the 1990s was that administrative reform leading to increased 'administrative efficiency' could itself alone produce improvements in care co-ordination, and that a service dedicated to that end, case man-agement, with low caseloads and specifically allocated field workers, was not necessary. The evidence from the latter part of the 1990s was that this was simply not the case. On the contrary, much of what transpired during this period of time simply proved that the more personalized approach to care offered by case management was essential, and that the general administrative reforms of the CPA and care management were no substitute.

Throughout the Conservative era mental health systems remained rel-atively starved of resources, and at no time did this government suggest clinical initiatives, with a view to directly improving the quality of care delivered to patients through new service initiatives. The 1990s also saw the closure of mental hospitals at an unprecedented pace, leading to the rapid reduction of mental hospital beds. In the 1990s, hospital bed num-bers had by 1997 reduced to no more than 37 000. This meant that the newly implemented administrative systems of the CPA and care man-agement were themselves under pressure to co-ordinate care of an increasing number of patients who were being discharged into the com-munity. These new systems of care co-ordination were struggling to cope with increased numbers of clients in the community at precisely the same time as they were experiencing severe constraints on expenditure. This resulted in annual increases in spending (of under 2%), which in real terms essentially meant a decline in resource levels for mental health services throughout the latter part of the 1990s (Sainsbury Centre 2000).

It is perhaps no coincidence then that around the mid-1990s public concern escalated. This was fanned by media 'outrage' over a number of tragic incidents in which members of the public or of the caring professions were killed by patients with severe mental illness who were 'at large' in the community. The incident that received most press coverage was the murder of Jonathan Zito by Christopher Clunis in 1992 (Ritchie et al 1994). The government's response was, rather than an allocation of resources to increase quality of care, yet more administrative monitoring. In the mid-1990s the overall balance of community care policy tipped much more explicitly towards the close monitoring and control of high-risk clients, particularly those likely to be violent. This led in 1994 to the establishment of a Supervision Register under the CPA in order to monitor the behaviour of high-risk clients more closely (NHS Executive 1994). In addition, new legislation was enacted in order to the make the mental heath services more responsible for control of risks to public safety. Supervised discharge orders made it possible for mental health services to call a review under the CPA for clients for whom there was major concern and to make their return to hospital more readily and speedily available (Department of Health 1995). Field workers and managers had to accustom themselves to year-on-year reductions in capital or revenue, in the name of ever greater efficiency savings; after a while, the effect was demoralizing and depressing.

1997 ONWARDS: THE ARRIVAL OF 'ASSERTIVE OUTREACH'

The advent of the Labour government in 1997 saw a remarkable transformation in the fortunes of case management. Essentially, case management was 'relaunched' or 'rebadged' as 'Assertive Outreach'. However, it is important to see this in the context of the major policy changes that the New Labour government was determined to bring in as a riposte to the Conservative government's changes in health and social care that had taken place throughout the 1990s. Two major White Papers (Department of Health 1997, 1998) on the NHS clearly signalled a new direction for the new government. An avalanche of new initiatives were announced, including the development of national targets, an expansion of the role of primary care through the launching of Primary Care Trusts and the improvement of quality of care through initiating two new national organizations (the National Institute for Clinical Excellence – NICE – and a Commission for Health Improvement – CHI). New procedures for monitoring clinical impact through clinical governance were also announced. Lastly, to address uncertainties over service shape and structure, a programme of National Service Frameworks (NSF) would be established based on the prototype for cancer services published in 1995. The first NSF was to be in the mental health area and was targeted for publication in 1999. The organizational structure within which this process would be embedded would involve each health authority making an annual performance agreement with its regional centre, covering all the key objectives for the year. This would lead to an annual accountability agreement containing key targets for the service as a whole and for specific components within it. If a particular mental health service, or strategically important element within it such as Assertive Outreach, were to be consistently missing its targets, or if a serious incident were to occur, then the CHI would take forward a service review, in partnership with the Social Services Inspectorate. This would lead to mandatory service improvement or restructuring.

THE NEW MENTAL HEALTH INITIATIVES: FROM CASE MANAGEMENT TO ASSERTIVE OUTREACH

After these two over-arching White Papers, which defined the focus for the NHS as a whole, there was a whole series of initiatives specifically in the mental health area. The first of these was the 1998 White Paper *Modernising Mental Health Services* (Department of Health 1998). The promised *National Service Framework for Mental Health* (Department of Health 1999) followed this about a year later. The *NHS National Plan*, published in mid-2000, contained significant mental health service developments (Department of Health 2000a). In April 2001, *The Mental Health Policy Implementation Guide* (Department of Health 2001) was published, which provided detailed guidelines for the implementation of all the new mental health services outlined in the previous policy papers. At the heart of these new initiatives there was a major emphasis once more on case management, now 'rebadged and repackaged', and known as Assertive Outreach.

Why has case management re-emerged as a major component of mental health policy under the Labour government? Firstly, and perhaps most importantly, the Labour government was prepared, unlike its Conservative predecessor, to spend more money on mental health services. With more resources available it became possible to think in terms of more clinical teams. Secondly, the incoming Labour government inherited major concerns over public safety with respect to the 'violent mental patient' and the apparent failure of community care to prevent the occurrence of violent incidents in the community. It would seem also that specialist mental health advisors at the Department of Health won a battle to convince ministers that case management was the most likely intervention available to control and manage the public safety agenda. (As Chapter 1 on the origins of and evidence for case management illustrated, there is evidence to suggest that case management can be highly effective in engaging severely mentally ill clients in the community.) However, for reasons that still do not appear obvious, the term 'case management' was dropped, only to be re-invented in the guise of 'Assertive Outreach'.

THE MENTAL HEALTH WHITE PAPER: MODERNISING MENTAL HEALTH SERVICES

This White Paper (Department of Health 1998) was arguably the most powerful and focused overview of mental health services in a quarter of a century, since the previous Labour government's White Paper on mental health services (Department of Health 1975). The 1998 White Paper is grappling for a balance between concerns with the public safety aspects of care in the community, on the one hand, and the commitment towards more patient-centred care on the other. The new policy initiative had to reconcile supporting people in the community with enabling them to be recalled to safer more restrictive environments when there was evidence that there was a threat either to their own safety or to the community at large. The 1998 White Paper set out the Labour government's vision of how it wished mental health services to develop over the next ten years, and announced a package of new measures, designed to balance extra support with greater security for the public. These included:

- Assertive Outreach teams to engage with and monitor at-risk users
- secure units in each region for the most seriously disturbed
- a 24-hour help-line and crisis intervention teams to respond to emergency needs
- extra acute inpatient care beds, hostels and supported accommodation
- the establishment of home treatment teams
- a NSF for standards of care.

The new mental health policy was summarized as follows (Department of Health 1998):

- Safe
  - Services should promote the safety of patients, users, carers, the staff and public.
  - Services should be delivered according to need including to those who are hard to reach.
- Sound
  - A full range of effective treatment and services should be available and accessible.
  - All available resources should be efficiently utilized in relation to need.
  - The workforce should be sufficient, supported, skilled and equipped for the task.
  - All agencies and professionals should be committed to working in partnership.
- Supportive
  - Patients, service users and carers should be informed, involved and empowered.
  - Service development and delivery should be responsive to the needs of minority ethnic groups.

These recommended service initiatives would seem to reflect New Labour's Third Way. Some, for example the emphasis on more acute inpatient beds or more secure or forensic accommodation, clearly reflect the policy requirement for services to prioritize public safety. Other recommended developments, for example Assertive Outreach or early and crisis intervention, seem more designed to encourage greater accessibility and responsiveness to services for users and carers. A concern raised by these proposals is that the government's suggested solution for severe personality disorder clients who are deemed to be violent may be 'therapeutic' incarceration, potentially on a permanent basis.

What is of particular note for the purposes of this chapter is the renewed emphasis on case management or Assertive Outreach. One of the centrally defining aspects of Assertive Outreach is the context in which it occurs, and the kind of client to whom it is offered. These important aspects are highlighted in the government's own definition in the White Paper (Department of Health 1998):

> "Assertive outreach is an active approach to treatment and care for those who are at risk of being readmitted to psychiatric hospital. Such people are typically hard to engage because of their negative experiences of statutory services. Assertive outreach… ensures that treatment is delivered early enough to prevent the patient's condition from worsening."

This definition gives a good indication of why Assertive Outreach had come back into favour, and why it was designated as one of the central planks of the new mental health strategy. The government was clearly concerned about public safety, and seems to have asked itself: How can the general public best be protected from those mental health clients most at risk in the community, particularly those most at risk of violence? The government's response to this issue was complex, and included new legislation, and more secure and forensic beds. However, it also included Assertive Outreach. This was seen as having a particular responsibility with respect to engaging with these high-risk clients, and to be providing a safety net for the public and the clients themselves.

The role the government saw for Assertive Outreach emphasized its proactive nature, and that it was designed to operate out of the office base and on the client's own 'territory' in the community. The White Paper would seem to assume that Assertive Outreach can be effective in engaging high-risk clients with complex needs who otherwise might have fallen out of contact with services and therefore provide 'safe, sound, supportive care', and thereby provide a safety net.

These pressures towards an increased emphasis on prioritizing public safety must give some cause for concern to mental health services. There is a risk that user perceptions of services may change. Users could be forgiven for becoming more cautious and more reluctant to engage with services that might be required at a crisis to prioritize public safety above user concerns. Paradoxically, the increased emphasis on public safety may have a negative effect upon another aspect of policy outlined in the White Paper, i.e. making services more accessible to users and increasing their engagement in them.

This White Paper was at the time an important development: it signalled that the Labour government was talking expansively about the development of badly needed new services – real services for real needs. There were, and will continue to be, arguments concerning the adequacy of the resources allocated but at least the argument is about how much additional resource is being given rather than about how much is being taken away.

THE NATIONAL SERVICE FRAMEWORK FOR MENTAL HEALTH

In September 1999, the NSF for Mental Health, promised in the 1998 White Paper, was finally published after a six-month delay. It built on the proposals contained in the 1998 mental health White Paper. The NSF set out the policy context, values, standards and implementation programme for mental health services. It addressed the full range of services responsible for mental health care of people of working age, spanning health promotion, specialist services, the NHS, Social Services and the independent sector. It articulated a set of seven standards that must be achieved locally and it recognized that full implementation could take up to ten years.

The NSF for Mental Health is a complex and comprehensive document. However, for the purposes of this chapter, attention is focused on its coverage of Assertive Outreach, which mainly refers to standards four and five, where the needs of clients with severe longterm mental illness are addressed. Standard four requires services to strengthen and deepen their approach to assessment, care planning, monitoring and review. This is to be achieved by integrating care management within the CPA. Also, the CPA is itself strengthened and deepened, through redefining it in terms of two main levels: standard and enhanced. The standard CPA is designed for clients who require relatively limited input, who pose no danger to themselves or others, and who will not be at high risk if they lose contact with services. The enhanced CPA is designed "for clients with multiple needs... this group needs more intensive support from a range of services, and who may have more than one clinical condition, or a condition which is made worse by alcohol or drug misuse. They will include those who are hard to engage, and with whom it is difficult to maintain contact. Some individuals would pose a risk if they lost contact with services." What is striking about the criteria for the enhanced CPA in particular is its focus on those at risk, or who would be at risk if they were to lose contact with services, or in other words precisely those clients to whom Assertive Outreach is most likely to be targeted.

Under standard five, the role and purpose of Assertive Outreach in the context of the NSF is discussed. It is clear that standard five is where the government addresses issues of safety, both for the client and for the community. "If personal and public safety and well-being are to be assured, it is essential that mental health services stay in contact with people with severe mental illness, especially individuals who are assessed as at risk of harm to themselves, or of posing a risk to others. Services should provide flexible help and outreach support in response to fluctuating need and risk." Assertive Outreach is seen as an outreach mechanism for mental health services as a whole, through which high-risk clients, whether a danger to themselves or others, can be engaged with services and their needs assessed. The NSF also emphasizes, in standard five, the importance of good service models for risk assessment, which involves "...ensuring that staff are competent to assess risk of violence or self harm, to manage individuals who may become violent, and to know how to assess and manage risk and ensure safety."

THE NHS NATIONAL PLAN

In July 2000, the National Plan for the NHS was published (Department of Health 2000a). This supported and built upon the NSF, and the 1998 White Paper before it. The National Plan, after restating the principles of the NHS, set out an ambitious modernization agenda for health and social care. So far as mental health services were concerned, the plan reinforced the standards set out in the NSF and articulated a comprehensive set of new service initiatives. It further added to the £700 million already committed to mental health services, by promising "an extra annual investment of over £300 million by 2003/04 to fast forward the Mental Health National Service Framework."

The plan contained details of new services in the spirit of but beyond the specification of the NSF. These included an additional 50 Assertive Outreach teams, in addition to the 170 teams implemented by April 2001. It was envisaged that these teams would be targeted at 20 000 highly vulnerable, high-risk, potentially violent clients nationally. Also planned were 335 crisis resolution teams nationally within three years, treating 100 000 people who otherwise would require admission to hospital. Round-the-clock cover, seven-days-a-week access would be offered by these teams, which would be targeted at clients with severe, longterm mental illness.

The plan also envisaged establishing 50 early intervention teams nationwide, with the aim of reaching (by 2004) some 7500 young people each year. These services would be aimed at first-episode mental health clients in their teens or early twenties, who are otherwise likely to develop a severe longterm mental illness such as schizophrenia. By intervening early in the course of the illnesses, and using techniques such as early signs monitoring and relapse signatures, it is hoped to alleviate the intensity of the course and duration of their illnesses. Also in the plan were:

- graduate primary care mental health workers
- a range of further community teams (see below)
- women-only day centres
- specialist support for carers
- appropriate community facilities for ex-secure patients
- adequate prison mental health aftercare.

The NHS Plan, certainly so far as mental health services are concerned, was an exciting and visionary document. It proposed a comprehensive package of local services, operating within an integrated CPA framework. The needs of clients are recognized, from those in primary care with common mental disorders, to those in secondary or tertiary services with more severe, longterm disorders. The need for greater service provision in the forensic services and in prisons is also recognized, and special arrangements are in place for personality-disordered clients. The plan had a bold preventive aspect to it by establishing 50 early intervention teams nationally. The 330 crisis resolution teams should prevent hospitalization for significant numbers of clients, thereby also reducing hospital costs. In this context, Assertive Outreach teams are clearly targeted at the 20 000 or so clients nationally who have severe, longterm illness and complex needs, and who are potentially violent or suicidal.

THE NEW LEGISLATION

The Labour government has been working on drafting and developing a new Mental Health Act since soon after it came into office. In 1998

Professor Genevra Richardson was appointed chair of a scoping committee to make initial recommendations for a White Paper on the subject. In December 2000 the promised legislative reforms were announced in the White Paper (Department of Health 2000b). Some of the key proposals were:

- Patients with severe personality disorder could be detained if judged a danger to the public.
- Patients in the community who refused treatment could be forcibly returned to hospital.
- Decisions to detain patients compulsorily for more than 28 days to be subject to scrutiny by the Mental Health Tribunal.
- Victims of attacks by mental patients to have the right to know when their attacker was due for release.
- A new Commission for Mental Health to monitor decision making and whether the new laws are being used properly.
- The abolition of the Approved Social Worker role.

When the draft Mental Health Bill was published in June 2002, these proposals were in the main confirmed but with some important modifications. The bill proposed a generic definition of mental illness: "Mental disorder means any disability or disorder of mind or brain which results in an impairment or disturbance of mental functioning." In addition, and of particular importance, the notion of a specific Community Treatment Order was abandoned but replaced with the even more far-reaching and draconian suggestion of a generic compulsory treatment order which would allow for transfer between settings. The draft bill confirmed that it was the government's intention to ensure that compulsory treatment or detention could be ordered in acute wards or in special units attached to prisons, and that there would be new powers to require service users to take their medication in the community – failure to do so would be sufficient grounds for a compulsory treatment order: "Orders will not be specific to the community, and clinicians will decide when it is necessary to move a service user to a hospital setting. Orders may apply in prison. This represents a potentially large increase in a professional's ability to intervene in the lives of service users. The proposal that treatment orders should be extended to prison seems particularly inappropriate. Prison is a wholly unsuitable environment in which to administer long-term compulsory treatment under the Mental Health Act. Prisoners distressed or ill enough to require compulsory treatment should be transferred to hospital" (Sainsbury Centre 2002).

The increased powers of the Mental Health Review Tribunal in the draft bill are both very welcome and entirely essential to counterbalance the massive potential intrusions into personal privacy and liberty caused by the compulsory treatment orders. There are however severe doubts as to whether the tribunal could cope under the enormous workload that would be caused by the implementation of the act. Under the draft bill's proposals the tribunal will no longer be optional. Whilst from a civil liberties perspective this is essential, it does raise serious cause for concern as to the overall viability of such a huge increase in workload.

Furthermore, timescales are likely to be shorter and the tribunal will have wider duties including involvement in care planning.

There are also recommendations for the abolition of the Mental Health Act Commission, and the integration of some version of its functions within the Health Care Inspectorate. This is a retrograde step. The Commission has served as a useful watchdog for mental health issues. To see it disappear into the amorphous mass of the Health Care Inspectorate is to lose an independent and influential observer of mental health issues precisely at the time when one is most needed.

The draft bill seems if anything to have further 'upped the ante' with respect to the introduction of controversial new powers, which threaten individual privacy and liberty. Treatable mentally ill people in the community will be obliged to take the medication prescribed in their care plan, or face compulsory treatment, either in the community itself, in hospital or for that matter in prison. It is currently possible to undertake compulsory treatment only in hospital but not in the community. This has meant people have had to harm themselves or others before they can be returned to hospital. If the draft bill becomes law, unchanged from current proposals, a possible scenario might be as follows:

Example

A patient prior to discharge from hospital agrees to compulsory care and treatment orders. This could include seeing a GP once or twice a week to receive medication. If the patient fails to follow the treatment plan, they could be forcibly readmitted to hospital to receive medication. An initial assessment would be made, which could result in compulsory treatment for 28 days. After that, further compulsory treatment or detention would have to be agreed by a Mental Health Tribunal, chaired by a judge or QC. The tribunal would be able to impose care and treatment orders for two six-month periods with subsequent orders of up to 12 months. As a counterbalance, patients would be able to get access to independent specialist advocates to protect their interests. Everyone detained under compulsory powers would have free legal representation and access to independent psychiatrists. They would also be able to request a review of their care and treatment by the tribunal during an order lasting more than three months.

The draft Mental Health Bill published in June 2002 generated a broad range of opposition from the Mental Health Alliance – a loosely disparate group made up of service user and mental health and legal professional representatives, in an unusual alliance against the intended changes to the Mental Health Act 1983. It highlights a number of ethical dilemmas where the government legislates for mental health provision. The biggest outcry appears to be against the dual potential of incarcerating people with a diagnosed dangerous and severe personality disorder indefinitely, for what they may do rather than for what they have done, and the potential for extending compulsory treatment into the community.

These two potential developments signify the intentions of government legislation to respond to the perceived needs of the public, as driven by the media representation of risk, to the relative detriment of the needs of the service users who experience the mental distress and who have a right to a range of appropriate services when required. Royal (2002) suggests that "The real worry about DSPD [dangerous and severe personality disorder] is that it is a very negative label and once you've been labelled it's very difficult to get out of hospital or prison as no services will have you." One of the serious dilemmas confronting the legal experts is to untangle the conflicting messages given by this potential legislation for detaining people who have not committed an offence, and the measures of the Human Rights Act 1998.

However, Lawton-Smith (2002) suggests that it is the holes in the proposed provisions that require our attention, most specifically "...the absence of any statutory right for patients to a comprehensive assessment of their needs and for those needs to be met with good quality services." This means that the legislation focuses almost entirely on control, to the relative neglect of care through providing the full range of services that people should be able to expect and find helpful when they become ill. With a radical agenda for changing the configuration of comprehensive integrated mental health services, there is a clear need for legislation that will support the provision of resources to implement the new improved services. This apparent lack in the legislation suggests that it may serve only to perpetuate people rapidly cycling on and off compulsory orders, without the provision of services to stabilize the support needed in the community when a person is released from a compulsory order.

With regards to the issue of capacity and incapacity Lawton-Smith (2002) raises the concerns that 'advance statements' have not received the support in the proposed legislation to make them legally binding. What this could mean in practice is that the person who has made a clear statement of how they would like to be treated should they become incapacitated can have those wishes overturned. The government would appear to be legislating that the only true statement of capacity is one that professionals determine to be best. This situation will be further compounded by the failure to legislate for access to independent advocacy until after the initial assessment for a compulsory order has taken place.

So far as Assertive Outreach is concerned, the new legislation has major implications. Assertive Outreach is targeted at those 'treatment-resistant' clients that services have found it hardest to engage. These clients are likely for a number of very good reasons to be suspicious and distrustful of services and therefore it is in any case a major challenge for an Assertive Outreach service to engage these clients. The new legislation is unfortunately likely only to increase the difficulty of engagement. Clients who in any case distrust and reject services are only going to be less inclined to engage with services such as Assertive Outreach, which risk being perceived by users in a highly negative light, as the agency par excellence for the execution of compulsory treatment orders, whether that implies compulsory treatment in the community, returning them against their will to hospital or for that matter to prison. We recognize (see Chapter 4) that under exceptional circumstances compulsory powers are sometimes necessary. Burns and Firn (2002) demonstrate convincingly that in those few cases where compulsion may be indicated currently existing powers such as supervised discharge are adequate to the task. The additional powers implied in the new legislation seem draconian and excessive, and likely only to undermine further the essential element of trust between service users and mental health practitioners.

CONCLUSIONS

This chapter has summarized a 15-year period of development in mental health policy and practice. There is no doubt that it has been a period of immense and at times bewildering change. At the end of the 1980s, case management was being favourably mentioned in the Conservative government's 1989 White Paper, and seemed set to become the backbone of mental health and indeed community care 'for the 1990s and beyond'. However, events rapidly overtook it. By 1991 it had sunk without trace from official government policy and had been replaced by two systems of administrative and organizational brokerage: the CPA for health services and care management for Social Services. In contrast, by the late 1990s the Labour government was signalling the need for massive service developments, in which case management, now rebadged as Assertive Outreach, was to play a strategically central part. This new role could be summarized by the one catchphrase 'safety'. There is much mention of the need to protect the safety of the client but few can doubt that the government has its eyes firmly fixed on protecting the safety of the public. Issues of care and control are hardly new to the health and social care workforce. For the new Assertive Outreach teams, this is a dilemma with which they are destined to become very familiar.

One of the potentially most damaging effects of the legislative climate, if the bill becomes law, is in terms of its obfuscation of a climate encouraging the engagement of trusting working relationships through openly constructive dialogue. Any requirement from the government that Assertive Outreach practitioners will deploy the mechanisms of compulsory treatment in the community runs a very considerable risk of shattering attempts to preserve a service based on working with the needs and aspirations of the service user. May (2002) points out that the very idea of compulsory treatment dehumanizes service users. He suggests that: "Compulsory treatment silences the perspectives and viewpoints of the person on the receiving end, designating them as unimportant." Despite assurances from government sources that it will not lead to enforced medication over the kitchen table, the constant threat of being removed from your home to a place where compulsory treatment will be enforced simply sets up legislation to undermine rather than underpin good ethical practice.

References

Burns T, Firn M 2002 Assertive Outreach in Mental Health: A Manual for Practitioners. Oxford University Press, Oxford

Challis D, Davies B 1986 Case Management in Community Care. PSSRU, Gower

Davies B, Bebbington A, Charnley H 1990 Resources, Needs and Outcomes in Community-Based Care. PSSRU, Avebury

Department of Health 1975 Better Services for the Mentally Ill. Cmnd 6233. HMSO, London

Department of Health 1989 Caring for People: Community Care in the Next Decade and Beyond. HMSO, London

Department of Health 1990 The Care Programme Approach for People with a Mental Illness Referred to the Specialist Psychiatric Services. HC(90)23, LASSL(90)11. HMSO, London

Department of Health 1995 Mental Health (Patients in the Community) Act. HMSO, London

Department of Health 1997 A First Class Service. HMSO, London

Department of Health 1998 Modernising Mental Health Services: Safe, Sound, Supportive. HMSO, London

Department of Health 1999 National Service Framework for Mental Health: Modern Standards and Service Models. HMSO, London

Department of Health 2000a NHS National Plan. HMSO, London

Department of Health 2000b Reforming the Mental Health Act. HMSO, London

Department of Health 2001 The Mental Health Policy Implementation Guide. HMSO, London

Lawton-Smith S 2002 Bad law. Mental Health Today, August: 10–11

May R 2002 Over our bodies. Mental Health Today, August: 14–15

NHS Executive 1994 Introduction of Supervision Registers for Mentally Ill People from 1 April 1994. HSG(94)5. HMSO, London

Ritchie J, Dick D, Lingham R 1994 The Report of the Enquiry into the Care and Treatment of Christopher Clunis. HMSO, London

Royal S 2002 Double jeopardy. Mental Health Today, August: 12–13

Sainsbury Centre for Mental Health 2000 Finding and Keeping: A Review of Recruitment and Retention in the Mental Health Workforce. Sainsbury Centre for Mental Health, London

Sainsbury Centre for Mental Health 2002 Briefing 18: An Executive Briefing on the Draft Mental Health Bill. Sainsbury Centre for Mental Health, London

Chapter 3

The purpose and principles of a 'strengths' approach

Steve Morgan

Take some time out now, to think about *what* guides you in doing good work

INTRODUCTION

Meaningful activity and a sense of purpose are vital for energizing all of us. Without them, we may feel adrift, disconnected from the lifeblood of the parts of society we exist within. It is economics that fundamentally underpins our ability to function in the mainstream of life. The job we do is seen firstly as a means to gain the money we need, but then becomes a definition of who we are and our broader value in society. Beyond accessing the basic means of survival, we then look to means of achieving the more complex needs.

It is worth reminding ourselves of two significant concepts from humanistic psychology proposed by Abraham Maslow: 'Hierarchy of Needs' and 'self-actualization'. In relation to the former, Maslow (1954) introduced a hierarchy that can most easily be visualized as a pyramid (Fig. 3.1). The base represents simple biological needs (hunger; thirst; personal security; love) that are essential to life, and the primary determiners of our actions until they are at least partially achieved. With these needs reasonably met our personal motives and actions may become more influenced by the higher levels of the pyramid representing more complex psychological needs (recognition; understanding; fulfilling potential).

Figure 3.1 The Hierarchy of Needs (based on Maslow 1954).

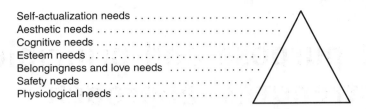

Self-actualization needs . . . .
Aesthetic needs . . . .
Cognitive needs . . . .
Esteem needs . . . .
Belongingness and love needs . . . .
Safety needs . . . .
Physiological needs . . . .

Table 3.1 Characteristics and behaviours of self-actualizers (based on Maslow 1967)

Characteristics

- perceive reality efficiently and are able to tolerate uncertainty
- accept themselves and others for what they are
- spontaneous in thought and behaviour
- problem-centred rather than self-centred
- have a good sense of humour
- highly creative
- resistant to 'enculturation' though not purposely unconventional
- concerned for the welfare of humanity
- capable of deep appreciation of the basic experiences of life
- establish deep, satisfying interpersonal relationships with a few, rather than many, people
- able to look at life from an objective viewpoint

Behaviours

- experience life with full absorption and concentration
- try something new rather than sticking to secure and safe ways
- listen to personal feelings in evaluating experiences rather than to the voice of tradition or authority or the majority
- honesty, and avoiding the pretence of 'game playing'
- prepared to be unpopular if views do not coincide with the majority
- assume responsibility
- work hard at whatever they decide to do
- try to identify personal defences and have the courage to give them up

Specifically regarding the attainment of the higher level psychological needs, Maslow (1967) reflected on the qualities of specific individuals considered to have made extraordinary use of their potential in history, in order to draw up a list of characteristics and behaviours of people considered to be 'self-actualizers' (Table 3.1). In subsequent conversations with selected groups of high-achieving college students, he reported the consistency of phrases that emerged: wholeness; perfection; aliveness; uniqueness; effortlessness; self-sufficiency; and the values of beauty; goodness; and truth (Maslow 1970).

A sense of purpose, principles and personal values underpin a strengths approach to working with people experiencing severe and enduring mental distress. These qualities should ideally be held by the individuals drawn into this type of work, and be applied by them to all levels of thinking about the people requiring the service, and indeed the organization of which the service is a part. In practice, a strengths approach is very much about promoting the actualization of the needs and personal aspirations of all people involved in mental health services (service users and practitioners).

A SENSE OF PURPOSE: WHAT ARE SERVICES FOR?

The most frequent context for working in contemporary mental health services is one of pace and pressure. Practitioners and managers alike are constantly 'in the moment', doing what is needed now, largely dictated by the crises or priorities at any given point. As the policy chapter (see Chapter 2) amply demonstrates, there has been an unprecedented amount of organizational change and development over the last 15 years in the mental health field. In consequence, all too often little time is available for devoting to reflection on the broader purposes of the work: how can we enable people who come into contact with services to express a personal view of their own needs and aspirations? How can we enable practitioners to feel more fulfilled in the way they are working? The strengths approach provides an organizing philosophical framework for mental health practitioners, and for their organizations. For people in contact with mental health services, the purpose of the practitioners within those services should be to help in accessing and sustaining the necessary interdependencies on others that promote the accomplishment of their personal aspirations.

By working with people to seek out and establish tangible resources, we are attempting to focus our purpose on enabling people to fulfil as many of their own aspirations through their own initiative and capabilities – to self-actualize to a level that they personally feel able to achieve, and to help raise people's own threshold of achievement. Consequently, in requiring practitioners to adopt a more challenging response to personal needs, as opposed to a more restrictive 'professional' assessment of need, the strengths approach taps into a more flexible and creative way of working which in turn enables staff members to feel more self-actualized in their day-to-day work.

A focus on resources that impact in areas of human occupation and daily activity challenges services to work more directly with environmental root causes of mental and social distress. Resources devoted to the treatment of medical signs and symptoms have their place but they frequently do little more than mask the causes through dampening down the acute reactions to stress and illness. The focus on 'cause', not just 'effect', brings the context of severe distress back into the realm of normal experience, by stressing the 'normally interdependent' character of human interaction. For some people this will mean the longterm connections with relevant parts of the mental health system; for others it will mean less connection with the system as other alternatives are sought and developed; and for many it will be a fluctuating combination of interdependencies.

Reflecting on the main purpose of delivering a mental health service need not be a theoretical exercise remote from the realities of practice.

Whilst this may not be a particularly frequent distraction from 'doing the job', or even a regular topic of conversation at the water cooler or photocopier, it nonetheless governs what we do and how we go about it. Purpose may appear abstract to the casual observer but it is translated into practice through adherence to certain principles, which will shape the nature of the human interactions and the way a service is presented to those who need it.

The originator of the approach, Professor Charles Rapp, states simply: "A strengths model of case management helps people achieve the goals they set for themselves" (Rapp 1993). As a straightforward purpose this statement recognizes that people most frequently can determine what their basic and more complex needs are, but the experience of mental distress presents a barrier, requiring some support from others in order to achieve their desired goals and aspirations.

He has elaborated the 'purpose' of the work in other sources: "... to assist consumers in identifying, securing, and sustaining the range of resources – both environmental and personal – needed to live, play, and work in a normally interdependent way in the community" (Rapp 1998). These statements of purpose represent a significant shift in the fundamental thinking that underpins the current mental health system, from placing issues of 'treatability' foremost in the determination of the service to be provided, to the notion of 'assistance'. This shift requires practitioners to move away from the more traditional prescriptive and interventionist approaches of service delivery, to something much more involving and led by the person in need. Furthermore, the shift is not one of rhetoric but of real action.

UNDERLYING 'PRINCIPLES' OF A STRENGTHS APPROACH

The original six principles of the strengths model of case management in a US context are documented by Rapp (1993, 1998) and have been articulated into a UK context by Morgan (1996). They will remain the foundation of the approach promoted in this book, with one further addition (Principle 5 of the following list):

1. The focus of the helping process is upon the service user's strengths, interests, abilities and capabilities, not upon their deficits, weaknesses or problems.
2. All service users have the capacity to learn, grow and change.
3. The 'service user–Assertive Outreach' relationship becomes a primary and essential partnership.
4. The service user is viewed as the director of the helping process.
5. Continuity and acceptance are essential foundations for promoting recovery.
6. The helping process takes on an outreach perspective.
7. The local neighbourhood is viewed as a source of potential resources rather than as an obstacle; natural neighbourhood resources should be considered before segregated mental health services.

Each of the seven principles will be discussed, and the Active Outreach team of the Julian Housing Support voluntary sector agency in Norwich will be used (Boxes 3.1–3.9) to provide illustrative case study material for each in practice.

A focus on strengths, interests, abilities and capabilities

The first defining principle of the strengths approach is its very focus on an individual's strengths as its primary aim. There is an inevitable pressure for all professional (and nonprofessional agencies) in contact with

---

Box 3.1   Julian Housing Support: background information

The organization was initially established in 1990, under the umbrella of a local Norwich charity (NORCI), with an annual grant from the Norwich Health Authority. The current name was adopted in 1994, in memory of a young black man who committed suicide whilst detained in a secure unit. Julian Housing Support receives joint funding from Norfolk Social Services, Norfolk Health (formerly through the Mental Illness Specific Grant), and other local sources. The philosophy of the organization is to:

- enable people with severe and enduring mental health problems to live within the community in accommodation suited to their needs
- build on people's existing strengths and skills in order for them to live as independently as they wish
- improve the quality of people's lives by focusing on what they feel are their housing and support needs, and accessing appropriate resources to help meet their needs.

Thus, the broad aim is to promote the social inclusion of people experiencing severe and enduring mental health problems. The method of achieving this is a specific focus on the stability of housing tenure, through the provision of appropriate levels of supported accommodation or outreach support.

The Active Outreach team was established in August 1995, with a remit to support people to sustain their own tenancies, through flexible and appropriately intensive levels of support. This was an attempt to develop an Assertive Outreach model of practice three years before the Sainsbury Centre for Mental Health publication *Keys to Engagement* (Sainsbury Centre 1998).

Team composition

A team manager (with active casework), five outreach workers (mixed nursing, social work and community housing support worker backgrounds), and a specialist dual diagnosis (mental health and substance misuse) practitioner.

The strengths of the Active Outreach team are in a combination of the professional and nonprofessional skill mix, but more importantly all team members demonstrate good personal skills, flexible and creative thinking around the challenges presented by their daily work, and negotiation skills (including with other agencies in statutory and voluntary sectors).

people experiencing severe and enduring mental health problems to be essentially problems oriented. People present to, or are referred to, mental health services because they have some identified problems that need to be resolved (for at least someone's agenda). The intrinsic rationale for most types of service is to identify and assess the nature of the problem(s), devise solutions, and monitor the success or otherwise of the prescribed solutions. The process should then ideally have a built-in system of revising the assessment to come up with alternative solutions if the original system has had little or no success.

A frequent problem with applying this approach in the context of Assertive Outreach is that the people being served have often been in contact with mental health services involuntarily. This contact may have been over some considerable time or they may pose particularly high-profile problems, e.g. violence, adding multiple stigma to their perceptions of self. The problems are more than likely obvious, well documented in historical notes or the referral, and repeatedly assessed every time the person has had contact with a new service provider.

From a service user's point of view, it is an extremely disheartening, deflating and ultimately depressing experience to be repeatedly discussed, referred to, described and attributed to as a long list of negatives. These are seen primarily in terms of the things you fail at, that you repeatedly 'screw up', the risks you pose to yourself and/or others, your deficiencies and deficits through life, and the repeated relapses and admissions to hospital. In our own lives we generally try to avoid the things we are not good at, keep failing at or simply do not catch our interest. If we have to engage in some such activity, we at least attempt to balance it with other more enjoyable activities in which we can succeed, in order to derive some sense of achievement and satisfaction. The maxim that practice makes perfect is fine but if we are predominantly being asked to work on a majority of things that we are not very good at, we run the risk of gradually adopting the persona of the 'failure'.

The strengths approach does not ignore the problems. It acknowledges they are there, and can possibly be resolved by using strengths and achievements, rather than focusing on the problems for problems' sake. It may occasionally involve a period of identifying the strengths first and then applying them to problem resolution.

The approach is closely associated with issues of motivation. We are often more concerned with a problems orientation that sets us up to create artificial motivations to work at an issue, when the person receiving the intervention does not perceive the situation in the same way as we do. The result is often a stalemate, where we quickly attribute the barriers to the lack of motivation on behalf of the other person, who does not follow our carefully constructed prescribed interventions. The strengths approach attempts to tap into the intrinsic sources of motivation held by the individual themselves, i.e. by focusing attention on what they like to do rather than trying to get them to do something that does not hold the same meaning or attraction.

It is important to note that the person may have their own reasons for wanting to focus on the problems (including a fear that if they just talk about positives, the service may be seen as unnecessary and withdrawn). In such instances, it is important not to deny the person their own identi-fied need but also not to lose sight of the need to keep coming back to an identification of the strengths as an important resource for challenging and resolving the problems. Rapp (1998) suggests that solving problems only really manages to bring us back to a state of equilibrium, whereas the using of strengths to exploit opportunities is the true way to promote growth.

What about the issue of risk? Service users can and do under certain circumstances pose a risk both to themselves and others. Assertive Outreach teams continuously do work with users who may be at very high risk of harming themselves, committing suicide or of harming others. A strengths approach must always prioritize issues of serious imminent risk or crisis. Nobody benefits from ignoring such extremes and allow-ing them to undermine the positive aspects of the work. However, the underlying principle is that of 'positive risk-taking' (see Chapter 11), one important element being the engaging and working with the service user's views and experience of risk. It enables risk to be managed through a greater appreciation of the available constructive resources, opening up more diverse options before the need for a restrictive response, and basing such a response, when it is deemed necessary, on a fuller reflection with the service user of their past history (Box 3.2).

Box 3.2   Julian Housing Support: Doug's story

The Active Outreach Team constructively use external practice development consultancy for a number of their needs, including several developments of a strengths assessment approach to their work. This has progressed from an initial appreciation of the strengths assessment tool from Morgan (1996) to the development of strengths within their comprehensive assessment tool – 'Day-to-Day'. More recently, they have been engaged in revising the original strengths assessment tool. The fruits of these developments can be seen in examples of the resulting work with service users referred to their service.

Doug (Active Outreach service user)

Doug is a 29-year-old man, born in the UK, who has lived in Norfolk most of his life. He spent some time in a drug rehabilitation unit during his late teens. He has never been in paid employment but is a talented musician. He loves to play his guitar and would like to be a performing musician in a rock band. He was referred to the Julian Housing organiza-tion approximately six years ago as one of the first people to be worked with by the Active Outreach Team.

Psychiatric history

Diagnosed with paranoid schizophrenia, Doug had several hospital admis-sions in his late teens and early 20s. Some of the admissions were under

box continues

sections of the Mental Health Act, and his presentation was complicated by frequent amphetamine and alcohol misuse. At the time of referral to Active Outreach, Doug was often greatly troubled by paranoid feelings, despite being on depot medication, which had not apparently been reviewed for some time. He was considered one of the people causing most concern for the local statutory sector services at the time.

Planned interventions

- steady 'non-judgemental' engagement
- reduce isolation by taking him to places he expressed interest in, including exploring options to meet his interests in music
- increase income through Disability Living Allowance
- look at alternative housing options
- advocacy via: reduction in medication dosage and physical health difficulties

Doug has become an essential part of a rock band formed with the help of the Active Outreach team! This has given him the confidence to play in other settings. The needs for co-operation in these endeavours have enabled him to listen to others at times, and to begin to make further social contacts. At the time of writing he has been off illicit substances for over a year and has considerably reduced his alcohol intake.

The capacity to learn, grow and change

As a principle underpinning routine practice, this statement applies most strongly to the attitudes of the staff within mental health organizations. However distressed and disabled a person may be by their experiences, we have to believe that everyone has the desire to change aspects of their lives and circumstances. Also, that they can change and grow, with the aid of appropriate guidance and support.

Stein and Test (1980) comment that: "This attitude is extremely important for staff to adopt in order to work effectively with patients as well as with the community. Staff must believe that the people they are working with are citizens of the community. That they are living in the community because they have a right to, and not because the community, through its good grace and kindness, is allowing them to be there; that they are indeed free agents able to make decisions and be responsible for their actions."

Staff not adhering to such beliefs may come to their work with a more narrow sense of purpose and hold predominantly negative attitudes, considering some people to be ill for life and unable or unmotivated to change. They may hold the view that some people derive intrinsic gains from the 'patient' status. Ultimately, this can lead to the concept of 'recovery' being denied to some individuals. If these are the predominant attitudes held by staff, they will be communicated through their work, and will be picked up by the people receiving the service. This will simply add an additional unnecessary barrier to potential achievement for people who already have enough distress to contend with. Rapp (1988) sees this as the service "institutionalising low expectations into people."

We need to acknowledge that there will be times when people feel a need to adopt a more passive 'patient' role, as we all do from time to time. We should not let this acknowledgement cloud our optimism – this is only a temporary state of mind, soon to return to one of hope for change, improvement and recovery as defined by the person themselves. At these momentary lapses, it is our responsibility to carry the torch of hope briefly relinquished. People do not lose their hopes and dreams because of a diagnosis or relapse of a condition. People should be encouraged to set realizable goals, as steps towards the achievement of greater wishes.

Rapp (1998) reminds us of the need for a 'can do' determination applied to all aspects of practice (Box 3.3). Language can be a significant indicator of attitude; for example, people are not schizophrenics, they are people with schizophrenia, i.e. it is just one aspect of their lives. In all

---

Box 3.3   Julian Housing Support: Marie's story

The 'can do' attitude is apparent through all team members' discussions about their work, accepting the reality of the service users' circumstances without losing a belief that people can determine the changes they wish to make for themselves, sometimes with the help of services.

Marie (Active Outreach service user)

Marie is a 57-year-old woman of Danish origin, who came to live in England approximately 20 years ago. Her parents are deceased. She is divorced and has lost contact with her son who now lives in Germany. She speaks English with a strong accent, which can occasionally make her difficult to understand. Previous employment experience is some time ago, generally in temporary jobs.

Health

Diagnosed with bipolar affective disorder, at the time of referral to the Active Outreach Team, approximately six years ago, Marie was an inpatient on a psychiatric unit under Section 3 of the Mental Health Act. At this stage, she had a 10-year history of contact with the psychiatric and criminal justice systems. She frequently felt that strangers were intending to harm her, and thus attacked them as her form of defending herself.

Marie has an arthritic hip and spine, and many other physical health problems. She had a habit of going 'walkabout', being found in various parts of the country in a dishevelled condition. Consequently, traditional services found it difficult to engage and manage her effectively.

Housing history

At the time of the referral to the Active Outreach team Marie's latest flat had been seriously neglected and damaged by flooding. She had longterm difficulties sustaining tenancies and large rent arrears.

box continues

Some residents of a local homeless persons' shelter were using her flat as a drinking den. She appeared to have poor self-care skills, unable to manage daily living activities and frequently neglecting to eat properly. She was generally isolated, with few friends.

Engagement and interventions

The team were committed to clearly focusing attention equally on interests expressed by Marie, and on urgent practical issues around her housing status. She needed much contact and support in all aspects of the work. Progress has been carefully planned and painstakingly slow, but is moving in the right direction:

- attending Bridge lessons at a local college
- joining a local 'Italian circle', supported by an Italian-speaking team member (to fulfil a desire to learn Italian)
- keeping parakeets
- exploring ways of renewing contact with her son
- support to return to her flat after the repairs were completed
- daily support to manage the simplest of tasks, until Marie develops her confidence
- increasing her income through Disability Living Allowance
- support through the stress of a hip replacement operation, and recuperation.

Outcomes

- no unplanned hospital admissions regarding her mental health, even through high-stress times when in acute pain from her hip (short planned respite admissions)
- no assaults on people, therefore no further contact with the criminal justice system
- housing stability for the past six years
- more structure in her life, with improved social contacts
- the possibility of reconnecting with her son in Germany
- increased income and reduced debts
- stress levels and anxiety dramatically reduced
- reduced vulnerability in the community.

Marie has expressed two future goals: to go abroad on holiday and improve her computer skills.

other respects, they are no different to anybody else, having a history of pain and of accomplishments, talents and foibles, dreams and aspirations.

The relationship as an essential partnership

This principle is essential to all work undertaken within mental health services, not only Assertive Outreach. We are working in the unpredictable field of human interactions, which require that our most valuable tool becomes a trusting working relationship. With this, we can have confidence in what is said and agreed between parties. Without it, we are working in the dark. We need to invest time and effort into developing a solid basis for trust from the outset, not to take that trust for granted. Therefore, we constantly need to be checking that the relationship continues to be a trusting one.

Deitchman (1980) suggests that what the service user needs is a 'travel companion' who will be there with them to share experiences, not a 'travel agent' who gives directions and then leaves them to get on with it.

When established on a basis of trust the work becomes deeper, more accurate and meaningful. If insufficient time has been devoted to the building of trust, or none exists, all other aspects of the work become undermined and flawed. Any assessment is necessarily incomplete, as it will lack the full co-operation and openness of the person themselves. Any attempt at monitoring progress will be dependent entirely on the information the person wishes to release, and with the accuracy they wish to offer. The quality of the relationship is crucial to working effectively together. As an approach it necessitates active work on behalf of the practitioner to engage the relationship through self-disclosure and offering a service that meets real identified needs (Morgan 1996).

Rapp (1998) suggests: "It is the relationship that buffers the demands of the tough times, anxious times. The relationship attenuates the stress and prevents or mitigates the exacerbation of symptoms. It is the relationship that supports the client's confidence in tackling the multiple requirements of the environment and other people."

Box 3.4   Julian Housing Support: being active

The local use of the term 'active' in the team's name reflects more accurately an emphasis on the role of workers to be active in their attempts to engage positive relationships with service users. This philosophy is reflected in the actual quotes of users of the service in a published independent user evaluation of the Active Outreach team (Graley-Wetherell and Morgan 2001):

"They asked me what I needed, just let me talk, I wasn't keen at first but they went at my pace, they waited to see what it was that I needed."

"I am offered all sorts of things, swimming or shopping etc, then I decide what I need, sometimes it's just tea and a chat, sometimes it's more if I need it. I want to do more but my medication makes it hard for me, they understand that."

"I worry they give me too much of their time, but they always say it's no problem."

"They are like friends, if I don't keep in touch they send little notes and cards. I get trapped in my environment but they stop me from being alienated. They are not intrusive; they talk about everyday problems not just mental health ... ."

"They seem to know how to handle me, they are not patronising or intrusive, they help me without me knowing I am getting help."

Directing the helping process

In the day-to-day working relationship, the challenge to service providers should be for them to demonstrate how they are working with the priorities set by the service user, rather than hearing what a person has said but still following a service-determined tangential line of priorities. Only in exceptions of high imminent risk and serious crises should such determinations be temporarily over-ridden. Where the practitioners and service user hold conflicting views, e.g. that monitoring mental state and medication are essential priorities, it is important to note that these functions can be openly discussed while engaging in activity that is more in line with the service user's expressed wishes, e.g. visiting a welfare rights agency to access information about maximizing income. In this way, the service priorities may come to be seen as less intrusive necessities by the service user, than if they are presented up front as the most important work to be done before moving on to the service user's wishes.

This primarily raises the issue of the potential for people to be truly empowered to take more control of their own lives, through determining the form and direction the helping relationship should most usually be taking. It upholds the function of 'working with' rather than a more paternalistic 'doing to' or 'doing for' stance (Morgan 1996). With the group of people frequently referred to as experiencing severe and enduring mental health problems, this principle may appear the hardest to grasp. How can a person who is experiencing serious psychotic symptoms, e.g. delusional beliefs about a family member trying to poison them, and possibly detained under a section of the Mental Health Act, really be the director of the helping process?

The initial response to the above dilemma is to ask ourselves to take an alternative look at how we view the role of 'directing'. We need to shed any one-dimensional views that may be held. At one level, the person is actually being directed by services to function in ways and places contrary to their own personal perceptions and desires. However, that is not to say that, while one part of the system is responding to the need for enforced containment of the perceived or real crisis, work cannot continue with the service user to remind them – and the mental health system itself – of the user's longer-term goals, for independent housing for example. It is the acknowledgement and active work in these other areas that will enable the person to keep giving some direction to the helping process.

Prance (1993) reminds us that: "This challenging approach stresses that therapeutic agendas should be set by what the client wants and should reflect the uniqueness of each client's circumstances. Each client has unique personal resources and should work towards his or her own goals. …"

Rapp (1998) expresses the importance of client self-determination as follows: "The client has the right to make the choices, but freedom may best be served by knowledge of the choices possible and the confidence that the person could successfully select from among these choices."

This principle recognizes that people need ongoing support in the community, but that the amount of support required may vary considerably.

Box 3.5   Julian Housing Support: evaluation

In the published independent service user evaluation of the service (Graley-Wetherell and Morgan 2001), the users of the Active Outreach team were asked about how much choice they felt they had within the service. The responses were:

"Never been a conflict or disagreement."

"They accept it's my choice."

"It's my choice, they wouldn't mind or take it personally."

"They persuaded me to go into hospital, but I would have been sectioned if they hadn't so it was okay."

In team discussions, members of the Active Outreach team recognize the importance of prioritizing service user choice through providing as much information as possible about the options available in specific circumstances. However, a balanced approach is achieved through the team checking out their understanding of the risks and resources required around particular choices. Sharing these and issues of difference with the person is equally important.

The task for practitioners is to be sufficiently responsive and flexible, delivering appropriate levels of support broadly in line with the wishes of the person themselves. This may be criticized for appearing an idealized approach to the working relationship. In reality, it is a necessity if we are to remain connected with people and not provide additional reasons for them to actively disengage.

Continuity and acceptance are essential foundations for promoting recovery

Continuity of care over an extended period of time is an essential principle of Assertive Outreach. Stein and Test's (1980) landmark research study found that service users receiving Assertive Outreach did very well over the first 14 months of the study but that when this service was withdrawn they did no better than the control group. Concerning the deterioration during this second 14-month period, Stein (1992) comments: "At first blush this deterioration in the second phase was a disappointment. However, on further consideration I believe that this was the most important finding of the study. What this experiment made clear is that we need to move from a time-limited model to a model that provides services indefinitely. In retrospect it seems obvious that when we deal with an illness that we do not know how to prevent or cure – and that is thus chronic in nature – the intervention must likewise be long term in nature." Service users vary enormously in the pattern or course that their illness takes. Allness and Knoedler (1998) express the point well: "Effective treatment and rehabilitation provided in a co-ordinated and continuous manner can have a positive impact upon the course of a mental illness so that episodes are less frequent and prolonged and functioning between episodes is improved."

In our view the principle of continuity applies equally to the staff of Assertive Outreach services. Mental health services are frequently organized to promote turnover of staff, e.g. six-month rotation placement posts, or they highlight the need for staff to change posts regularly to avoid 'burnout'. The other structural difficulty is the lack of continuing financial recompense for people who remain in the same post for a long time, thus encouraging ambitious staff members to rapidly seek promotions through changing jobs. The recurring theme is that staff remain fresh and vitalized by seeking change, and will tend to stagnate if they remain constant in one place.

For the groups of people who require longterm care and support in response to their conditions and experiences, discontinuity of staffing frequently presents a barrier to progress. Many people complain of having to repeat their somewhat negative life story to a never-ending succession of staff. For every step forward, they seem to have to take a step back at best. Just when trust and confidence is established in a person they move on.

The emphasis seems to be on a service orientation as a first priority, and service user orientation as a second. Services are not specifically thought through with a view to working with a small number of complex people over extended time, e.g. at least years. The strengths approach aims to attract people who specifically believe in longterm continuity as a foundation for recovery, and seeks to support the nature of individual and team practice in a way that provides rewarding experiences for those who stay for the longterm.

An important feature in Assertive Outreach practice is a *team approach* (see Chapter 5). Its advantages include the likelihood of continuity in the delivery of services, in that if one worker is on leave or sick another can take over. It can increase the creativity in care planning and it can improve the possibilities of avoiding burnout, as well as encouraging the development of staff morale (Box 3.6). Witheridge (1991) puts this point well: "the burdens of the work become 'ours', not just 'mine', and the accomplishments – including those that might seem inconsequential to outsiders – likewise belong to everyone."

One of the important innovations in promoting continuity of service delivery has been to extend the concept of normal working hours. Crises are not limited to the 'nine-to-five' working pattern, and hospital admissions generally are over-represented after five at night, at weekends and on holidays – periods of time when the normal support system is unavailable. Twenty-four hours per day availability of crisis responses ensures that a support system can, potentially, always be available, to promote recovery through responsiveness at the point of need.

This principle is actively working against the inconsistent UK 'discharge culture' that anecdotally appears to hinder case closure in the overburdened community mental health team (CMHT) sector of community services, while constantly pressuring the Assertive Outreach sector to be looking to move people back into the CMHTs!

Box 3.6   Julian Housing Support: team mental health

Sustaining longterm intensive work with people experiencing severe and enduring mental health problems is assumed to induce burnout in staff, and rapid turnover. This has not been the case for Active Outreach team staff, and this is a tribute to the ability of all the team to address its collective mental health. Anecdotally this is attributed to a number of factors (not in any particular order of importance):

- good quality individual and peer supervision
- a recent innovation of user involvement in staff selection
- good internal communication, including the use of a message book
- flexibly available and responsive to support each other's needs
- a culture that encourages creative 'out-of-the-box' thinking
- a sense of humour
- impromptu lunches and planned outings together
- external facilitators who believe in the work of the team
- checklist on the office wall, of early warning signs of *staff* stress
- looking out for each other's levels of stress
- feeling supported by the 'host' organization's culture
- tolerance of difference, in staff members' ideas and service users' choices.

The size of team may be a significant factor to add to this list. It is easier to achieve some of the above with a group of five or six people than it would be with 12 or more.

Developing an outreach perspective

Lack of motivation and social withdrawal are very frequently observed aspects of the secondary, ongoing effects of schizophrenia. Moreover, many clients with perhaps several painful experiences of compulsory hospitalization may be actively seeking to avoid services. This creates a dilemma for office-based community services, since clients with longterm mental health problems are often not very good at turning up at the office and keeping appointments. For this reason, traditional community services often have trouble keeping in touch with longterm clients.

At its most fundamental, this principle highlights the importance of working in the person's own environment and social network. In this way, we are more able to get a clearer idea of what contributes to their distress, of what works or does not work in relation to relieving the distress, and promoting positive change towards recovery. It underpins the promotion of empowerment by handing more control to people about where and when the helping relationship will happen. It is not simply a question of doing home visits for some, and encouraging others to attend the service base if they can!

Rapp (1998) reminds us that the nature of the priorities and work cannot be completed by an office-bound approach: "An outreach mode offers rich opportunities for assessment and intervention. Office-bound assessment limits the sources of data to what the client says, the case manager's observations of the client, and the 10-inch stack of paper referred to as a case file. This is simply not enough for a variety of reasons." Skill development needs to be carried out in the environment where the person is actually encountering problems of adaptation. Hence, the person can be encouraged to develop coping skills in the precise location where they are likely to be of most benefit. Skills learned in a natural setting can be used later with little or no additional requirement to generalize. Thus, unlike skills learned in institutional settings such as hospitals or day centres, skills learned 'in vivo' immediately begin to make a difference in a person's actual living environment.

We ultimately put service organization pressures at the top of the agenda, by requiring the service user to fit into our appointments system at our locations. What does this achieve? In some circumstances, anger, frustration and disengagement from the whole process. The rhetoric says service user involvement and empowerment but reality says we are too busy for anything other than a service-centred approach to the organization of our work. 'Our work' takes higher ground over 'service users' needs and aspirations'.

Adopting an outreach perspective also helps to move the balance of power more towards the service user. Much has been discussed in terms of the 'difficult to engage client'; there is far less discussion about the 'difficult to engage service'. The essential priority for Assertive Outreach services is to adapt to situations and circumstances of the service user, and to put *their* convenience above those of the service. The service user as expert in their own experiences becomes a more dominant model when outreach requires that professionals travel out beyond the confines of their service bases.

Box 3.7   Julian Housing Support: initiative in practice

One example of initiative in practice is the development of a 'video group'. The idea arose from a service user suggesting that workers should see what service users really experienced. At the time, one person was dealing with their paranoid ideas by erecting a video camera outside their own front door. The idea evolved into commissioning an independent film-maker, with no experience in working with mental health difficulties. The results have been that a small group of service users have written and produced their own video 'Give Us a Minute', and are receiving commissions for other video projects, e.g. videoing a conference, and potential 'training' materials for the local statutory sector services. The use of an independent facilitator is felt to bring an entirely different focus and perspective – the project feels less like a mental health group, and the external person has learned and disseminates a much less stigmatizing view of service users' capabilities.

Risks do pose a realistic note of caution, as personal safety remains paramount when offering an outreach service function. Information about the carers and others in the local environment is just as important as the potential risks that service users could pose. Conversely, some people when offered the choice may decide to conduct more meetings at the service bases, rather than have too much perceived intrusion into their own home.

The neighbourhood as a resource

This principle challenges us to think more carefully about what we mean when we talk of integrating people back into the community. Most frequently, mental health services achieve little more for the individual person than to establish a new community-based mental health institution around them. At the point of hospital discharge the more usual plan consists of an outpatient appointment at a mental health service base or clinic, a regular appointment at a depot medication clinic where appropriate, a referral to a mental health day centre or similar resource. We say we have discharged a person back into the community, when all that has really been achieved is to shift them from an 'inpatient' psychiatric community to an 'outpatient' psychiatric community.

When considering the local communities in which people with mental health problems reside, the service providers most frequently arrive at the early conclusion that there is nothing but barriers to acceptance. We must not fall into a trap of ignoring the difficulties, stigma and dangers that frequently confront people with mental health problems in local communities. Equally, we should not use these as convenient barriers for not accepting the more challenging task of genuine integration of a person into their own neighbourhood. We need to look closer at their own locally available resources and potential or real networks of support. Developing individual strengths should lead us on to developing unique links to meet individual needs – what Rapp refers to as niches.

The underlying challenge should be to identify the resources that we or anyone else uses, before falling back on segregated community mental health resources. Having identified what is possible, it is then a responsibility for a strengths approach service to recognize the barriers to full access and integration for a person with a mental health problem, and to work with negotiating these barriers.

There are people and resources waiting to be tapped in local neighbourhoods. The problem is often that local people receive their knowledge of mental health from the misguided reporting in the media. Service providers do little or nothing to challenge the misconceptions, or to offer alternative intelligence around the subject. "As with all aspects of this work, it is time-consuming, risk-taking and will not always be successful, but it extends the bounds of knowledge way beyond what can be achieved only at a service base" (Morgan 1996).

Rapp (1998) reminds us not just to attend to the strengths of the individual, but also to the strengths of the environment. The community is the source of mental health and opportunities. The presence of community-based mental health resources can act as an obstacle to real neighbourhood integration.

> **Box 3.8   Julian Housing Support: local connections**
>
> The 'active' focus of the work requires the team to hold a wider vision of what is available in the local community. Their focus on housing issues, combined with their place outside of statutory sector services, requires them to be more active in pursuing links with local community resources and other voluntary services. This is reflected in the words of the service users in the independent evaluation of the team (Graley-Wetherell and Morgan 2001), where they talk of swimming, the rock band, attending local football matches and horse racing, local churches, and other 'community' resources not linked to mental health services in any way.

Our task is to work to create neighbourhood collaborators. Blaming the 'community' for its lack of resources only leads to paralysis, frustration and impotence. Each community boasts a unique combination of assets, capabilities and skills, and these should be carefully mapped.

An effective programme of community support needs to be aware of Maslow's Hierarchy of Needs. The starting point should be ensuring that people have access to the basic material resources required to survive in their neighbourhood – food, shelter, clothing and so on. In addition, these should be considered in a culturally sensitive way, appropriate to the particular setting in which the person resides. Assertive Outreach services frequently prioritize their connections with local housing and benefits agencies (neighbourhood resources, not mental health resources) and as such they are naturally inclined towards working with the resources of the local neighbourhood.

FREQUENT PRACTITIONER RESPONSES TO THE 'PRINCIPLES'

The types of comment from practitioners in response to these principles have generally ranged between two extremes. Negative reactions include:

- I/we already do it.
- It represents nothing new.
- It is all too obvious.
- It is far too simple.
- It is just positive reframing, without any change in the fundamental delivery of services.

It is difficult to challenge deep-rooted attitudes with only a few words. The real test of these challenges is for an experienced 'strengths' practitioner to spend a longer spell of time working alongside the doubters to demonstrate the differences of approach; or to closely monitor and constructively critique the practice of those who believe they already do it in their work. The authors felt this way, when Charlie Rapp and Wally Kisthardt first introduced it to them in 1991. The authors have one suggestion to offer to those who feel they already practise a strengths approach to their work: "You might think you do... we thought we did, until we did... then we realized we weren't... so maybe you aren't either!"

Furthermore, one of the authors has co-hosted strengths workshops with an experienced service user consultant trainer (Steve Morgan and Roberta Graley-Wetherell), where the audiences were encouraged to be equal numbers of service users and their care co-ordinators. A number of practitioners alluded to practising this way early on in the workshop, only to have the claims unanimously refuted by the service users. One outcome of the workshops was a much stronger mutual understanding of how to take the ideas forward in the working relationships.

Positive reactions include:

- This is how I like to think I should work, but how can I work with this approach more completely?
- How can these principles become more integrated into the wider team/service?

The principles outlined above are considered to be a set of rules governing the consistency by which a range of practitioners may apply a strengths approach to their work. Their application in practice also requires adherence by individual service providers to the intrinsic attitudes of Assertive Outreach staff. These would include attention to the quality of the working relationship, through acceptance of 'difference', commitment to individual needs and wants, collaborative and friendly styles of working that cross the artificial boundaries commonly favoured by most mental health services, patience to work with the often slow incremental pace of change, creativity and optimism.

Organizational development of the principles

It is one thing to develop a strengths approach to individual practice, or even to develop a small team espousing the principles into a unified approach to practice. However, it is quite something else to apply them more widely across a whole service. We do not have any current UK examples of a 'strengths organization' in mental health, though the Julian Housing Support voluntary sector agency, used as an illustration throughout this chapter, is a rare example actively working towards this goal. How can these principles become a service philosophy, i.e. what would a 'strengths organization' look like? A workshop facilitated with a management team in Julian Housing Support (Morgan 2002) produced the following application of the strengths approach to the management functions (Box 3.9).

Box 3.9   Applying 'strengths' principles to the management team purpose

The following principles guide a collective accountability for all levels of staff to promote standards of good practice within the current mission statement of Julian Housing Support.

---

box continues

> **Principles**
>
> 1. The focus of the supportive management process is upon developing the team members' strengths, interests, abilities and capabilities. Individual deficits or weaknesses are addressed constructively and positively in a safe environment.
>
> 2. All team members have the potential to be reflective, to enable learning, growth and change.
>
> 3. The team member–team manager relationship is an essential partnership.
>
> 4. The collaborative management relationship promotes appropriate levels of autonomy and skills.
>
> 5. Commitment to openness and opportunities are essential foundations for promoting staff development.
>
> 6. The supportive management process takes on an outreach perspective.
>
> 7. Promoting the 'housing support' perspective will enable staff to be an essential part of multi-agency working.
>
> 8. Team members will be encouraged to view the local neighbourhood as a source of potential resources. These should be considered as well as more segregated mental health resources (Morgan 2002).

CONCLUSIONS

In the day-to-day demands of mental health practice, we can easily become consumed by the everchanging requirements of top-down service development, the interprofessional rivalries, and the personal crises of service users and carers. The world of mental health service delivery is a complicated web. On one side, the managers are entangled in a plethora of government directives and a need for perpetual audit. On the other, practitioners are entangled in an ever-increasing requirement for bureaucracy and administration. The result is that we all quickly lose sight of the original purpose for services to be established in the first place: care and support for service users.

In this web, it is easier for burdened practitioners to revert to type without particular thought: they adopt a seemingly noble and paternalistic medical approach of 'saving people'. Service managers may be seen to adopt a leadership role in the saving culture, by delivering policy guidance and reviewing incidents of failure. On all accounts, we fail to hold on to the important values and principles that help to clearly define our purpose. The strengths approach upholds the purpose of supporting service users to capture and use their own positive resources, to counter the negative experiences of severe and enduring mental distress. It encourages the service user to define their own personal definition of recovery, and the goals to achieve its direction. The seven principles cut through the complex web we manage to create around us. It is the responsibility of all practitioners and managers to remind themselves of the principles that underpin their real purpose.

References

Allness D, Knoedler W 1998 The PACT Model of Community-Based Treatment for Persons with Severe and Persistent Mental Illness. NAMI, Virginia

Deitchman W S 1980 How many case managers does it take to screw in a light bulb? Hospital and Community Psychiatry 31 (11): 788–789

Graley-Wetherell R, Morgan S 2001 Active Outreach: An independent service user evaluation of a model of assertive outreach practice. Sainsbury Centre for Mental Health, London

Maslow A H 1954 Motivation and personality. Harper & Row, New York

Maslow A H 1967 Self-actualization and beyond. In: Bugental JFT (ed) Challenges of Humanistic Psychology. McGraw-Hill, New York

Maslow A H 1970 Motivation and Personality, 2nd edn. Harper & Row, New York

Morgan S 1996 Case management responses. In: Morgan S Helping Relationships in Mental Health. Chapman & Hall, London, p 45–67

Morgan S 2002 Julian Housing Support: A Manager's Practice Development Programme. Workshops facilitated for the newly emerging management team. November 2002, Norwich (unpublished)

Prance N 1993 Travelling companions. Nursing Times 89 (5): 28–30

Rapp C A 1988 The Strengths Perspective of Case Management with Persons Suffering from Severe Mental Illness. University of Kansas and NIMH, Lawrence

Rapp C A 1993 Theory, principles, and methods of strengths model case management. In: Harris M, Bergman H (eds) Case Management: Theory and Practice. American Psychiatric Association, Washington, DC, p 143–164

Rapp C A 1998 The Strengths Model: Case Management with People Suffering from Severe and Persistent Mental Illness. Oxford University Press, New York

Sainsbury Centre for Mental Health 1998 Keys to Engagement: Review of care for people with severe mental illness who are hard to engage with services. Sainsbury Centre for Mental Health, London

Stein L 1992 Innovating Against the Current. New Directions in Mental Health 56: 5–40

Stein L, Test A 1980 Alternatives to mental hospital treatment: conceptual model, treatment program and clinical evaluation. Archives of General Psychiatry 37: 392–397

Witheridge T 1991 The 'active ingredients' of assertive outreach. New Directions for Mental Health Services 52: 47–64

PART 2

A guide to practice

The larger section of the book is focused on issues of daily practice, where service users are more directly involved, in contact and out of contact, with services. This is where people can be encouraged to express their aspirations in relation to their health and social circumstances, and where they may have opportunities to consider their talents and achievements in relation to potentially resolving areas of difficulty they may be experiencing. For practitioners, this is where they too may express their creativity and talents, finding potentially new solutions to challenging situations.

A strengths approach is designed to capture the achievement of goals by individual service users, and the imagination and potentials of the staff. It is a means of enabling vision, rather than restricting the sight of what can be achieved through individual and collective relationships, and permissive working processes and practices. It enables individuals (service users and practitioners) to find their personal niches, and to develop real networks of support not just mental health service connections.

The chapters in this section will focus on the following areas:

- Understanding some of the ethical dilemmas unearthed when a new and potentially contentious method of service delivery is introduced to engage people who have possibly chosen to disengage from mental health services.
- Considering different ways of configuring positive 'team working'.
- Helping to define the groups of people that Assertive Outreach services are more likely to be working with.
- Considering the meaning and processes of 'engagement'.
- Developing strengths-based 'assessment' and 'care planning'.
- Examining the effectiveness of what the working relationships and interventions aim to be providing through this method of service delivery.
- Considering the constructive role and mechanisms for achieving positive risk-taking in the lives of service users.
- Examining the roles that research, training, practice development and reflective group supervision can play in implementing good strengths practice.

Chapter **4**

Ethical dilemmas

Steve Morgan and Peter Ryan

Why call people service users, when they do not want to use the service?

INTRODUCTION

The ethics of care is a particular minefield, and throughout the complex considerations and debates of bioethics nowhere is it a more thorny issue than in mental health. The debate puts into sharp focus the boundary between free choice and reduced responsibility, the examination of human rights, the accessibility and appropriateness of services, issues of consent to treatment, personal and professional boundaries, and of confidentiality. Discussions about ethics in mental health frequently get bogged down in issues of professional codes of conduct. As important as the latter are for directing guidelines for good practice and monitoring practitioner performance, too narrow an appreciation of their purpose risks losing sight of the specific values that underpin practice. The whole issue that value diversity, as held by different people, may enrich our perspectives of the individual dilemmas faced in routine practice may be lost. An urge to adhere to a universally agreed set of values will only result in the loss of any sense of value diversity.

We must avoid the temptation of looking to ethics for a prescription of answers to the many dilemmas. We need to adopt a more pragmatic stance, looking to develop more ethical processes that promote recognition of the diversity of values held by different individuals in different situations (Dickenson and Fulford 2001, Williamson 2003). Right and wrong may apply on occasions, but such a black and white approach is inappropriate and obstructive to our consideration of the issues. This shift of emphasis is referred to by Williamson (2002), where he proposes an ethical basis for supporting the delivery of Assertive Outreach services focused more on the clients' values, and areas of assistance with which they express genuine appreciation and satisfaction. This direction is very much in line with that upheld by a strengths approach.

This chapter will attempt to explore an ethical approach to practice by following a structure that primarily examines the 'ethics of practice', working through the clinical process from engagement to discharge. The debate begins with an overview of the civil liberty issues of privacy and freedom, given their centrality to the operation of Assertive Outreach. There has been a great deal of emphasis in the National Service Framework (NSF) and elsewhere on Assertive Outreach targeting the 'hard-to-engage client'. However, the various ways in which services themselves, from a user perspective, may be hard to engage or resistant to change has been almost entirely neglected. This chapter attempts to correct this imbalance.

PRIVACY, FREEDOM AND CONFIDENTIALITY

Assertive Outreach infringes individual rights to privacy and freedom of choice, or so it is often alleged by many of its critics. It is interesting to note that when mental health services were still primarily configured around the mental hospital, issues of privacy and confidentiality received scant attention (Skull 1993). However, care in the community has highlighted a whole series of moral dilemmas and ambiguities in terms of balancing the care of those who need it with the broader concerns of the possible implications and impact of such care upon the community as a whole. 'The community', when translated into its specifics in terms of a particular neighbourhood, or family, is inevitably involved either as an observer or as a participant, in the care of those who, two generations ago, were out of sight and out of mind. Equally, there are ethical ambiguities for the service user:

- To what degree is the mental health service user simply a citizen with all the rights and duties of anyone else living freely in the community?
- To what degree does the fact they are deemed to have a major and severe illness cut across their rights to privacy, freedom and freedom of choice?

Nowhere are these ethical ambiguities more apparent than with Assertive Outreach. Normal custom and practice offers the choice to attend an appointment for assessment and intervention where indicated. These are precisely the conditions that are *not* operative in Assertive Outreach, which in the UK is established with the brief to provide a service for those who are highly unlikely to attend an appointment, and who may be positively hostile to receiving any service at all: "Problems may occur because of discrete circumstances or a combination of factors involving *where* the care occurs, *who* delivers the services, and *what* those services entail" (Backlar 2001).

There is an important sense in which privacy is culturally determined – we happen to live in a society in which privacy is very highly valued. Imagine a situation in which we have a medical condition for which we have been prescribed medication. For a while we take it and then, because it has unpleasant side-effects, we stop taking it. One day someone knocks at our door and, amongst other things, asks us if we are taking our medication. We reply that it is none of their business, go away and do not come back. The person replies politely but firmly that they understand what we are saying but that they will come back tomorrow to see how we are getting on. The next day, the same scenario repeats itself, and the day after, etc. We may be forgiven for thinking that we do not need to see the film 'Ground Hog Day' since it is happening to us in real life! Yet it is precisely this kind of consistent and persistent intrusion that Assertive Outreach visits upon its clients as a matter of routine, indeed essential, practice.

Clearly, government policy as enshrined in the *National Service Framework for Mental Health* (Department of Health 1999) and the *NHS National Plan* (Department of Health 2000) have come to the conclusion that such intrusion is not only warranted but desirable in terms of good practice. Yet perhaps it serves a useful purpose here to step back and consider some basic issues: on what ethical and moral grounds has the government (and mental health services) legitimized such intrusion on privacy for a particularly vulnerable client group? Are these grounds justifiable? If they are not, then the case for Assertive Outreach falls at the first hurdle.

Perhaps a good starting point is defining what we mean by 'privacy'. According to Dworkin (1993), privacy can have three connotations or domains. Firstly, there is 'decisional privacy', denoting that we are free to direct our own lives. Clearly, from a strengths perspective, this value is fundamental to the whole approach and is defined in this book (see Chapter 3) under Principle 4 as: "The service user is viewed as the director of the helping process". The strengths approach is therefore dedicated wherever and whenever possible to optimize, re-enforce and develop the decisional privacy of the individual service user. However, Burns and Firn (2002) rightly state that: "Issues of free will and personal autonomy are at the heart of all mental health practice… In psychotic disorders, the perception of the world we live in is changed – the familiar becomes threatening, neutral acquaintances become persecutory and random irrelevant events become charged with personal meanings." It is precisely under these circumstances that a strengths approach has a major role to play. Its challenge is to assist the user to maintain in these terms a sense of self, which is as fully capable as possible of 'decisional privacy'.

Secondly, privacy can be understood in terms of personal space and the individual's right to protect it. Nozick (1974) refers to this as: "An area in moral space around an individual." For many Assertive Outreach clients, this can be in any case very fragile and easily lost. For some clients, living precariously in the community, it may sometimes feel as if the only area in their lives in which they can actually exercise a degree of choice is with respect to their medication, i.e. whether to take it all and, if so, how much. The ethical dilemma here of course is that almost by definition Assertive Outreach challenges consistently the boundaries between freedom, consent to treatment and the right to refuse treatment (for consideration of the issue of the right to refuse treatment).

The third domain of privacy according to Dworkin (1993) refers to information about ourselves or our situation that we are not required to divulge to anyone else: "We do not have to disclose to others what we are thinking, how we cast our political ballot, what religious beliefs we hold – or except to the taxman – how much money we have in our bank accounts" (Backlar 2001). It is probably this third domain that lies closest to the issue of confidentiality. Bok (1983) refers to confidentiality as pertaining to "...the boundaries surrounding shared secrets and to the process of guarding these boundaries..." Fulford (2001) states that a major paradox of confidentiality is: "This double bind on healthcare practice – to disclose and to keep secret, to expose and to hide..." This has been achieved for several reasons, including the shift from closed institution to more open community, the emergence of multidisciplinary and multi-agency collaborative practice, the requirement under the Care Programme Approach (CPA) to share information across services and agencies, and the risk and safety agenda. Engaging a meaningful working relationship has always been based on the issue of trust. For a person experiencing mental distress, in a climate that predominantly stigmatizes and excludes people with mental health problems, this requires the client to confide in the practitioner. This confiding of personal information is entered into on the assumption that it remains confidential, i.e. it will not be put out and shared in a wider domain than the therapeutic relationship.

Szmukler and Holloway (2001) remind us of the recent structural and procedural changes in community mental health, with the risk agenda leading to a greater emphasis on co-ordinating care in a more dispersed and fragmented service landscape. To achieve successful co-ordination will require a greater degree of information sharing. This is completely at odds with the rules of confidentiality, which are still largely concerned with regulating the one-to-one relationship. Recent writers have agreed that the rules governing confidentiality in mental health have become outdated and impractical (Fulford 2001, Szmukler and Holloway 2001). They also agree that the way forward lies with a greater focus on individual diversity, whether that be of client values or expressed wishes set out in advance of the situations that may give rise to withholding consent.

One of the principles of strengths Assertive Outreach is to view the wider community, beyond mental health services, as a potential reservoir of resources to meet individual need (see Chapter 3). This requires a more sophisticated understanding of a person's needs, and of the community as a whole. As such, Assertive Outreach will be at the forefront of confidentiality considerations, always facing the dilemma of weighing up the benefits of strict confidentiality with the benefits of appropriate disclosure of information in order to access other resources. The principle of upholding confidentiality needs to remain a foundation of routine practice, but the greater openness of discussions with people can be the best guide to working with individual differences in values, in order to come to the most appropriate outcome in each set of circumstances. Maybe we put too much emphasis on trying to achieve the definitive criteria for confidentiality that will satisfy all circumstances – the 'confidentiality yardstick' that does not really have to exist. Cordess (2001) deals with the complexities of 'confidentiality' in much more depth than can be covered here.

Finally, the concerns for risk and danger dictate that there will be occasions when Assertive Outreach and other services have to breach confidentiality without the consent of the individual. Szmukler and Holloway (2001) remind us that as long as disclosure without consent is carried out responsibly the two broadly agreed criteria are:

1. Risk to the person, in a situation where they lack the capacity to give consent.
2. Risk to others resulting from nondisclosure.

In respect of these relatively rare circumstances, it is important for Assertive Outreach practitioners to be aware of how their own values diverge from those of the person they are working with (especially where different values are held by different professionals or teams resulting in tensions or conflicts within and between organizations).

A further issue of confidentiality surrounding some people who are in contact with Assertive Outreach is that they may be *very* well known locally as people with mental health problems, to neighbours and to generic services, e.g. housing or the police. This has the potential to make the confidentiality issue more complicated where secrecy is highly valued. Conversely, at a pragmatic level of trying to find out where or how someone is, and occasionally accessing more support, confidentiality could become a simpler issue.

ETHICS OF PRACTICE

Holloway and Carson (2001) propose there is a close correlation between the ethical issues of Assertive Outreach and those previously experienced in traditional rehabilitation services. They particularly highlight issues of 'empowerment versus neglect', 'care versus control' and 'respect for autonomy versus intervention'. Whilst there are some undeniable similarities in the types of dilemma experienced, the fundamental nature of Assertive Outreach services implies they will experience them more intensively. Unlike Assertive Outreach, rehabilitation services were not primarily established to work with such a negatively and narrowly defined group of people. The service context in which Assertive Outreach is located throws open a greater opportunity for more challenging debate of the true aims and purposes of mental health service delivery.

ETHICS OF ENGAGEMENT

The 'hard-to-engage' client

A significant impetus for establishing Assertive Outreach services has been an expectation of working more intensively and consistently with a group of people who were disengaging from the services they were deemed to need. The phrase 'hard to engage' is strongly associated with the definition of the client group. Descriptions of this group of people generally attribute negative connotations to them, such as 'resistant' to services or 'unreachable' (see Chapter 6). The use of such terminology can only lead to negative attitudes about the people concerned permeating the thinking of practitioners, policymakers and public alike. Within services, it may inevitably creep into everyday language, serving a dubious purpose of a quick indication of the client group appropriate for referral to Assertive Outreach services. The inherent danger of relying on verbal shorthand is the strong possibility that the negative sentiments filter through to the group of people concerned. The obvious implications are that engagement becomes more difficult, through the introduction of an additional barrier of negative perceptions held by the service providers.

Little attention is paid to why people become so hard to engage. It may be conveniently attributed to their personality, the convenience being that services do not have to reflect on their own culpability in this respect. From a service perspective, it is much easier to think in terms of the person lacking insight or failing to comply with the advice and interventions prescribed. It is less easy to think about the lack of insight and the failure of the services to identify and respond to the true needs in a flexible manner.

The 'hard-to-engage' service

How often do we think about the hard-to-engage service? What might it look like? In its most blatant form, the hard-to-engage service is one that perpetuates a stigmatizing view of people experiencing severe mental distress, largely 'medicalizing' their experiences, and compartmentalizing their needs and potential service responses in a way that is barely recognizable to the person in need. These types of service are more likely to attract practitioners who believe in the expert stance – that they are professionals and, as such, know the needs and possibilities better than the people using the service. This type of service is most often identified through a 'doing to' and 'prescribing for' approach, accompanied with attribution of blame on the user of the service if positive outcomes are not achieved. They may know and use the politically correct terminology of involvement and inclusion, but their actions do not demonstrate the real meaning in practice.

A person's right to refuse a service

Ethical debates have a habit of throwing up more questions than answers, and the issue of right to refuse is no exception. This issue becomes particularly acute in relation to the previous outline of the potentially hard-to-engage service. In this scenario, people may be seen to be exercising their right of refusal based on a previous experience of services they did not feel were appropriate or responsive to their personal perceptions of need.

In most areas of medicine people opt in to treatment. They also have the freedom to opt out of treatment, or ignore the advice they have been offered. In situations where emergency services are involved treatment is delivered to people – considered an urgent or life-saving need – with little question of choice, rights or discussion (though Jehovah's Witnesses would hold strong disagreement with this line of argument). In mental health services, people opt in to a degree, but once in find the services taking much more control. It is possible, but not so easy, to opt out of contact. For a minority of people the initial opting in was not an issue of choice either.

What happened to the right to refuse? Why is it such a difficult issue in the field of mental health? The answers to these questions are much more intricately woven into the broad sweeping views and fears of society, which possibly makes the situation more difficult and intangible for the individual wishing to oppose such views. The service providers' defences can be quickly raised against some people who attempt to exercise a right to refuse, based on professional assessments of lacking insight and impaired judgement and decision-making abilities. The mechanics of mental distress and processes of mental illness are largely deemed to impede the very basis on which a refusal of service is based – it's Catch 22!

When do we reach the point that it is right to make decisions for others? Is it ever right, or perhaps more accurately seen as 'humane,' to intervene in the decision-making processes of another person? Perhaps the most difficult dilemma is justifying a service and individual clinical practice where you have neither a mandate from the person receiving the service or a specific legal mandate. Duty of care and the apparent requirements of the CPA feel very flimsy in this respect. Any perceived clarity on this issue becomes shrouded in divisions of opinion when we examine exactly who is making the judgements of when to over-ride the wishes of another, and by what criteria these decisions are being made (Perkins and Repper 1998). Professionals, whether doctors, nurses or social workers, can make arbitrary judgements of mental capacity, without full possession of the facts and without sufficient consultation, not necessarily paying sufficient attention to social considerations or alternative views. Is a decision thus reached a right or full one? At the very least, decisions thus taken could be regarded as overpaternalistic and even coercive (Stovall 2001).

Those taking control of the decision-making process are predominantly coming from a 'professional' viewpoint. As informed as this frequently is, it does not equate with the reality of experiencing the conditions and distress that people sometimes find themselves in. It is also often only one part of a broader professional spectrum, not necessarily giving equal validity to all the pieces of information potentially influencing the decision. It is often a different matter when people as 'patients' are assessed to be making a fully informed and rational judgement, e.g. in physical illnesses. The case of Diane Pretty in 2002, regarding the right for assisted suicide in a terminal stage of motor neurone disease, went all the way to the European Court of Human Rights (Pretty 2002) but still resulted in a judicial decision over-riding her own expressed wishes.

When an individual's decision may have serious consequences of risk, to self or others, how free should they be to make such decisions? Suicide, for example, is no longer illegal. However, are we providing people with the best service by simply accepting their decision to inflict potentially fatal harm to themselves, when we consider them to be mentally unstable and not thinking in a clear and fully informed way? And what about the many service users who have thanked service practitioners or carers after the event, for taking control of decisions, even when it was against their apparent wishes at the time?

Inflicting harm on others is a crime. Are we right to attempt to prevent crimes, or should we be giving people freedom of choice to take chances and deal with the criminal justice system if they are caught? What about the victims of crimes we could reasonably predict but took no action because it would infringe the apparent rights of the perpetrator? In the reality of mental health service delivery practitioners cannot win. There are too many opposing positions – requiring action, upholding freedom and demanding someone's blood when something ultimately goes wrong. The liberal viewpoint, supporting individuals' rights to make choices and to refuse services, is an important voice for shaping better mental health services. However, the Not In My Back Yard (NIMBY) mentality is just as likely to apply to incidents as it does to physical proximity, e.g. if it was your child or partner who would be at serious risk from someone else's freedom of choice, however liberal your attitudes, how free would their choice be then?

What value do we place on preventive rather than reactive support and interventions? There has to be a reasonable position that upholds rights as well as providing support at times to those in need, even when they do not agree with the need at the time. In the case of Assertive Outreach services, we need to ask a specific question: does the person really know the service that they are refusing, or are they basing their refusal on an assumption that Assertive Outreach is the same type of service as they have previously experienced? It is our contention that a strengths approach to Assertive Outreach is not the same type of service, as it promotes a stronger focus on the person's expressed needs (which are more often social than mental health oriented), although assertive community treatment and the government's intentions for Assertive Outreach may well be similar to previous negative experiences.

It is our view that Assertive Outreach operates at the very limits of health and public policy, and should be expressly set up with the expectation of providing a different, user-focused and user-centred experience of services, both for people delivering and for those receiving them. Therefore, the right of refusal should be an informed right relating to what a person knows, not just accepting refusal at face value. It is important to take any appropriate opportunities to explore what a stated refusal is based on, and to negotiate where differences of opinion clearly arise (Box 4.1). Persistence is a key requirement of people working in Assertive Outreach. However, Burns and Firn (2002) remind us that

Box 4.1   Case study

John had a history of 20 years' contact with mental health services, predominantly diagnosed with psychotic depression. He had been living alone since his wife and child left him nearly 17 years ago. He experienced frequent episodes of feeling very low with suicidal ideas, and on each occasion the services offered little support other than medication, and then responded by taking him into hospital, apparently for his own safety. John always disliked the hospital admissions and felt that they contributed nothing more than making him feel worse; so he decided to try to avoid all contact with the community mental health services by failing to attend appointments and through not answering the door when people called. He was referred to the Assertive Outreach team with the aim of re-engaging him with the mental health services.

The initial written contact with John briefly outlined an idea of the new team trying to work differently with him, suggesting that the first visit to his home may only be to ask him where he would prefer to meet up. John opened the door for a couple of minutes to suggest he did not need a mental health service. The two Assertive Outreach workers accepted this initial statement but asked if they could meet him somewhere to talk about what services had been offered previously, and whether there was something else that would meet his own view of his needs. John suggested they may find him at his local pub, where he goes two or three times a week for an hour. The workers joked that they may be drinking non-alcoholic drinks for a long time waiting for him to arrive if he could not give a more specific time.

At the local pub a few days later John again expressed the view that he did not need a mental health service. The Assertive Outreach workers asked him if he wished to talk more about his negative experiences of services, suggesting that they did not wish to make any unfounded guesses about why he wished to refuse contact. They both acknowledged and accepted his account of being controlled through hospital admissions when he felt he would be better placed to stay at home and 'ride the storm'.

Over the next few weeks John accepted regular short visits to his home, and other contacts in the pub. He met a third worker from the team during these contacts. He began to explain that he had been feeling very low again, thinking a lot about the child he had not seen since she was three years old, who would now be 20. He suggested that he would be ashamed for her to see him the way he is, and even though he had suicidal ideas he did not want services taking him back into hospital. The Assertive Outreach workers responded by encouraging him to talk more about his feelings for his daughter and ex-wife, and what he felt he had lost. Whilst checking out his suicidal ideas and plans with him, they did not discuss hospital admission but did offer to see him at home daily if he wished.

John interpreted the increased interest and proposed contact as a precursor to a hospital admission, and asked the team to stop working with him. Their initial response was to acknowledge his concerns and reassure him that hospital is not necessarily always the best solution. They negotiated for John to keep in daily contact with a trusted neighbour, and for the neighbour to maintain contact with the team in case John felt the intensity of his feelings might cause him to contemplate acting on his suicidal ideas. They suggested that they would spend more time within the team thinking about alternatives to hospital admission, and would communicate these to him via the neighbour or in writing, as a demonstration that they respected his wishes not to fear the outcomes of increased face-to-face contact.

The Assertive Outreach team in this instance contemplated the use of potential 'community treatment orders' as an order placed on the service rather than the client, requiring the service to acknowledge an important deficit in the range of service provision. It actively pursued the idea of crisis/respite accommodation as an alternative to hospital admission for people in extreme distress with potentially suicidal ideas. Simultaneously, they used a more flexibly negotiated approach to monitoring John's suicidal potential. His right to refuse a service was considered important but not absolute, as they assumed a responsibility to help him

through a difficult time emotionally without suicide as the eventual outcome.

John engaged more with the Assertive Outreach team following this episode. He subsequently had one mutually negotiated hospital admission lasting two days, at a time when he developed plans to end his life by jumping in front of a train. The team still pursue the idea of a reasonable 'crisis house' as an alternative to hospital admission, based on the experiences of John and a number of other people they are currently working with.

what the service provider sees as persistence can easily be seen as harassment by the person on the receiving end. However, Phillips et al (2001) suggest that people who do reject Assertive Outreach should be offered alternative services.

Rights come with responsibilities and choices come with consequences. Promoted correctly they are positive, but if negatively motivated they may become destructive.

Assertive versus aggressive

Some critics of Assertive Outreach claim it to be 'aggressive' outreach, as a reference to the coercive nature of a service that persists against the wishes of the recipient at an individual level, and as social control through the imposition of an oppressive biomedical model (Spindel and Nugent 2000). A paternalistic approach has undoubtedly been delivered within the remit of some Assertive Outreach services, particularly through a failure to develop treatment plans in conjunction with service users, and the over-riding of personal autonomy on the grounds of benefiting both the client and the wider community (Williamson 2002).

Aggressive implies the service dictating to people what their needs are, and prescribing the necessary steps in response. As an example, Stein (1992) and Witheridge (1991) both give accounts of how some assertive community treatment teams in the USA make handing over the user's welfare benefit cheque contingent upon taking the prescribed medication. A user's refusal to comply can be interpreted by the service as a symptom of the illness, adopting the 'professional judgement is right' approach, as opposed to devoting time to the more challenging but rewarding activity of creating and negotiating alternative responses. For example, a strengths approach to the above issue would focus more on separating the issues of welfare rights and needs for medication, promoting the rights of the individual to financial support, and the right to refuse medication.

In a strengths approach, the term 'assertive' is taken to mean requiring the service to be flexible and creative in its engagement and response to people's needs; it is not about being assertive about a narrow set of prescriptive interventions. It is more of an insurance that the service will do all in its imagination and power to remain engaged with the individual's perspective, and to work with their perception of needs rather than dismissing them. An Assertive Outreach team will also openly acknowledge and work with the issues of 'difference' this approach could give rise to, rather than shirking some of the more intricate issues of service provision by hiding behind a 'professional' shield. The term 'assertive' also acts as a reminder to the service not to give up just because there has been a failure to engage constructive contact in the early phase. Persistence can be more easily interpreted as harassment when it is presented more as harassment, but it can be constructive care for a person's needs (Box 4.2).

FROM PERSUASION TO COMPULSION: THE ETHICS OF CONTROL IN ASSERTIVE OUTREACH

Much of the debate around the new legislation (see Chapter 2) revolves around the proposals for compulsory treatment. It can therefore easily be assumed that various grades or degrees of compulsion do not or cannot occur in current mental health practice. However, Burns and Firn (2002) usefully remind us that: "Much of the current debate about compulsion in the community oversimplifies both the nature of decisions and the nature of human relationships. Most of the important decisions we make

---

Box 4.2   Case study

Derek was flagged up as a major concern to mental health services by the primary care team who were caring for his elderly mother, with whom he shared a flat. He was believed to be severely agoraphobic and psychotic, occasionally preventing access to the District Nurses who called to his mother daily. On a thorough check of service records it was understood that Derek had been in the care of the psychiatric inpatient unit 12 years previously, but had been completely lost to all contact since.

The Assertive Outreach team was requested to make contact with Derek to offer an appropriate service, and to help in assessing and managing the risks to his mother. Their first point of contact was with the District Nurses, but it was then decided not to put their accessibility to the flat in further jeopardy by linking them with the mental health system. It was determined that Derek could read sufficiently well, so the team made their first approach by informal letter announcing a time they would visit.

However, Derek refused to allow the Assertive Outreach workers into the flat for 15 months but did occasionally talk with them at the front door, sometimes face to face and sometimes through a closed door. The manner of the acceptance of his control over the situation enabled the team to maintain a fragile contact with Derek, while continuing to support the concerns of the primary care team. Derek permitted access to the flat for the Assertive Outreach team worker at a time when his mother had a stroke. The team worker was the first person to visit after the tragic event, and Derek confronted his own degree of trust in the worker at a time of serious crisis. Derek's mother died shortly after the emergency admission to hospital, but he continued a more open working relationship with the Assertive Outreach team from this point onwards. Persistence had paid off in the long term.

as adults involve elements both of freewill and compulsion... It is important to be honest in confronting the power relations that do exist within mental health practice... we delude ourselves if we pretend that everything apart from compulsory admissions are entirely free and voluntary."

Wilen Berg and Bonnie (2001) and Szmukler and Applebaum (2001) both outline a spectrum of interventions, all within current mental health practice and all of which are aimed at changing or altering the expressed view and preference of the service user. They discuss various gradations in what they term 'treatment pressure' as follows:

- persuasion
- leverage
- inducement
- threats
- compulsory treatment in the community or as an inpatient.

Persuasion

It has been made clear in several places in this book that the strengths approach does not equate simply (and simplistically) to giving the user what they want. Wherever this is feasible this indeed should be the driver of the relationship between the service user and practitioner. However, there will be some occasions when the seasoned professional view of the practitioner may differ from that of the user. Under these circumstances, persuasion is an essential element of the strengths approach. The essence of persuasion is well summarized by Szmukler and Applebaum (2001): "The discussion with the patient revolves around an arguably realistic appraisal of the benefits and risks of treatment. There is a respect for the patient's arguments, and the treatment is discussed in the context of his or her value system. The process does not go beyond a debate."

The strengths approach promotes people's access to all the available information so that personal choices and decisions can be based on open discussion and negotiation. It also recognizes the reality that there may come times when a service user will not be fully in control of their decision-making abilities, and that the Assertive Outreach team may, in situations of high risk, have to make choices that over-ride the preference of the client. In other cases, service users may not be making the choices or lifestyle decisions that the team would endorse or agree with, but if there are no obvious immediate serious risks it is our role to maintain contact, support user decisions and keep discussions open.

Leverage

An Assertive Outreach practitioner will, under most circumstances, have engaged with and developed a therapeutic alliance with their service users. A practitioner can exercise leverage or 'interpersonal pressure' by using the relationship itself as a bargaining counter or instrument with the service user to remind them, with varying degrees of subtlety, of its importance to them. Therefore the practitioner can persuade the service user of the desirability of doing something that the practitioner wants or thinks advisable, and with which the service user does not necessarily agree.

Inducement

Inducements refer to contingencies: if you are prepared to do this (which you do not necessarily want to do) then I will do this or provide that. An inducement does not intrinsically imply taking away a right or a privilege from a service user. Arguably, it is an important, tried and tested element in engagement. At the engagement stage, the message to a service user is: 'Look at all these things which are useful to you (like sorting out your flat or welfare benefits) which I can do to help you – it would really be to your advantage to learn to trust me and the service I represent'. Wertheimer (1993) makes a useful distinction between an inducement and a threat: "The crux of the distinction between a threat and an inducement is that A makes a threat when B will be worse off in some relevant base-line position, if B does not accept A's proposal; but that A makes an inducement when B will be no worse off than in some relevant base-line position if B does not accept A's proposal." Thus an inducement accepts the situation, rights and privileges that the user is currently experiencing, and offers to materially or substantially add to the situation the user is in, whilst a threat works with the possibility of removing it.

Threats

A threat indicates an intention to take away or remove, unless the user complies in specified ways, aspects of privacy, place of stay, etc., which the user values and of which he or she would be reluctant to be deprived. Szmukler and Applebaum (2001) make the important point concerning the community-based mental health services within which care of various kinds and gradations is offered to service users: "Defining the moral baseline requires that a mental health service defines a patient's entitlement to various components of health care as well as help to be offered in accessing social and other forms of care." Thus, paradoxically but necessarily, the fact that we are moving towards a legislative landscape in which threats and compulsion are more in evidence places upon us a far greater requirement to be clear about the rights and access to services a user should expect from mental health services.

Compulsory treatment

In their chapter on engagement, Burns and Firn (2001) outline an overall framework for Assertive Outreach consisting of three strands or approaches: constructive; informative; and restrictive. These describe a spectrum of approaches from those that build a genuine therapeutic alliance (constructive), to monitoring strategies designed to keep a close watch on the user (informative), to those concerned with using the ultimate legal sanctions 'where all else has failed' (restrictive). By a constructive approach they seem to mean a strengths approach: "While the strengths model has its limitations as the foundation for a whole service, its concepts (and in particular its emphasis on the patient's agenda) provide an excellent philosophy for engaging constructively." They discuss a restrictive approach in the context of discussing the powers currently available such as long leave, supervised discharge, guardianship and appointeeship: "The power is about persuading the persuadable… it is valuable for a small group of patients with whom one has some relationship, and who can agree to it. It is of no value whatsoever in the absence of a basic therapeutic relationship. It is not a *substitute for engagement* but a *tool for engagement*. The patient who says 'no' will still say 'no' even if on an order." They go on to mention that they have successfully worked with around a dozen users using supervised discharge.

A case illustration will be used to distinguish between the different levels of 'treatment pressure' (Box 4.3).

Box 4.3   Case study

Eileen is aged 35 and has been in contact with mental health services since aged 19. She has been hospitalized on four different occasions with severe mental illness, once for over nine months. She tends to binge-drink and can become threatening and violent under those circumstances. She was discharged from hospital four months ago, into a hostel, but was discharged from that four weeks ago after a series of fights with other residents and staff. She has two children aged five and nine, who are in care with Social Services. She dislikes taking medication and is currently refusing to do so. On leaving hospital she was referred to the Assertive Outreach team but it is very early in the engagement process. The Assertive Outreach worker has found her a bed-sit, but she is not currently looking after herself or it very well. The practitioner has established that her main aim and aspiration is to re-establish contact with her children and provide a home for them.

Persuasion

The practitioner keeps her aim in focus and shows respect for that intention. He decides that the first step really has to be to persuade her to take her medication, since not taking it seems to have been clearly linked in the past to her previous admissions. He goes over the past pattern of what seems to have led to her being re-admitted, and establishes that on every previous occasion when she was admitted she had stopped taking medication

some time before. Over a number of sessions he goes over the advantages and disadvantages of medication and side-effects. She continues not to take medication and is still binge-drinking when the opportunity arises.

Leverage

The practitioner begins to point out that the likelihood is, if things continue the way they are looking, a return to hospital is a definite possibility. He continues to reassure her that he is committed to helping her stay in the community and help her to realize her hopes and aspirations. His message is that he will continue to do everything he can do to help her, and help her to realize her aspirations, but she will need to start working on the behaviour that he thinks is causing problems for her: her binge-drinking and not taking her medication. She still does not show much sign of stopping the behaviour, which is likely to lead to a return to hospital. She continues not to look after herself or her bed-sit very well. She is hearing voices, which are increasingly intrusive.

Inducement

The practitioner reminds her that she holds the hope of seeing her children again very dear – how can going back to hospital, which still seems likely, help her move towards that? If, however, she started to take care of her appearance and began to keep the bed-sit tidy, maybe that would be a small step in the right direction? (She seems a little more responsive to that than to taking her medication.) She responds that she can see the point of that. The practitioner works on an agreement with her. If she will start to take care of herself and look after the bed-sit, then perhaps he could begin to make arrangements for her to visit her children, and he would accompany her. She does after a while begin to look after herself better and begins to make efforts to keep the bed-sit tidier. However, she is still drinking and not taking her medication. Her overall condition continues to deteriorate.

Threats

By now the practitioner is very concerned with her overall condition. He explains that a compulsory section back to hospital is looking increasingly likely. She really does not want to go back to hospital and is determined to see her children again. She agrees to accompany the practitioner to outpatients the following week to see a psychiatrist and to a review of her medication.

Compulsory admission

Her condition continues to deteriorate and before the outpatient appointment a compulsory admission is facilitated by the practitioner, who stays with her through the admission process. Her hospitalization is brief, and the practitioner is able to stay in touch with her while she is in hospital and afterwards. Her medication has been reviewed whilst in hospital, and she is now experiencing fewer side-effects. For the moment at least, she is taking her medication. The fact that the practitioner is involved in her compulsory admission does not permanently damage her relationship with him. She is able to see now that something has to be done and she appreciates the practitioner's honesty in facing her with the issues, and his commitment to her in staying with her throughout the process. The practitioner continues to work with her to reduce her drinking, continue medication and to keep herself and her accommodation tidier. They are working towards a visit to her children.

What are we to conclude from this discussion on the ethics of control? Firstly, issues of the use of various kinds of treatment pressure, whether it be the use of persuasion, leverage, inducement, threats or compulsory use of powers, are around us all the time: they are not just issues relevant to the implementation of the new legislation. Secondly, the strengths approach is compatible with the use of various degrees and levels of control, provided:

- They are applied appropriately in terms of the level of risk involved.
- The practitioner is in full awareness of the rights and duties to which the user is entitled.
- They are carried out with honesty, integrity and in full communication with and respect of the user.
- They are carried out in the context of a longterm commitment to the fulfilment of the user's aspirations.

It may seem strange or abhorrent even to use such terms as 'threat' or 'compulsion' to describe work undertaken with a service user. However, it has to be remembered that from a civil liberties perspective if, for example, we are facing a user with the possibility or probability of compulsory removal to hospital, then whether or not we ourselves like to see it that way, the user in all likelihood will.

ACCESSIBILITY AND CHOICE

We are proposing that a strengths approach to Assertive Outreach involves a comprehensive, inclusive approach to user involvement and user-centred care. Does this necessarily mean that every service user should have access to Assertive Outreach? The simple answer would be that all components of comprehensive mental health services should apply the principles of a strengths approach. However, the adherence to caseload sizes of approximately 1:10 inhibits widescale implementation on economic grounds alone. Whether we promote access or not, there remains a concern about the use of inclusion and exclusion criteria within local services that are insufficiently sensitive to identify the priority people to be engaged. There is a temptation to suggest that some services are playing God in their role of determining who does and does not access more responsive services.

ETHNIC AND GENDER SENSITIVITY

Accessibility of services comes into sharper scrutiny when we consider issues of race, culture and ethnicity. It is vitally important to promote access to 'culturally' responsive services. However, the 'ethnicity' arithmetic in most community mental health and Assertive Outreach teams

---

Box 4.4   Case study

Gladstone is a 62-year-old man of Jamaican origin, who has lived in the UK for approximately 45 years. His wife has recently died from a heart condition, and he was referred to the Assertive Outreach team based on his long history of persistent psychotic experiences, and the loneliness and isolation precipitated by his recent tragic loss. He has had many long hospital admissions under the Mental Health Act, and high doses of antipsychotic medications have dampened but not eradicated his paranoid ideas of persecution by neighbours and the mental health system. He still retains a very strong accent of origin, and though he has an excellent command of English his verbal communication can be difficult for some people to understand.

Following a team discussion about the lack of workers of similar ethnic origin, it was determined that a white male would make the initial contact with Gladstone. From information given by a voluntary sector agency that he frequently visits, the worker felt confident about asking Gladstone to repeat anything that was not easily understood.

After the initial few visits Gladstone was able to confide in the worker that he appreciated being asked to repeat himself these days, because it meant there was a better chance of his real needs and wishes being heard and understood. He recounted that many services had previously assumed that he should be allocated 'black' workers, without any real consideration that black people are not a homogeneous race. He often felt that some young black workers did not share the same cultural experiences and values as himself. Yet the assumption still held that black workers knew best what Gladstone needed without spending sufficient time to check out his wishes. On one occasion he recalled being allocated a young black woman as his social worker; his resistance was interpreted as a symptom of decline in his condition without checking the fact that he had lost his last meaningful job some 35 years earlier through wrongful allegations made by a young black female colleague. He was cleared of all the allegations but the damage was done.

does not match up between service providers and people using the services. Some teams may be working in a catchment area populated with numerous different ethnic minority groups. No team could possibly reflect this in its staffing. The primary issue is the widescale ignorance or neglect of racial, cultural and spiritual needs of the client group within services, which fundamentally needs to be addressed. The absence of a staff member from the same cultural background does not necessarily mean a person cannot receive a responsive service (Box 4.4). Two principles should be adhered to, in order to reflect the diversity of values characterized in a multicultural society:

- All Assertive Outreach team members are to be open to and listening to what the individual service users actually want and need.

- All Assertive Outreach team members are to be aware of the diversity of community resources, in order to support culturally sensitive responses to individual needs. It is about being willing to learn from the person themselves, and their own unique community and cultural support network.

BEING AN ASSERTIVE OUTREACH CLIENT

Once a person is engaged with an Assertive Outreach service, the service needs to be aware it cannot meet all needs in isolation. Further issues of accessibility and choice arise out of attempts to link people with other more appropriate sources of support for identified needs. The potential and real stigma that may accompany the badge of being an Assertive Outreach client may act against ease of access to other services. Judicious editing of information in order to influence access to another service carries significant dangers, not least that the person will experience subsequent prejudicial treatment from the service to which the user is referred. Conversely, the Assertive Outreach team could become tagged with the unwanted label of lying to get their clients into other places.

The service could lie to its own clients, saying that the other service was not really so appropriate to their needs, but this stores up the real potential for undermining any hard-earned trust. A quote from a recent study (Ryan and Green 2001) on implementing Assertive Outreach illustrates this point: "The assertive outreach worker would often discover to their dismay that their comprehensive, holistic understanding of, compassion towards, and commitment to, the user was not necessarily shared by the rest of the service. So far as other elements of the service were concerned, the user might be perceived as 'high risk', or 'dual diagnosis', or some other partialising view of the client, which reduced their understanding of the client as a whole. Perhaps service perceptions were coloured by particular traumatic or distressing events or episodes in which the user had been involved. Often it was only the assertive outreach worker who had a unique sense of the user's complexity and individuality. This could lead to a distancing or alienation of the worker as well as the client from other parts of the service, which had a much more shallow and partial appreciation of the user and their needs." One member of Team 1 commented: "Housing benefit are the worst people of all to work with. I was waiting for two years for the claims of one client to be processed… it creates such uncertainty, and causes endless problems of eviction or the threat of it."

An overemphasis on the negotiating skills could result in the Assertive Outreach team developing a blind spot to the impact of its unique ways of working, and consequently pushing other services into territory or decisions they feel uncomfortable with.

The middle ground lies somewhere in the territory of working with the person's preferred choices and decisions, but maintaining transparency of information, so that the reasoning for any over-riding of choices is usually more apparent, however unpalatable the effects of stigma may be. This approach should be accompanied by the Assertive Outreach team flagging up the stigma of restricted accessibility to the other services employing these practices, as well as to appropriate managers.

BOUNDARIES IN THE CARING RELATIONSHIP: FRIENDSHIP OR NOT?

Mental health services have an ability to create issues and dilemmas where they do not necessarily have to exist, e.g. the frequent claims by personnel in other parts of the system that Assertive Outreach is straying over the line from professional relationship into friendship with clients. To paraphrase a critique that is often made: 'Assertive Outreach portrays itself as a friend to the client rather than as a professional service'. Clearly, to stray over such a boundary would cloud the objectives of professional judgement and delivery of a service. This is generally fully understood within Assertive Outreach services, as the issue of friendship and service delivery is an area that would have been debated within the team as a part of its initial team-building and operational policy development. Rapp (1998) reminds us that: "…case managers are not friends. In fact, case managers should devote considerable effort to clients building 'real' friendships with others. On the other hand, the relationship should be friendly. The relationship should be characterized by warmth, acceptance, caring, respect, and even fun."

Graley-Wetherell and Morgan (2001) report the views of people engaged in an active outreach service in Norwich, where the views expressed are a more accurate reflection on the working relationship. Some people using the service were able to clearly articulate that they did not see the workers strictly as their friends, but they felt that a significant difference from previous experiences was the friendly face and manner in which the Assertive Outreach service was presented to them.

The authors reported: "The service users all felt that the team delivered a service that was different to other services they received, or had received in the past. A large majority of them said it was about attitude, they felt they are treated with more respect, that they are listened to and that they are given more time to express what their problems are. Some of them said that the workers are like friends, but that they understood that there are boundaries and it is their job. However, they certainly felt much more comfortable with the friendly approach and they expressed a willingness to engage with this model of working."

One respondent said: "They are like friends, if I don't keep in touch they send little notes and cards. I get trapped in my environment but they stop me from being alienated. They are not intrusive; they talk about everyday problems not just mental health. They also help with the practical stuff like washing, etc. When I almost lost all my possessions they tried to stop that happening."

Within the creative remit of Assertive Outreach it is possible to see how some of the working practices may become misconstrued as friendship, rather than professional intervention, e.g. one-to-one swimming sessions. Again it is the individually held value system that processes events in different ways – with the staff member on a volatile ward or the community mental health team member with the caseload of 35 people only interpreting the actions of other services though their own current experiences. So the swimming session at the local pool with one client looks like a luxury they could not even contemplate. The Assertive Outreach worker, and team, would have a clearly thought-out plan for engagement and working that reflects a complex mutual assessment of needs and wants. The swimming session may be many things: an ideal vehicle for connecting engagement through sharing mutual interests; a confidence-boosting activity that has been a personal goal for the client for many months or years; part of a graded plan towards longer-term goals; an opportunity for both parties to check out part of a strengths assessment; current mental state; and planned risk-taking and social interactions. Ultimately, it may have proved to be the most effective vehicle for holding any number of important discussions and observations that may have been hindered for the client in a more formal appointment-based service-centred interview. The fact that the activity is taking place should also be an indicator that risk and safety have been carefully considered by the team and with the individual client concerned.

Stovall (2001) identifies 'boundary diffusion' as one of the many ethical dilemmas that are qualitatively different in the context of Assertive Outreach as opposed to other parts of the mental health system. It can be closely associated with a further conflict of allegiances set up by the risk agenda – being with the client or for the safety of the wider community. The value system observed by Assertive Outreach workers and teams will primarily uphold the rights of the individual but within a context of fully appreciating the manifestations of risk. It is generally understood that no individual client benefits from a 'negligent' service ignoring the potential consequences of allowing risks to play themselves out to a disaster. Similarly, there are therapeutic risks that any individual, within identified personal circumstances, would benefit from being supported to take.

The challenge to Assertive Outreach workers is to clearly identify risk and safety factors with the individual involved, and to set personal and service boundaries that enable desired goals to be achieved without a cost to the safety of anyone. Transparency of discussion, based on sharing appropriate information, will be the key to each individual situation. However, these considerations may occasionally trespass into the territory of 'collusion', where Assertive Outreach workers are criticized for going along with a person's denial of possibly psychotic experiences because they appear more determined not to have their symptoms challenged, or even wishing to have their own views affirmed. The orthodox service response is to challenge or even deny the person's view of their experiences.

For example, the person who feels their neighbour is causing them severe physical symptoms by transmitting electrical waves into them through their false teeth may become irresistibly fixed in this explanation of the experience. The traditional approach would be to assess the psychotic symptoms, and to deny the validity of the preferred explanation. This may be the correct response for the majority of people but in rare circumstances it could result in developing a barrier to trust and a reason for disengaging from services. Strengths-oriented Assertive Outreach services may assess the primary need for engagement, in order to open up new ways of managing the experiences of physical symptoms, to monitor and manage other possible risks, and to ensure a more accurate assessment of the mental state. In this situation, the service may not overtly agree with the individual's explanation but may engage ways of caring for the false teeth, even agreeing to temporarily take possession of the teeth, with the individual's agreement. This more creative approach holds the potential to open up discussions about other causes for the perceived sensations, without causing unnecessary alienation. Does this constitute unhelpful collusion?

ETHICS OF DISENGAGEMENT

Even though the implementation guide for Assertive Outreach (Department of Health 2001) recommends continuity of care, because of pressure on services it is often current practice to consider discharging a service user once their condition has stabilized. The current perceived wisdom is that we now return people to the very services they may well have originally experienced, and subsequently disengaged from!

Is it ethically sound to remove a service from a person that may have been a hard fight to engage in the first instance, and has come to be seen as meeting their needs? This question opens up a number of important issues that a comprehensive mental health system needs to get to grips with:

- Is the function of 'discharge/case closure' one of the reasons why people become disenchanted with services?
- Are we creating an unnecessary dependency if we view a part of the system as 'a service for life' for some individuals?
- If the value base of one part of the system connects with people who have disengaged from other parts of the system, should these other parts be required to change their value base and practices?
- Is there such a thing as a positive disengagement from a service?

THE ETHICS OF 'DISCHARGE' AND 'DEPENDENCY'

Discharge has a finality about it, which seems at odds with the concept of severe and enduring mental health problems. If the perceived wisdom in psychosis research is that a group of people will experience chronic and/or recurring episodes, which will significantly affect their ability to function in the ordinary demands of daily living (Stein and Test 1980), how may we justify withdrawing services from people in need?

Many of the people who are recently being referred to, and taken up by, the proliferating Assertive Outreach teams in the UK have been known to mental health services for many years, with variable histories of contact. The reasons for disaffection with services are likely to be many and varied but the procedures and experiences of discharge are likely to be high among them. For people who accept they have problems, there may be a degree of discontent at being seen for a specific period of time, or for a specific series of interventions, and then discharged. They may also disagree with the assessment of their more significant problems, feeling they are being discharged following resolution of service-determined priorities above their own. For many other service users, the issue may be more to do with the inflexibility of the service, in terms of the times of contact, places of contact or a 'three strikes and you're out' approach to failed attendances.

In such instances, any gains made through work with a more flexible and creative Assertive Outreach team may be rapidly lost at the prospect of 'discharge' back to other parts of the system. This may be an issue to do specifically with the other parts of the system, or it may be intrinsic to the emotions generated by discharge as an entity. The limited research that exists into the outcomes postdischarge from intensive services such as Assertive Outreach are not good. Generally, people have been found to resist discharge, or the gains made over a number of years rapidly regress (Stein and Test 1980). A strengths approach incorporates a notion of 'recovery', whereby some people do 'get better' (hopefully as a result of Assertive Outreach input) and therefore no longer need the service, or continue to meet the criteria for such intensive input. The challenge in these circumstances is to promote more of a positive sense of disengagement that supports the gains achieved (see Chapter 7).

It is also important to acknowledge that a small number of people successfully resist *all* attempts to engage with them and/or are consistently hostile towards Assertive Outreach services, whatever their approaches, over a long period of time. Assertive Outreach sometimes has to give the person the benefit of the doubt, particularly if they are not coming to the attention of services elsewhere due to their mental health problems, and consider discharging someone in these circumstances (without precluding them from being re-referred at some point in the future, if needs or desires change). And, of course, sometimes psychiatry gets its diagnosis all wrong in the first place, and Assertive Outreach services end up picking up the pieces.

The natural assumption following the difficulties with moving people on from Assertive Outreach is that it becomes a service for life. This mode of thinking generates negative emotions in clients and practitioners alike, of creating an unmovable dependency. Indeed, a frequently made allegation about Assertive Outreach services is that they create a dependency in people, as if to say that discharging people for not attending a few successive appointments manages to gain some moral high ground! It is just as unhelpful to think of a service for life as it is to use the idea of discharge as a time-limiting factor on service contact. Neither concept acknowledges the reality of individual experience and needs, placing potential quantity of service above potential quality of service.

Most commentators on Assertive Outreach raise the organizational concerns of scarce resources, requiring teams to move people on, in order to create the space for new referrals to be taken on. Burns and Firn (2002) lean heavily on the medical language and perceptions of a health care-oriented culture, talking of "patients needing to be discharged back to the care of community mental health teams". Whilst they propose a low level of transfers, suggesting relatively long periods of contact in Assertive Outreach, they still justify the need for discharge from a rather narrow existing orthodoxy of statutory service medical care. The justification is not only from a perception of establishing continuity of care through reducing the Assertive Outreach frequency of contact down to the level achievable by community mental health teams, within a loosely defined timescale of three to six months, but also from a need for Assertive Outreach team throughput in order to sustain levels of worker vitality.

From a strengths perspective there are a number of difficulties with discharge viewed purely as return to statutory services. Firstly, it fails to recognize that people may not wish to return to the type of care they had previously experienced, and this may be a cause for an apparent shift from hard-to-engage at the outset to hard-to-discharge later on. Secondly, it fails to demonstrate how Assertive Outreach services are developing more creative working practices, for sustaining their staff as well as meeting the needs of people using the service.

References

Backlar P 2001 Privacy and confidentiality. In: Thornicroft G, Szmuckler G (eds) A Textbook of Community Psychiatry. Oxford University Press, Oxford

Bok S 1983 SECRETS: On the Ethics of Concealment and Revelation. Vintage, New York

Burns T, Firn M 2002 Assertive Outreach in Mental Health: A Manual for Practitioners. Oxford University Press, Oxford

Cordess C (ed) 2001 Confidentiality and Mental Health. Jessica Kingsley, London

Department of Health 1999 National Service Framework for Mental Health: Modern Standards and Service Models. HMSO, London

Department of Health 2000 NHS National Plan. HMSO, London

Department of Health 2001 The Mental Health Policy Implementation Guide. HMSO, London

Dickenson D, Fulford K W M 2001 In Two Minds: A Case-Book of Psychiatric Ethics. Oxford University Press, Oxford

Dworkin R 1993 Life's Dominion. Vintage, New York

Fulford K W M 2001 The paradoxes of confidentiality: a philosophical introduction. In: Cordess C (ed)

Confidentiality and Mental Health. Jessica Kingsley, London, p 7–23

Graley-Wetherell R, Morgan S 2001 Active Outreach: An independent service user evaluation of a model of assertive outreach practice. Sainsbury Centre for Mental Health, London

Holloway F, Carson J 2001 Case management: an update. International Journal of Social Psychiatry 47: 21–31

Nozick R 1974 Anarchy, State and Utopia. Basic Books, New York

Perkins R, Repper J 1998 Dilemmas in Community Mental Health Practice: Choice or Control. Radcliffe Medical Press, Abingdon

Phillips S D, Burns B J, Edgar E R et al 2001 Moving assertive community treatment into standard practice. Psychiatric Services 52: 77–79

Pretty D 2002 www.justice4diane.org.uk or http://news.bbc.co.uk/1/hi/health.stm

Rapp C A 1998 The Strengths Model: Case Management with People Suffering from Severe and Persistent Mental Illness. Oxford University Press, New York

Ryan P, Green D 2001 Implementing Assertive Outreach. Middlesex University internal report

Skull A 1993 The Most Solitary of Afflictions: Madness and Society in Britain 1700–1900. Yale University Press, New York

Spindel T, Nugent J 2000 Polar opposites: empowerment philosophy and assertive community treatment (ACT). Ethical Human Science Services 2: 93–101

Stein L 1992 Innovating against the current. New Directions in Mental Health 56: 5–40

Stein L, Test A 1980 Alternatives to mental hospital treatment: conceptual model, treatment program and clinical evaluation. Archives of General Psychiatry 37: 392–397

Stovall J 2001 Is assertive community treatment ethical care? Harvard Review of Psychiatry 9: 139–143

Szmukler G, Applebaum P 2001 Treatment pressures, coercion and compulsion. In: Thornicroft G, Szmukler G (eds) A Textbook of Community Psychiatry. Oxford University Press, Oxford

Szmukler G, Holloway F 2001 Confidentiality in community psychiatry. In: Cordess C (ed) Confidentiality and Mental Health. Jessica Kingsley, London, p 53–70

Wertheimer A 1993 A philosophical examination of coercion for mental health issues. Some basic distinctions: analysis and justification. Behavioural Sciences and the Law 11: 239–258

Wilen Berg J, Bonnie R 2001 When push comes to shove: aggressive community treatment and the law. In: Dennis D, Monahan J (eds) Coercion and Aggressive Community Treatment – A New Frontier in Mental Health Law. Plenum Press, New York

Williamson T 2002 Ethics of assertive outreach (assertive community treatment teams). Current Opinion in Psychiatry 15: 543–547

Williamson T 2003 Enough is good enough. Mental Health Today, April: 24–27

Witheridge T 1991 The 'active ingredients' of assertive outreach. New Directions for Mental Health Services 52: 47–64

Chapter 5

The foundations of creative collaboration

Steve Morgan

"None of us is as smart as all of us"

Bennis and Biederman 1997

INTRODUCTION

The most significant challenge laid down for Assertive Outreach is that which is heavily implied but rarely made explicit – to do things differently. The traditional ways of delivering mental health services have clearly failed to respond effectively to the needs of a small but significant population of service users, with the result that they disengaged from the mainstream for a variety of personal reasons. Challenging the orthodoxy requires not just individuals with the right attitude for change but teams with attitude! Such requirements do not come without a price, and within local mental health systems that price usually emerges through conflict.

The more frequent reactions in response to the innovations of Assertive Outreach are, unfortunately, for community mental health team workers to assume the changes represent a criticism that they have not been doing a good job. Rather than integrating with the newly forming Assertive Outreach functions to provide a broader range of options, existing services usually appear to move through a process of feeling threatened and questioned before they can get to a mutually beneficial point of redefining their own speciality alongside the new service. Mental health services generally appear to have poorly developed immune systems, preferring to initially attack 'friendly' incursions, as opposed to accepting the potential for positive change and integrating with them.

The emergence and historical development of case management through to Assertive Outreach has initiated an examination of what we mean by the concepts of 'team' and 'team working' in contemporary mental health. The parallel development of the service user movement has also caused this examination to fundamentally challenge our ideas of service user responsibility, and to place them squarely at the centre of the whole process of needs assessment and care delivery. It is no longer sufficient to claim professional credibility as the foundation of service delivery decisions. A strengths approach fully embraces the power shift of the 'expert stance', moving, as it should, away from the service provider to the service user in a flexible collaboration that reflects individual abilities and circumstances.

THE SHIFTING POLITICS OF COLLABORATION

The most fundamental notion of collaboration is of two people working together in a process aimed at combining their skills to achieve a desired outcome. In community mental health services, this has largely become aligned to mechanisms that support and promote ideas of expertise. The service user or patient has their needs assessed, and this process establishes the signposts for linking the person to the specific experts who specialize in working to resolve their compartmentalized concerns. At the apparent pinnacle of clinical responsibility lies the doctor–patient relationship, whereby the psychiatrist is able to make a medical diagnosis and prescribe the appropriate medical interventions (medication; ECT; hospital admission; therapy) and additionally defer to a 'lesser' level of professional expertise offering a multidisciplinary menu of assessment, monitoring and interventions.

Realistically this is collaboration only in name, largely based on the notion of the majority buying into the supremacy of the minority, with the service user generally in a passive role as recipient of the available expertise. A significant deficit of this type of collaboration rests in its narrow medical determination, even where socially oriented issues are clearly identified as being prominent influences. However, the importance of expertise within the individual relationships was still recognized by promoting a 'brokerage' model of identifying needs and linking the person to the experts in meeting the different needs (Brandon and Towe 1989). Similarly, in the UK care management (NHS 1990, Burns 1999) and care co-ordination (Department of Health 1990, 1995, 1999) have attempted to sharpen the focus onto the individual practitioner, with a consequent resistance based on a range of fears from blame to loss of skills.

The compartmentalization of mental health needs, as described above, has continued to fail a small but significant minority of service users. The result is that models of intensive case management and Assertive Outreach have had to completely rethink the narrowly defined 'signposting to expertise' approach. Early developments of case management in the USA attempted to promote an equal recognition of the social welfare and health-related needs of the individual (Intagliata 1982, Harris and Bergman 1987, Rapp and Chamberlain 1985, Kanter 1989). Services have had to be delivered in more imaginative ways, with fresher ideas on how expertise may be delivered more creatively through collaborations – not just how service providers collaborate with the individual service user but how service providers collaborate with each other, within and between teams.

When we think of creative collaboration it is most important to think of the relationship between the service and the service user, through positive engagement and user-led interventions. Consideration of our roles and relationships with significant carers will also contribute enormously to this end. However, Assertive Outreach has been a significant catalyst for making us rethink what we mean by working together in teams. The basis of creative collaboration in this chapter will be through accessing the necessary tools for sharing and developing ideas within effective team working.

THE REALITY OF TEAM WORKING

Most of us work in teams… or do we? We claim to work in teams; we may find ourselves to be part of something called a team, or often define our role as being part of a team: inpatient team; community mental health team; medical team; social work team; Assertive Outreach team; crisis response team; early intervention team; or Trust management team. The notion of team permeates the language of service delivery, often without much thought; however, do we really work as a team and, if so, how?

The current context of mental health policy and service development reflects a need for team working (Onyett et al 1995) yet still places the fundamental emphases of structures and responsibilities squarely on the shoulders of the individual worker. The cornerstone of contemporary UK mental health service delivery is the care co-ordinator/care manager, with all other connections and specialist contributions revolving around this core component of the system (Department of Health 1999). Have we achieved little more than teams in name only – collections of individuals hampered by the fear of getting it wrong? The challenges of a blame-oriented culture will be explored in more detail in Chapter 11 but they need to be acknowledged here for their potential impact on the ability of workers to collaborate effectively as teams.

So, what is being in a team all about in the strictly functional sense? For many people, the workload pressures and structures largely dictate that they get on with their own business most of the time. They share an office base and meet together for specific purposes, e.g. the team meeting. However, they probably do not function as a team much beyond these. The recent emergence of the care co-ordinator appears to have taken on more of a bureaucratic role, which often mitigates against effective team working. Whilst this was not the intention in theory, it probably seems to be more the case in practice. Practitioners become more blinkered through a focus on their own personal administrative workload and responsibilities, with less time to fully appreciate the skills and work of other members of the team.

Assertive Outreach emerges as a distinctive style of working, very different from the traditional approaches developed through community mental health teams (Ford and McClelland 2002). It requires practitioners to adopt attitudes and practices that challenge their more usual ways of thinking and working and to respond to complex needs in more flexible and creative ways. It is not about assuming traditional professional roles under a different team name, neither is it about losing the uniqueness of personally and professionally aligned skills. However, the concept of team alone may be quite limiting in this context. What is more productive when considering the tools of truly creative collaborations is to explore factors that contribute to making an effective team.

What makes an effective team?

Put simply, we may define a team as a collection of individuals with different skills, abilities and strengths working towards achieving common goals.

To identify a strengths approach to what we want out of the concept of Assertive Outreach teams we will take an uncharacteristic starting point of failure! Start by identifying some contemporary examples of where team working is not, or recently has not, been seen to function effectively. Identify some of the elements of what is not working, then draw the messages from these about what effective team working would possibly look like (Box 5.1).

Box 5.1   Fluctuating team fortunes

French football team

Expectations of success coming into the 2002 World Cup were high, with France as current world champions and one of the competition favourites. On paper, they presented a formidable collection of individual talents, with some of the top goal scorers of the domestic national leagues present in their team. Having lost two and drawn one of their first group matches, with no goals scored and three conceded, they were the first but not the last of the big names to fall at the first hurdle. Implications for Assertive Outreach teams:

- Brilliant individuals may not always gel as a team.
- Unreasonable and high expectations are placed on a small group of people.
- 'Complacency' – failure to see beyond international research successes, to the current local resources.

Railtrack

At the centre are the moral and ethical political debates of privatizing the maintenance and safety of a public utility. Overall spending on safety almost doubled in the first six years but the fragmentation of the subcontracting arrangements made overall control and accountability for quality of maintenance work difficult to monitor. Many small firms made their profit margins with little overall improvement in safety.

As a result, the organization failed to manage the external pressures and expectations placed on it. The safety record was very good in comparison with the road accident statistics but it could not shake off the criticisms of its safety record following a relatively small number of fatal rail accidents.

Implications for Assertive Outreach teams:

- Clear accountability of new teams is needed within the overall structure.
- External influences are acting on team and practice development.
- Demands for short-term cost-effectiveness are deflecting from service user needs.

Consignia

The Post Office may have faced many problems but the clarity of its name was not one of them. An attempt to re-brand the image most famously through a name change is doomed to failure where it primarily serves to confuse customers and employees alike, particularly if it then deflects attention from other structural changes being imposed without a clear and open rationale. In this instance, 'Consignia' proved to be a short-lived and much-maligned name change.

Implications for Assertive Outreach teams:

- Re-branding existing workers as Assertive Outreach is not enough.
- Poor management structures, namely lacking consistency of understanding about Assertive Outreach throughout the organization, important decisions affecting the team made from outside the team, feeling remote within the organization, and not drawing on the recognized skills and resources of the workers, leading to a lowering of morale.

Marks & Spencer

A market leader for many years still has to move with the times, particularly in the fickle world of fashion. Whilst the company had built itself an apparently secure niche, it did not sufficiently account for fluctuating market trends. A dramatic fall in market share and share price was followed by gradual revival after some management changes and the introduction of new fashion lines.

Implications for Assertive Outreach teams:

- Applying the messages from research in imaginative ways that reflect local resources and needs.
- Always needing to be innovative in practice delivery, based on 'reflective practice' and review as essential components of team working.

Lessons on achieving effectiveness can always be drawn from the experiences of others. The collection of individuals is important but it is as much about their shared values and attitudes towards the function of the team as it is about their individual strengths and skills (good individuals need to gel as a team). This presents a difficult conundrum for constructing anything approaching the ideal team: it should be possible to match up the need for a group of people with shared values towards the work with the client group, while still aiming to broaden the base of different skills, knowledge, personal backgrounds, personalities, interests, lifestyles, and political, religious and spiritual beliefs. The trick is to uphold the vision of an ideal whilst accepting that you can only blend so much with a small group of the people available to you.

The function and style of leadership will also play a significant role in defining the tasks of the team, and supporting its individuals to achieve them collectively. The size of the team in relation to the functions it is expected to perform will influence the way everyone's input can be valued as a creative collaboration, and how they may be involved in the decision-making processes of the venture. Teams always need to be open to the need for change but resist the re-branding that may be imposed largely by external forces and expectations without sufficient consultation of those involved in its subsequent implementation.

Clarity of team objectives

The research literature on Assertive Outreach strongly establishes the concept of 'fidelity to the model' (Sainsbury Centre for Mental Health 1998, Teague et al 1998, Hemming et al 1999). As a concept it is frequently used but equally misunderstood. There is not only one model for service development and implementation of good practice. An implicit danger of adopting a prescriptive approach, from the research or central policy, is the inherent failure to take account of local structures and resources. Core components of effective practice are clearly indicated in the research but these can be adapted in different ways to reflect local needs. What fidelity means in practice is that a local model should clearly articulate how it proposes to implement the essential components, and that it adheres to its stated model of implementation. Organizations that simply set up a team and then expect 'fidelity to the model' to be implemented, with little understanding or local interpretation of what it means, will frequently have their lack of vision rewarded with a group of confused and frustrated practitioners.

Team working is more likely to be effective where the organizational management responsible for implementing Assertive Outreach sets clear aims for the team and the client group it is intended to serve. The service can then be specifically designed to deliver those aims. The reality is more frequently a situation where the management of the organization are not clear why they are establishing an Assertive Outreach function, other than a response to government directives. Consequently, it is set up with a loose vision, where expectations are altered without involving or even informing the workers who have themselves accessed more information and experience of what works effectively. For example, there are teams that are set the primary aim of engaging resistant and disengaged individuals but are then wholly measured on their short-term impact on hospital admission. The workers are likely to have tried to engage people who have been out of contact with services, and have a higher potential need for hospital admission in the short term. Failing to meet unexpected and elusive short-term expectations may quickly result in Assertive Outreach services becoming confused and demotivated by a lack of clear leadership from the organization.

Leadership

Leadership from the organizational management structure has the potential to restrict creative capability, being more concerned with structures and hierarchy. Innovative leadership must be permitted from above but driven from much closer in to the team. Bennis and Biederman (1997) suggest that leaders of creative groups are not necessarily 'creators' but are 'curators', i.e. they give the group what they need and free them from impositions as far as they can. They shelter outreach workers from the demands of management and bureaucracy. Creative groups and creative leaders can make each other; they feel they are on a shared mission and they are often more optimistic than realistic, as a means of pushing the boundaries in search of new solutions to problems.

A strengths approach recognizes that an important function of developing teams to implement innovative practice will be the risk of accepting the challenge to the operational thinking of the organization. Asking a new part of the organization to function differently will necessarily have a ripple effect. As the team manager is often at the interface of operational and organizational responsibilities, it is clear that he or she will require considerable skill and understanding of the demands of creative and collaborative practice if the person is to be a credible leader of the people he or she manages. The team manager also has to be skilled at delivering the requirements of higher management, albeit in new or unorthodox ways, e.g. matching a team approach to the requirements of care co-ordination.

Playing the numbers game

Generally, whenever numbers of staff and service users on caseloads are introduced into the discussion, an element of game playing ensues. Comparisons and limits become set in concrete, and statistics take on their unique ability to prove equal and opposite arguments simultaneously. Numbers do play an important function in setting some boundaries for realistic practice, thus providing a barrier for particular services, helping them to avoid the inevitable failure associated with being 'swamped' or 'dumped on'. This line of argument should apply equally to all other components of the service system, not just Assertive Outreach.

A study of the literature and research on Assertive Outreach is far less conclusive about team size than it is about caseload size. Many of the reports prefer to focus on the skill mix, including types of specialist input on the team, rather than what would be the optimal size of team.

The most comprehensive description of team composition found in the literature is Allness and Knoedler (1999), providing a companion of revisions to their Program of Assertive Community Treatment (PACT) standards manual of the previous year. They recommend the following minimum standards for team staffing:

- Urban services: 10–12 whole time equivalent (WTE) plus one administrative assistant and 16 hours of psychiatrist time/50 clients on the team.
- Rural services: 5–7 WTE plus half-time administrative assistant and 16 hours of psychiatrist time/50 clients on the team.

They break these staffing levels down further for specialities required. However, the important point is that this staffing level covers two shifts per day, and on-call overnight.

The Sainsbury Centre for Mental Health (1998) echoes these standards, claiming a minimum of 10 staff on the team, with requirements to employ some people for their specialist input, e.g. psychiatrist, substance misuse specialist and vocational rehabilitation. Stein and Santos (1998) advocated the deployment of 10 core staff serving around 100 clients.

The danger with the potential interpretation and implementation of the above figures is that one simply provides a community mental health team by a different name. Higher levels of staffing become more unmanageable when considering models of a team approach. Information becomes more difficult to communicate effectively to larger numbers of people. It also becomes more difficult for any one staff member to hold information in their head about increasingly large numbers of service users seen by the team. Too much time becomes invested in the functions of team communication, and less on its most important creative outcomes.

Other references to team size have stressed lower numbers but not necessarily being as explicit about hours of operation. Mueser et al (1998) provide what is widely seen as one of the most definitive reviews of the research literature into case management and assertive community treatment (ACT). However, they make little reference to team size other than that ACT should have one psychiatrist, one nurse and 'at least' two case managers. Marty et al (2001) review the 'experts'' opinions on the essential ingredients of a strengths model. In a supplementary question they found an overwhelming agreement on team size to be four or five case managers, a team leader and one administrative support person.

Onyett (2003) concludes that the ideal for ACT is therefore to achieve small focused teams of between five and nine people. Careful consideration needs to be given to the diversity of skills and experience that small teams can offer but this may be complemented by improved links with other specialists. Larger numbers only make it more difficult to co-ordinate and achieve the benefits of a team approach for knowing all the clients accepted into the service. A team smaller than five hands-on workers will find it harder to provide sufficient cover when workers are on holiday or sickness leave.

Attitudes and experience: skills and knowledge

A great deal of emphasis has been placed in the literature on the skills mix required to staff an Assertive Outreach team adequately, usually focusing on permutations of professions and other specialists (Allness and Knoedler 1999), with a substrata of unqualified support worker input (Sainsbury Centre for Mental Health 1998). The knowledge and skills agenda is important but is often promoted to the detriment of paying sufficient attention to the need for people with the right kind of attitudes and experience to work with the complex needs and risk presentations of the client group.

Creative collaborations frequently require thinking laterally to the established patterns of practitioner behaviour. Assertive Outreach, as a specialized and demanding area of work, needs to ensure, as much as possible, that it attracts staff with the personal attitudes and qualities that equip them to work in different and challenging circumstances. Simply appointing existing staff within the service to a new area of work is no guarantee that they can achieve the change of values and attitudes required to deliver a different service. It is more a function of trying to attract people with specific interest in the challenges of the new and the different, some of whom may very well be from staff currently within other parts of the organization. Beyond this, there is also the challenge of blending the different personalities together into a coherent functioning whole unit.

Not just any group of people can be brought together and be expected to truly perform as a team. There is something in the attitudes and commitment that certain individuals display towards specific challenges or ways of working. Most of all, the much clichéd concept of a user-centred service needs to be taken beyond the convenient rhetoric, to its real meaning in practice. There is something unique and different about the way some people think and talk about service users and their work, a way which conveys an inner belief about the value and respect for people whatever their experiences and occasionally challenging behaviours. It is an indefinable quality that some workers have but many do not; and it is one of the most difficult things to put across through the medium of training. Try asking a question in a job interview to elicit it? What would that question be? What would be a right or wrong answer?

Assertive Outreach workers need to be able to adopt a positive and persistent approach to seemingly intransigent circumstances. The Sainsbury Centre for Mental Health (1998) suggests that staff have to:

- demonstrate a needs-led approach
- have the right style to engage with the client group (including being of similar ethnic group or with experience as a service user)
- adapt to working in informal settings
- demonstrate low expressed emotion
- hold realistic expectations of the scope for improvement
- be committed to longterm therapeutic relationships.

Bennis and Biederman (1997) remind us that a characteristic of creative groups is their desire to believe in optimism over realism, with a healthy attitude towards mutual support and persistence in search for new ideas, when one line of inquiry falters. They need to feel comfortable working outside the traditional expectations of their role, cutting across artificial boundaries established by the systems within which they more commonly work, in order to create appropriate solutions, e.g. across primary–secondary care and health–social care, and networking and co-ordinating diverse provider agency contributions, e.g. housing, social security and the criminal justice system.

Team meetings

How often have you experienced the rush of the massed agenda, where if it is your turn this week to have a slot, or you manage to keep enough people awake to appreciate the significance of your thinly disguised panic-stricken call for help, you have little more than two minutes to eek out and articulate your pain quickly and coherently? A few seconds of wisdom may be dispensed from the gallery of equally beleaguered colleagues, directing you to do the very thing that you have tried several times before, with failed outcomes. Does it really have to be this way?

Imagine a place where the team meetings were so productive and enjoyable that you felt like you had missed out if you could not be there – now wake up from the dream! A strengths approach to the function of meetings aims to promote the full participation of all people present, by tapping the well of ideas, expertise, experience and feelings. It introduces a greater element of reflective interaction, with less of a business-like rush to complete everything. It is important to remove from the meeting the content that can be efficiently managed elsewhere in the team structures, thus reducing the clutter and enabling more in-depth discussion of matters pertinent to the whole team.

These meetings still require a structure and skilled chairing, to keep a focus on the important priorities for times when the whole team is together. Their frequency, structure and function should be determined and regularly reviewed by the whole group, not by what tradition dictates should more usually happen.

Daily handover meetings

These may take place at the beginning of each day or shift. The purpose is to briefly update all staff on the current progress, issues and needs of all the service users. It is not an in-depth discussion, because it happens every day (similar to inpatient unit and crisis team shift handovers) – 45 minutes should be a carefully managed maximum length of time for such a meeting, with all service users mentioned by name, even if it is only for someone to say 'OK, nothing to report'. Meeting time efficiently used saves valuable time in other functions of the work. The primary tool for this meeting, and other aspects of team functioning, is the white board, a large board on the office wall containing:

- the names of all current service users
- locally determined priority columns of information, e.g. next CPA review, risk issues, type of medication
- the days of the week, with an indication of preferred visiting arrangements, and any routine structures of note to the team
- a section for the distribution of the day's task assignments for staff on shift
- other information and messages.

It is vitally important for the whole team to keep the white board immediately up to date as it is the guiding mechanism for the work of staff most frequently working out of the office. It becomes one of the most essential and indispensable tools for facilitating creative collaboration within teams.

Clinical review meetings   These are to be weekly or monthly. They are opportunities for more in-depth discussion of a few service users and involve people from outside the immediate staffing of the Assertive Outreach team, e.g. the psychiatrist in cases where they are not an integral member of the team. They are a function of the team, and may be used more specifically for discussing and agreeing the 'team' care plan, rather than the CPA review of the wider network of care.

These meetings provide opportunities for team reflection, on practice and service development issues, as much as service user-oriented reviews.

Alternatively, beyond the daily handover, the team may wish to set up monthly meetings covering a range of purposes and functions, potentially organized in the following rotation:

Week 1 Team business meeting
Purpose:

- to discuss team business in a multidisciplinary context
- to provide a forum for the development of team processes, systems and structures in relation to the operational policy
- to support and develop team working practices
- to facilitate the development of the team approach.

Attendance:

- full Assertive Outreach team.

Week 2 In-depth case presentation meeting
Purpose:

- to provide the opportunity for team members to be able to present a client in depth and facilitate a multidisciplinary review of the case in more detail than that discussed in the weekly clinical case review meeting
- to support team systems and decision making with respect to the referral process
- to clarify and further develop team approaches to clinical care planning and risk management.

Attendance:

- the 'full full-time equivalent' (FTE) and sessional Assertive Outreach team, including a consultant psychiatrist
- representatives from relevant local community service providers
- representative from an inpatient service.

Week 3 Team training meeting
Purpose:

- to provide a forum for team training in relation to research and development of Assertive Outreach, and related topics of interest to the team

- to bring in external trainers to focus on priority areas of skill development
- to provide the opportunity for individual team members to share skills, knowledge and experience
- to support multidisciplinary team working and the cross-fertilization of ideas
- to support and promote team development.

Attendance:

- the full FTE and sessional Assertive Outreach team, including consultant psychiatrist
- representatives from relevant local community service providers
- representative from an inpatient service.

Week 4 Team supervision

Purpose:

- to provide a formal forum for team supervision and support, in addition to individual clinical supervision

Attendance:

- closed group – the full FTE and sessional Assertive Outreach team, including a consultant psychiatrist.

Recommendation   That the team develop a well-organized, clearly structured series of meetings which cover:

- the capacity for daily review
- weekly clinical case review
- screening, referral and allocation
- team support and supervision
- indepth case review
- team business.

Team 'mental health'

Sustaining longterm intensive work with people experiencing severe and enduring mental health problems is assumed to induce burnout in staff and rapid turnover. This need not be the case for an Assertive Outreach team developing an ability to address its collective mental health. For an example of ways in which this may be achieved, the Active Outreach team in Norwich (Graley-Wetherell and Morgan 2001) anecdotally attributed a number of factors that contributed to it sustaining its own mental health (not in any particular order of importance):

- personal investment by all team members in the co-working model of practice
- shared personal values about the work with this group of service users
- good quality individual and peer supervision
- a recent innovation of user involvement in staff selection
- good internal communication, including the use of a message book

- flexibly available and responsive to support each other's needs
- a culture that encourages creative, 'out-of-the-box' thinking
- a sense of humour
- impromptu lunches and planned outings together
- external facilitators who believe in the work of the team
- checklist on the office wall, of early warning signs of staff stress
- looking out for each other's levels of stress
- feeling supported by the 'host' organization's culture
- tolerance of difference, in staff members' ideas and service users' choices.

The size of team may be a significant factor to add to this list. It is easier to achieve some of the above with a group of five or six people, than it would be with 12 or more.

Developing teams with 'attitude'

Innovation is a key output of creative collaborations but it frequently requires a great deal of risk taking by Assertive Outreach teams to push the known boundaries of how we usually do things in community mental health. This approach does not sit easily with the existing service structures, and will often be achieved only through teams with 'attitude' (Onyett 2003). The individual with attitude is commonly seen as the loose cannon, not playing the same tune, the person who either has to be brought back into line or is ostracized for their views and beliefs. Such people are seen as a danger and a threat. The team with attitude may eventually stand a better chance of promoting change than the lone voice. Such teams are frequently characterized by strongly held beliefs and principles, driving a level of positive dissent, and persistence in challenging traditionally held views. They have a desire to change the way they work, and to influence positive change in the system they operate within.

The very reasons why Assertive Outreach services are established require that innovative solutions to apparently intractable problems should be found. To this end, we need practitioners and teams that are able to think independently and urgently in crises. This influences the need to look within the team to create a reflective space; reflection in such teams frequently looks beyond the team. The reflective team has an acute awareness of its organizational context and the barriers it faces. The team adapts to these barriers but also sets about attempting to modify them through communicating its beliefs and ideas in a rational way.

A team dissenting from the views of the majority in the wider organizational context, e.g. other providers, parts of the system or the management of the host organizations, has to have a strong belief in its ideas. It also has to have an inner belief that the creative persistence that works with its service users can also bring about change in organizational attitudes through sustained debate or even conflict. Dissent from the majority view can at least initiate debate of the minority view. It makes the organizational majority examine the issues and problems more thoroughly, and potentially think more creatively around the topic. It creates more divergent thinking.

Pushing the boundaries should ideally be about routinely seeking out feedback from users of the service on their experiences, by using valid techniques that take due account of the reality of the power relationships (Graley-Wetherell and Morgan 2001). The process of team reflection has the ability to provide new and challenging information, promoting innovation within a well-managed process.

CONFIGURING COLLABORATIONS

Once the need for an Assertive Outreach service has been locally established, there are three key steps involved in setting up the service:

1. Deciding on the model of service delivery, based on the findings of a local needs assessment.
2. Identifying the most effective recruitment process for staffing the new service.
3. Building support for the new service, and enabling its integration within the existing network of service provision.

Each of these is likely to have a significant influence on the ability of the Assertive Outreach service to develop creative collaborations.

The Sainsbury Centre for Mental Health (1998) set out a rationale for identifying the characteristics and needs of the client group nationally. Within its wide-ranging recommendations, it identifies 100 to 150 people as a significant local client group that would justify setting up one or more Assertive Outreach teams. Where the numbers are not sufficient to justify separate teams, the report concludes that other arrangements need to be made for identifying workers to take on the role, most significantly suggesting that this function may be contained within the community mental health teams.

Morgan and Juriansz (2002) reflect that the community mental health team (CMHT) is not necessarily the best place for establishing Assertive Outreach workers. CMHTs have traditionally failed to offer the kind of service required by this group of people, resulting in the need for Assertive Outreach. The reasons why an effective service was not offered by the CMHTs are many and are justifiable within the context of the lack of specialist direction offered to this foundation of community services. However, without any attempt to apportion blame, the reality is that CMHTs and Assertive Outreach services think and work very differently. They are established to meet very different remits. The placing of the latter within the structure of the former serves to produce far more tensions than creative solutions. Ultimately, the Assertive Outreach function can become undermined by pressures to conform more to the rules of the CMHT, and even to cover for the constant sense of insufficient resources that so many CMHTs feel in relation to the expectations heaped upon them.

Assertive Outreach as a service

Based on experience of working alongside Assertive Outreach workers in the Kettering and Wellingborough sectors of northern Northamptonshire (UK), one of the authors proposes a 'dispersed team' model for developing and delivering Assertive Outreach for a semi-rural area (Morgan and Juriansz 2002). Kettering, Wellingborough, Corby, Rushden and East Northants consist of local populations and needs, to be served by local 'small' teams, outside of the CMHTs. Collectively, the Assertive Outreach staff across the north of the county could identify with a unified service, sharing principles, attitudes, working practices and policies, and ongoing training and development needs. Their working differences are only a minority, mainly reflecting knowledge of specific local population needs and community services.

Multidisciplinary staffing can be achieved across the service, where it is not so easily achievable within the smaller local teams. The individual Assertive Outreach worker still retains a close identity with the service users and local needs of their sector, but the wider service identity would avoid small numbers of people becoming an isolated function with little organizational impact. Specialist expertise, professional or personal, can be accessible across the service, without the fear that individuals would have to move between teams and get to know too large a number of service users. Negotiation of medical input would be responsive to needs, where a dedicated psychiatrist post is not formally attached to Assertive Outreach. Importantly, the application of a purer team approach may be possible within the smaller units. The 'service lead' would play a crucial role in balancing the separate elements and the overall unity of the service across the geographical area. They would also be required to have a hands-on practice development role within all functional parts of the service, rather than a role devoted more to the functioning of senior management within the organization.

Assertive Outreach as a team

Assertive Outreach has become synonymous with the concept of a team approach as one of the crucial components of effective service delivery. Though it appears to be widely referred to as an essential component of effective practice, it is difficult to find detailed descriptions of what it is in the main research literature on Assertive Outreach. However, what is meant by 'team approach' has been increasingly debated within mental health services. It can be delivered in a number of different ways (Navarro 1998, Mueser et al 1998, Allness and Knoedler 1999).

What is generally agreed, by practitioners across different types of Assertive Outreach team, is that the team approach is a necessary reaction to the more traditional functioning of CMHTs through the 'individual' key worker or care co-ordinator (Navarro 1998, Onyett 2003). The key worker is seen as an approach where workers provide all one-to-one contact themselves. It avoids defining skill mix and preserves the myth that everybody is equally competent to work with a wide range of issues. The unwritten informal rule is that if one assessed an individual one either became the key worker or turned the referral down on behalf of the team. This encouraged reluctance to take up unattractive referrals for assessment because it was known that other workers would not get involved. The service user becomes dependent on one service provider. Inevitably workers move on, and the service user has the frustrating experience of going back almost to square one, to recount the failures of their life history to yet another stranger. Even periods of annual leave or worker sickness can have a negative impact on the continuity for the service user, and other agencies involved in the network of care (Navarro 1998).

A 'whole' team approach

Onyett (2003) suggests that the adoption of the team approach to team work is one key element that differentiates ACT from case management. The idea appears to have originated in the early 1980s with the Thresholds service in Chicago, for street homeless people experiencing serious mental health problems (Witheridge et al 1982, Witheridge and Dincin 1985). As an approach it is well suited to a transient population, which would be extremely difficult to follow up on an individual key-working basis. The approach was studied in Chicago and subsequently implemented by the Tulip Project in Haringey, London, with a mainly African Caribbean population of people experiencing severe and enduring mental health problems (Navarro 1998, Gauntlett et al 1996).

The idea of the team approach is one of all workers acting together, thinking together in decision making, and sharing responsibilities toward all clients. It is based on the premise that continuity of service is best offered through shifting the fostering of dependency of the service user, from the individual worker to the team as a whole. Through greater role clarification and accountability to peers, staff burnout can be reduced, and reflective practice can be enhanced (Navarro 1995). It is essentially about all workers on the team appropriately engaging and working with the whole team caseload, such that all staff are effectively interchangeable. However, it is primarily about enabling the collective skills and experience of a whole team to be made available to all the people accessing the service.

An evaluation of the Tulip Project by Gauntlett et al (1996) generally demonstrated the stated advantages of a team approach to be:

- good engagement with users, in that few lost contact with the service
- good peer support and consultation
- high job satisfaction and low burnout among staff
- improved continuity of care within the team.

However, some workers missed the opportunities to develop individual responsibility for a holistic approach to their work with users. Others encountered practical difficulties, e.g. in establishing effective liaison with other agencies.

The implementation of such an approach needs to be constantly reviewed and monitored. There are some intrinsic difficulties by the very nature of the service users that Assertive Outreach is set up to work with: they are commonly referred to as 'resistant to services' or 'hard to engage'. Reasons for this are often to be found in their previous experiences of workers changing and moving, undermining the concept of a trusting relationship. People damaged by such a system find it difficult enough to trust one worker, let alone a whole team. In reality, some people may be helped to engage equally with all team members whilst for others it is quite realistic to expect them to engage more readily with some members of staff, and that these alliances may shift across the whole team in certain circumstances. This latter situation can be negatively dismissed as just a further deficit of the individual, or it can be accepted and worked with in a practical way. Enforcing a dogmatic approach to engaging with the whole team may have detrimental effects of promoting disengagement in some circumstances.

Some users of the Tulip service preferred to develop individual relationships with fewer staff. They complained of having to tell the same story to different staff and experienced a lack of continuity among staff in the way they managed tasks over time. Workers forgot tasks and users had problems remembering the names of everyone visiting them (Gauntlett et al 1996). Spindel and Nugent (1999) criticized the American ACT evaluations in the same vein:

> "...it is much more difficult, if not impossible, for any human being to establish warm, supportive, and trusting relationships with a 'team'."

Spindel and Nugent (1999) also argued that the whole team approach creates a very negative image of mental health service users, implying they were so different and abnormal they required a whole team to work with them. Some ACT evaluations report a high rate of drop-out (McGrew et al 1995), despite their supposedly positive evaluation by service users. The nature of the team response may also risk usurping natural supports provided by community, family and friends. Teams are not necessarily easy for family and friends to work with; high-profile professional responses may lead others to drop out of their involvement assuming that the team is 'taking care of it' (Spindel and Nugent 1999).

The role of care co-ordinator also poses some difficulties for the ways in which a team approach is implemented. Within this role, most individuals feel they have to do most of the engaging and delivering of services for the people they work with (Department of Health 1999). How can a whole team be the care co-ordinator? It may be a function performed under a single name for administrative purposes, e.g. the team leader, but the whole team approach enables all staff of a relevant seniority/grade to perform the role interchangeably. Other parts of the system contain workers who are not thinking and working in this way and do not wish to have their understanding of bureaucracy challenged in a way that makes them have to think differently to what is usual for them. Assertive Outreach has a habit of throwing up such challenges to the orthodoxy, and becoming an uncomfortable relative to have around, not always abiding by the house rules.

However, it is not wise to see the team approach in restrictive terms – it is as much about the way the team manages its own administrative and support functions as it is about the delivery of care to the individual service user. Thus, it offers opportunities for creative capability through its mechanisms of team meetings, communication and facilitated reflection.

Box 5.2   Kettering Assertive Outreach team: a team approach handover meeting in practice

The place is the Assertive Outreach team office. The time is 9.00 am and the kettle has boiled. Present are five members of the team and any visitors that particular day. Sue reminds the visitors that it's 'handover', a time when the team discusses an update of all the service users, so visitors will remain quietly ignored. All attention is focused on a whiteboard covering most of one wall of the office. For the next 45 minutes the current needs of the whole team caseload will be updated, then a 15-minute focus on planning the work for the team across the whole day will be negotiated – not a difficult task when a whole team is focused in its belief in the service users, the value of the work and support for each other. Then all you need is for the interlopers to know their place, and not interrupt the process with inane questions about 'the what and the how'.

Any member of the team calls out the name of the first service user represented on the board. In this instance, Diane calls out the name of the first person on the white board. Sam updates the Sports Group attendance, and plans for enrolling at a local gym. Tony adds that this individual is drinking less alcohol than previously. Diane remembers this is a good sign of personal motivation improving and Nigel explains how their mood seemed much calmer when he and Sue visited yesterday afternoon to deliver weekly medication supplies. Sue suggests this individual appreciates the help the tablets can offer, since more information and discussion about medication issues is happening and Tony suggests the early signs chart needs reviewing by whoever plans to do the next visit.

It's 9.02 am and Tony calls the second name on the board. Nigel smiles, Sam smiles even louder! Diane has had a couple of days' leave and looks puzzled. Sue explains that yesterday the person in question took the decision to set up a bank account to manage their own finances more clearly. Viv, the team administrator, describes the initial phone call to her from the service user, and Tony says it is fabulous to see them taking this on as a personal decision, showing how much they have progressed in confidence.

At approximately 9.24 am Sue reminds the team that time is moving on and there are a further 14 service users to mention. She calls out the next name on the list and outlines the individual's desire to see the psychiatrist quickly for a review of medication. Tony states that the service user went with him to the pharmacy to collect the latest prescription but suggested that the service user would stop taking it altogether if there was not a reasonable discussion about changing the tablets. Diane suggests that the risk is real from previous experiences, and asks if the team feels its ideas about early warning signs of relapse and contingency plans are in place. Sam says he updated the relapse signature with the service user in recent weeks but will bring it to the 'team reflection' meeting for further discussion later in the week. Sue suggests she will phone the psychiatrist as a matter of urgency to set up a home visit.

> At 9.49 am the service user update is complete and the team set about allocating the visits, the administrative needs and other team functions for the day.
>
> The team approach is in full swing but the effective application of the team approach is what continues to go on for the rest of the day and beyond. It is not just a meeting, it is all aspects of the team's work and functioning. A team approach is also about different personalities gelling with each other, in a way that recognizes their individuality, and that they are even better for being able to respect and work with each others' strengths and personal qualities. The meetings and the ongoing work continually reflect a melting pot of the problems, strengths, successes, mental state, social and psychological needs of all the service users.

Co-working

In this model of working a minimum of two workers are encouraged to engage with each service user referred to the team. A flexible development of the approach enables the team to allocate more than two people to work with a service user where the need is identified but never just a single key worker. The co-workers are charged with the responsibility of arranging regular meetings between themselves to discuss the ongoing work with the service users they share responsibility for, and to review and develop team care plans for discussion with the wider team. Such an approach can become a complicated patchwork of different team members forming co-working arrangements. It requires all members of the team to be equally committed to the mechanisms for meeting together, and to arrangements for monitoring effective implementation.

Key working within teams

The approach identified as key working shares the aspirations outlined in effective team working above but differs markedly in its need for each service user to have an identified key worker, charged with the responsibility of initiating engagement and the necessary service co-ordination (Allness and Knoedler 1999), particularly with respect to CPA responsibilities. Shared teamwork, in whatever model, will include responsibility for individually assigned activities that will necessarily reflect different personal skills and abilities as well as the needs expressed by different service users. The task of the key worker is not to do all but to ensure that all is done (Hemming et al 1999). In this sense, the key worker will build a small team of three or four workers around the identified needs of the service user, based on the skills of the workers.

For the service users who identify more closely with one or two workers as their primary contacts, the key working or co-working approaches offer flexibility, whilst still working to help the service user connect with the team to establish service continuity. Sight is not lost of the need to work with the dangers of dependency on the individual worker, who is likely to move on at some point in the future. However, individual key working presents a specific danger where isolated outreach workers are appointed to deliver a service. This is as much an issue of isolation

Box 5.3   Norwich Active Outreach team

Team composition

This is voluntary sector team, established in 1995, with a strong service user evaluation of services (Graley-Wetherell and Morgan 2001). There is a part-time team manager (with other managerial responsibilities in the organization). There are five outreach workers (mixed nursing, social work and community housing support worker backgrounds).

The strengths of the Active Outreach team are in the combination of the professional and nonprofessional skill mix. More importantly, all team members demonstrate good personal skills, flexible and creative thinking around the challenges presented by their daily work, and negotiation skills (including with other agencies in statutory and voluntary sectors). The weakness lies in the limitations of skills and expertise that a small number of people can be expected to possess, e.g. around issues of dual diagnosis (mental health and substance misuse).

Model of team working

The model of care is inevitably shaped by the beliefs and personalities of the people who make up the team. Consistency of workers has been an important factor in the ownership of the philosophy and model of care. For the Active Outreach team, the dominant method of practice is a 'co-working model'. The team currently works with 53 service users. Each service user has at least two but up to five workers in contact depending on what works best for the individual person at any point in time.

Primary responsibility for overseeing the individual package of care and support offered by the team is managed by outreach workers on an approximately one in ten allocation. This is very much in line with the recommendations in the research. As a voluntary sector agency Julian Housing staff do not carry CPA care co-ordinator responsibilities. However, they do adhere closely to the principles of care co-ordination within the scope of their practice. This includes identifying daily and weekly tasks, and ensuring that they are followed through. Each member of the team takes responsibility for ensuring records are kept up to date and that other services are informed about the needs of the service user when appropriate.

The team operates a flexible structure around the hours of 8.30 am to 6.30 pm. They cover seven days a week, but because of the small size of the team only one person will be on duty at weekends. This lone worker will primarily offer social visits, but in the case of risks and crises can call for back-up from Oak House staff (this is the housing assessment unit part of the Julian Housing organization).

A duty system, known as front-line afternoons, is managed on a rota basis by the team. This involves one member of staff being office bound each afternoon, to deal with any service user visits or telephone

> calls to the office. It can also be a time for catching up on note keeping.
>
> The co-working model is facilitated by two types of meeting:
>
> - Wednesday pm – planning the work of the whole team for the following week.
> - Co-worker meetings – for updating information and care planning, flexibly arranged through the mechanism of the Wednesday pm meeting.

within an Assertive Outreach team that does not adopt any form of team approach, as it does the identification of individual outreach workers within community mental health teams. The danger is one of potential staff burnout, as well as the more likely issue of losing the focus on the core components for effective delivery of a creative and intensive service.

The failure to adopt a system of key worker responsibility may undermine the necessary network co-ordination role, particularly within the responsibilities of the CPA. Engagement and practical support will be a primary focus but the broader range of identified needs will only be successfully achieved by accessing the resources developed through a wider network of service relationships.

A team approach can fulfil these functions, as long as it operates effective team systems of communication and a managerial overview that does not lose sight of the external service connections. In these circumstances, a key worker function is still necessary for providing essential administrative and liaison roles. If the relationship between service providers relies on one service acting as an outreach service, but an entirely different service providing the key worker co-ordination, then the frequently occurring dangers of poor communication may be exacerbated.

GROUP SUPERVISION

"Clients presenting with long-term problems and high degrees of risk are a very needy group of people, who present the practitioner with a complex range of issues and tasks and intense emotional demands… supervision becomes a valuable part of taking care of oneself, maintaining a commitment to learning and addressing the issues of self-awareness and on-going professional and personal development…" (Morgan 1996). In a strengths approach supervision and reflecting on practice are always considered constructive and positive experiences, whether conducted individually or in a group.

The definitions, purposes and skills of individual supervision are widely covered in the literature (Hawkins and Shohet 1989, van Ooijen 2000) so will not be examined further here. In proposing a model of group supervision Rapp (1998) states:

> "Strengths model case management is a demanding job that requires high levels of skills and energy in the face of heretofore incorrigible situations to achieve ambitious ends… Group supervision is a mechanism

for case managers to feel connected to a group sharing the same mission and challenges. Its aim is to affirm case managers: their efforts, their ingenuity, their accomplishments… and exchanging feedback… The central task is the generation of promising ideas to more effectively work with clients… To facilitate learning, by placing individual client situations under the microscope, case managers have an opportunity to learn things that would apply to similar situations… Group supervision provides information on community resource alternatives that could be useful for other clients."

In developing the earlier work of Rapp into a UK context, Bleach (1996) suggests that group supervision is specifically designed to achieve four goals that are related to successful meetings:

1. Affirmation – to receive recognition of the work you are doing.
2. Information – to share and clarify details about your work.
3. Ideas – to generate new thoughts for ways forward.
4. Fun – to have a good time with your colleagues whilst working.

Group supervision is basically a peer-based sharing process, intended to provide mutual reinforcement and development of the day-to-day practice of strengths-based work. It can easily replace a great deal of the time spent in one-to-one case supervision and the time spent in informal sharing, support, information seeking, etc. If working effectively it will free more time than it uses, and will enhance the team and working environment.

Do not confuse or mix this group supervision with other processes. For example, it should be kept separate from professional or line-managerial supervision. Also, do not intermix it with meetings to sort out the day-to-day business of your team, allocate cases, etc., unless you carry out the processes entirely from the same strengths perspective. Remember this is a strengths-focused process. Your conduct should reflect the process. The same perspective will be applied to each other as is applied to service users; this helps to improve both approaches.

Within the context of the group supervision meeting Rapp (1998) suggests: "The presentation should include:

– A statement of the difficulty or problem.
– A statement of what the case manager would like to see instead (desired state) and how the group can help.
– A complete list of strategies and efforts already tried to achieve the desired state.

"The presentation is then followed by questions from the group and brainstorming solutions or alternatives. Statements of empathy and support are often exchanged."

The guidelines for participation in group supervision sessions are (Bleach 1996):

• When someone says something, listen to them, validate, encourage and build on what they are saying. This form of supervision may provide 'critique' (i.e. careful and constructive analysis) but it does not criticize.

- If someone is saying or doing something you disagree with, be clear about separating respectively what you and they say, do, think, want – both should be recognized and validated, *e.g. there is a world of difference between telling a colleague, or user "You were wrong to do that" or "You should not do that" and limiting yourself to "I would not do that".*
- Keep it personal. Avoid abstract or 'professional' speech unless it is very pertinent, *e.g. to state that "this person's psychosis is very florid" says much less about the issue than "I can not follow what they are going on about".*
- Stay personal, concentrate on the user's own unique individuality, wants, aims, *e.g. "She is a Jamaican housewife with post-natal depression" says very little compared with "I know she moved country 10 years ago, feels isolated now, used to be considered quite a wit, but is very sad and under a lot of pressure and wants to do the best for the baby and thinks she is not good enough".*
- Allow yourself and others to 'brainstorm' – to generate new and creative perspectives and ideas. This means both giving permission for people to throw in wild ideas and not criticizing them for doing it or judging their ideas for 'validity'. Share your information and experience.
- Keep this as a peer process not a supervising one – if you get too much "Why don't you…", "Yes, but…" going on then you are probably getting distracted into professional problem orientation rather than generating ways forward.
- Join in and encourage others to join in – if you do not have any 'professional' input to make, allow your own personal curiosity, empathy and inventiveness to contribute.
- Allow feelings into the picture – if someone makes you angry, scared, sad, happy, as a worker or as a human being, it is going to affect what you do, so recognize it in this process.
- Keep it positive – focus on the strengths in what is being done, *e.g. If someone has made a mistake, or failed at something, the chances are that they will learn more and move on faster if you recognize their positive motives, good intentions, making the effort, taking the risk. If someone has done something that has turned out well they may not usually recognize and celebrate it with peers – recognize that small steps towards change are vitally important in this work and encourage, if necessary, an atmosphere of false immodesty.*

The checklist for 'monitoring' whether group supervision is achieving its aims (to be used by all participants periodically) (Bleach 1996):

- Do you look forward to the group supervision meetings?
- Do you leave the meeting feeling energized, validated, optimistic and hopeful?
- When discussing a specific situation did you receive several creative ideas that you could bring back to discuss with the people involved?
- Do you feel that you can share an idea when the group is brainstorming without being judged by others in the group?
- Did the discussion focus more on deficits and disorders rather than ideas to help people get what they want and need?

- Does everyone in the group participate by asking questions and suggesting possible helping approaches?
- To what extent has the group integrated work and fun during the meeting?
- How does the group celebrate and validate successful efforts, and less successful efforts?
- Has the group fostered an atmosphere of openness, collaboration and learning?
- Is the group helping you learn more about community resources, especially resources that are public rather than specialist?
- Is the group identifying occasions within the organization, or within other agencies, that require an advocacy role?
- Does it appear that members of the group believe that this time together is a priority?
- Do you meet in a comfortable place, free from interruptions?
- How much of what was said about individual service users would you be comfortable about repeating to them?
- Was there a 'can do' attitude or a 'yes, but' atmosphere?
- Were service users talked about in terms of their own uniqueness, individuality and personal interests?
- Were 'problem' areas analysed into wants, aims and motivations?
- Were potential resources/people in the community identified?
- Was there a discussion of possible 'niches' in the community where service users and resource people would benefit from each other?
- Was there laughter in the meeting?
- Were ideas generated when discussing service users that could be shared with them?
- Does the agenda wander into other business, e.g. team dynamics, managerial issues or team rotas?
- Were general goals broken down into concrete and achievable steps?

Rapp (1998) summarizes the 'power of group supervision' as:

- generating ideas/creative alternatives
- potential for wider cultural perspective
- support, affirmation and understanding
- sharing successful helping efforts and success stories
- different perspectives
- sharing/consensus on difficult decisions
- time-efficient
- team approach
- support in face of opposition, e.g. family
- enjoyment and fun
- generalized learning
- respite from other work demands.

In reality, group supervision and reflection may form a part of most team meetings, daily handover or weekly/monthly case reviews, and in some models of practice group supervision will form a regularly identified team meeting in its own right. For services wishing to explore the technique it is strongly recommended that it should be focused on one type of meeting to begin with, namely the case review.

CONCLUSIONS

Together

Everyone

Achieves

More

(Kettering Assertive Outreach team: acronym devised within the team, and placed on their white board)

Creative collaborations may be facilitated through a team approach in the pure form, all workers working with all service users referred to the service. It may take the form of co-working individual service users or it may be a 'clinical' team of professionals built around the needs of the specific individual service user. Each of these will have its in-built degree of flexibility. However, we cannot assume teams will be effective unless we very specifically design them to be effective, and recruit and train their members to be effective.

In general, the need for flexibility and the avoidance of dogma is paramount. The over-riding principle of adjusting the service response to meet the needs of individual service users should also apply to the model of team working adopted. Indeed, it is perhaps most productive to think of the user as the central team member and then design the rest of the team around them as a functioning network where each element has a relevant task to perform.

Within such a team, individual service users may gradually establish trust and confidence in a few members of the team, whilst their awareness of others may lead to a curiosity for meeting with them. In some instances, the service user who gets to know the team reasonably well may request certain individuals on the team to help them resolve specific needs – the service user dictating the functioning of the team approach! This is the dominant approach established in the initial development of the Wellingborough Active Outreach team. However, the true team approach operates through management mechanisms agreed within the team, whereby staff are able to monitor and support the positive reasons underpinning the service user directives. As Spindel and Nugent (1999) state:

> "It is … perfectly natural that some case managers may gravitate to particular clients and vice versa. This is a reasonable outcome, since it stimulates a more trusting relationship, when client and case manager have an affinity for each other"

Creative collaborations are not static – they are flexible arrangements in response to needs! A good team recognizes differences of approach, ideas and individuality. It celebrates and works with these differences, rather than suppressing them. It instils all its work with a 'can do' attitude – thinking the unthinkable and then doing it! Much of this style of working requires a smaller size of teams. A true team approach is not something that can be easily achieved with groups of 12, 15, 20 or more people. How many service users can any of us hold significant amounts of detail about in our heads? Working as a team is something we too often claim to be doing but we can rarely justify the claims in practice.

This is likely to work where the whole team is focused on, and values work with, people with severe mental health problems, and where the team as a whole can maintain an awareness of each member's caseload. It becomes problematic when it encourages staff to spend most of their time working with the more socially rewarding users who are perceived as having more tractable difficulties.

References

Allness D, Knoedler W 1999 Recommended PACT Standards for New Teams (revised 3/31/99). National Alliance for the Mentally Ill, Virginia

Bennis W, Biederman P W 1997 Organizing Genius: The Secrets of Creative Collaboration. Nicholas Brealey, London

Bleach A 1996 Unpublished exercise sheets for developing strengths based group supervision. Sainsbury Centre for Mental Health, London

Brandon D, Towe N 1989 Free to Chose: An Introduction to Service Brokerage. Good Impressions Publishing, London

Burns T 1999 Case management, care management and care programming. British Journal of Psychiatry 170: 393–395

Department of Health 1990 The care programme approach for people with a mental illness referred to the special psychiatric services. HMSO, London

Department of Health 1995 Building bridges: a guide to arrangements for inter-agency working for the care and protection of severely mentally ill people. The Stationery Office, London

Department of Health 1999 The National Service Framework for Mental Health. Modern Standards and Service Models. The Stationery Office, London

Ford K, McClelland N 2002 Assertive outreach: development of a working model. Nursing Standard 16 (32): 41–44

Gauntlett N, Ford R, Muijen M 1996 Teamwork: Models of Outreach in an Urban Multi-cultural Setting. Sainsbury Centre for Mental Health, London

Graley-Wetherell R, Morgan S 2001 Active Outreach: An Independent Service User Evaluation of a Model of Assertive Outreach Practice. Sainsbury Centre for Mental Health, London

Harris M, Bergman H C 1987 Case management with the chronically mentally ill: a clinical perspective. American Journal of Orthopsychiatry 57 (2): 296–302

Hawkins P, Shohet R 1989 Supervision in the Helping Professions. Open University Press, Buckingham

Hemming M, Morgan S, O'Halloran P 1999 Assertive Outreach: implications for the development of the model in the United Kingdom. Journal of Mental Health 8 (2): 141–147

Intagliata J 1982 Improving the quality of community care for the chronically mentally disabled: the role of case management. Schizophrenia Bulletin 8 (4): 655–674

Kanter J 1989 Clinical case management: definition, principles, components. Hospital and Community Psychiatry 40 (4): 361–368

Marty D, Rapp C A, Carlson L 2001 The experts speak: the critical ingredients of strengths model case management. Psychiatric Rehabilitation Journal 24 (3): 214–221

McGrew J H, Bond G R, Dietzen L et al 1995 A multisite study of client outcomes in assertive community treatment. Psychiatric Services 46: 696–701

Morgan S 1996 Helping Relationships in Mental Health. Chapman & Hall, London

Morgan S, Juriansz D 2002 Practice based evidence. Openmind 114: 12–13

Mueser K T, Bond G R, Drake R E et al 1998 Models of community care for severe mental illness: a review of research on case management. Schizophrenia Bulletin 24 (1): 37–74

National Health Service (1990) NHS and Community Care Act. The Stationery Office, London

Navarro T 1995 Tulip Team Approach: A Working Paper. Tulip, Haringey, London (unpublished)

Navarro T 1998 Beyond keyworking. In: Foster A, Roberts V (eds) Managing Mental Health in the Community: Chaos and Containment. Routledge, London, p 143–153

Onyett S 2003 Teamworking in Mental Health. Palgrave, London

Onyett S, Pillinger T, Muijen M 1995 Making Community Mental Health Teams Work: CMHTs and the people who work in them. Sainsbury Centre for Mental Health, London

Ooijen E van 2000 Clinical Supervision. Harcourt, London

Rapp C A 1998 The Strengths Model: Case Management with People Suffering from Severe and Persistent Mental Illness. Oxford University Press, New York

Rapp C A, Chamberlain R 1985 Case management services to the chronically mentally ill. Social Work 30 (5): 417–422

Sainsbury Centre for Mental Health 1998 Keys to Engagement: Review of Care for People with Severe Mental Illness who are Hard to Engage with Services. Sainsbury Centre for Mental Health, London

Spindel P, Nugent J A 1999 The Trouble with PACT: Questioning the Increasing Use of Assertive Community Treatment Teams in Community Mental Health. http://www.madnation.org/pacttrouble.htm

Stein L I, Santos A B 1998 Assertive Community Treatment for People with Severe Mental Illness. Norton, New York

Teague G B, Bond G R, Drake R E 1998 Program fidelity in assertive community treatment: development and use of a measure. American Journal of Orthopsychiatry 68 (2): 216–232

Witheridge T F, Dincin J 1985 The Bridge: an assertive outreach program in an urban setting. New Directions for Mental Health Services 26: 65–76

Witheridge T F, Dincin J, Appleby L 1982 Working with the most frequent recidivists: a total team approach to assertive resource management. Psychosocial Rehabilitation Journal 5: 9–11

Chapter 6

Targeting: who is the client?

Peter Ryan and Steve Morgan

Who wants to be a target anyway?

INTRODUCTION

This chapter addresses the issue of targeting: who is Assertive Outreach for? It explores the tension between what government policy requires Assertive Outreach to focus on, and what the research evidence suggests is the client group with which it is most effective. The implications for the wider care system are then discussed. The chapter goes on to look at 'targeting' from a historical perspective, and observes that in fact the kind of client that Assertive Outreach has worked with has changed substantially over the years, and that the current 'target group' for Assertive Outreach services is a determinant of government social policy. The chapter then switches perspective, and considers the issue of targeting from a service user's point of view. What is it like to be a 'target' for mental health services? Is this indeed a helpful concept? The chapter then explores a user-centred approach to defining and selecting the 'target group', which includes an examination of the selection criteria for Assertive Outreach. The chapter ends with some reflections as to the risks and pressures Assertive Outreach services themselves run, given that their 'official' target group is not one with which the research literature would suggest it is optimally effective.

THE TARGET GROUP FOR ASSERTIVE OUTREACH

Throughout the 1990s perhaps the most important trend in mental health policy was towards targeting the severe longterm mentally ill. Community psychiatric nurses and social workers in the 1980s and early 1990s had been able to choose who they wished to work with, but suddenly found under the Care Programme Approach (CPA) (Department of Health 1990) that this was no longer the case. Under the Conservative government (1979–97), the overall balance of community care policy tipped much more explicitly towards the close monitoring and control of severe longterm clients, particularly high-risk clients likely to be violent. This had led in 1994 to the establishment of a Supervision Register under the CPA (NHS Executive 1994), in order to monitor the behaviour of high-risk clients more closely. When the Labour government was returned to power in 1997, it continued this trend; even though it abandoned Supervision Registers, it replaced them with an explicit emphasis on targeting high-risk clients.

It has been estimated that this relatively circumscribed high-risk group of people in need of intensive support accounts for 80% of the direct costs of mental hospital treatment and care for people with schizophrenia. An influential report from the Sainsbury Centre (Sainsbury Centre for Mental Health 1998) concluded that Assertive Outreach was the 'treatment of choice' for the most 'problematic' of the severe longterm client group. In overall terms, the report estimated the prevalence of this group as likely to vary considerably from 200 per 100 000 in the inner city to as low as 14 per 100 000 in rural areas. The report estimated an average prevalence of 45 per 100 000 or a maximum of 15 000 nationally. Some of this group may be causing anxiety or concern in their local communities through their history of violence against others; many more will be at risk of suicide or severe self-neglect. To put this in perspective, about 50 homicides and 1000 suicides per year are likely to involve people with longterm severe mental illness (Appleby 1997). Many clients in this group will have experienced frequent re-admissions to inpatient care or will have experienced extended periods of time of a year or more as inpatients. Some may be caught up in the judicial system as minor offenders, whilst others might be homeless or frequently change address. Many others may be experiencing problems with drugs or alcohol as well as experiencing longterm mental illness. A recent study found that more than 80% of clients on the caseloads of the Assertive Outreach teams had at least one of the following criteria: "History of self-harm, history of violence, non-compliance with medication, non-co-operation with mental health services, or at least one admission in the past two years" (Ryan et al 1999).

These high-risk clients slotted neatly into the two-tier standard and enhanced version of the CPA introduced by the Labour government (Department of Health 1999a). The clients that Assertive Outreach is designed to work with seem to be clearly within the criteria for the enhanced CPA:

- clients with multiple needs
- intensive involvement of more than one agency required
- more than one diagnosis, or indications of substance misuse

- hard to engage
- risk to self or others.

A comprehensive assessment and care plan is required for clients in the enhanced CPA, which should include:

- psychiatric, psychological and social functioning
- risk to the individual and others, including previous violence and criminal record
- needs arising from co-morbidity
- personal circumstances including family or other carers
- housing, financial and occupational status
- physical health needs
- user and carer views.

It would seem therefore that in the UK government mental health policy has added political and social control impetus to the issue of targeting. Money has been allocated, Assertive Outreach teams implemented and arguably the term itself invented to deal with a particular social concern. That concern is well expressed in the Labour government's National Service Framework for Mental Health (Department of Health 1999b):

> "If personal and public safety and well-being are to be assured, it is essential that mental health services stay in contact with people with severe mental illness, especially individuals who are assessed as at risk of harm to themselves, or of posing a risk to others. Services should provide flexible help and outreach support in response to fluctuating need and risk."

These policy statements are noteworthy both in terms of what they emphasize and for what they overlook or ignore. They clearly emphasize Assertive Outreach as focusing on the 'difficult-to-engage' clients, and underline its contribution to safe care and treatment. The intended legislation is clearly designed to optimize the public safety aspects of this role. Assertive Outreach is tasked therefore to engage with the politically sensitive issue of 'care in the community' for a group of people who offer a potential threat either to themselves or, more pertinently, to the community at large, i.e. service users with a severe and persistent mental illness, and who are at risk of self-harm or violence towards others. It is very clear that Assertive Outreach in the UK does not have the freedom to work with the client group with which the research evidence suggests it is most effective. It must work with a client group which government policy requires it to, whether or not this is the group with which it is necessarily most effective.

This is clearly reflected in the Implementation Guidelines for Assertive Outreach (Department of Health 2001) which point Assertive Outreach towards a very specific kind of client, namely adults between the age of 18 and approximately 65, with the following:

- A severe and persistent mental disorder (e.g. schizophrenia; major affective disorders) associated with a high level of disability.

- A history of high use of inpatient or intensive home-based care (for example, more than two admissions or more than six months' inpatient care in the past two years).
- Difficulty maintaining a lasting and consenting contact with services.
- Multiple, complex needs including some of the following:
  - history of violence or persistent offending
  - significant risk of persistent self-harm or neglect
  - poor response to previous treatment
  - dual diagnosis of substance misuse and serious mental illness
  - detained under Mental Health Act 1983 on at least one occasion in the previous two years
  - unstable accommodation or homelessness.

In summary, it would seem from examination of the 1998 White Paper, the National Service Framework standards four and five (Department of Health 1999b) and the Assertive Outreach Implementation Guidelines (Department of Health 2001) that there are certain areas where Assertive Outreach is as it were expected to 'deliver' but other areas where there is no particular 'pressure to perform'. The primary task for Assertive Outreach, from a policy perspective, is clearly to engage high-risk clients with severe mental illness who are resistant to contacting services, to keep them out of hospital if possible, but to prevent them above all from harming themselves or others. No particular emphasis is placed on other areas of clinical outcome such as symptomatic improvement, increased social adjustment or improved quality of life. What this discussion would seem to argue for is that the targeting of Assertive Outreach is as much determined by social policy and service context as it is by the research evidence. It further follows therefore that the target group for Assertive Outreach in the UK is an artefact engineered by government social policy, rather than an evidence-based fact.

Asking a different question: what is Assertive Outreach for?

What is the target group for Assertive Outreach? As Burns and Firn (2002) say in their useful account of this issue: "This is the wrong question to start off with. The fundamental question should be 'what is assertive outreach for?' In other words, what treatments and procedures, of proven worth, can we not provide currently that we could with an assertive outreach service? From the answer to this question comes the answer to 'who is it for'?".

It is commonly said that Assertive Outreach works best with 'psychotic' clients (Burns and Firn 2002). It is certainly true that the great majority of research studies have focused on a client group that could generically be called 'adult severely mentally ill with a primary diagnosis of schizophrenia' (Mueser et al 1998). It also needs to be acknowledged that a wide variety of other client groups have been targeted, including those with learning disability and mental illness, dual diagnosis clients and the homeless. Also, clients have been selected at widely different parts of the life event cycle including prior to admission so as to prevent admission, relocating the 'old long stay' into the community, working with young 'first admission' clients so as to mitigate against a longterm 'career' in mental health services, and working with young black male service users.

However, what seems to be insufficiently recognized is that there have been wide variations over time in the severity of the clients with whom Assertive Outreach services have worked. What is assumed in one social and political context as being the 'ideal' client for Assertive Outreach is not necessarily the same in another. This can best be demonstrated by looking at some of the classic studies in the field, which are now over 20 years old (Stein and Test 1980, Hoult et al 1983). It is important to recognize that mental health services 20 years ago were faced with a very different set of challenges and were working with very different kinds of clients.

Target groups: the early classic studies

In 1970, when Dr Leonard Stein took up the post of Director of Education and Training at Mendota State Hospital in Madison, Wisconsin, mental health services were in a very different condition and stage of development. Essentially, community-based mental health services in Wisconsin, as in most other places, were either non-existent or in a very early and primitive stage of development. There was not the plethora of community services we frequently see today. The challenge for Stein in Wisconsin, and shortly thereafter for Dr John Hoult in Sydney, was to kickstart the development of effective community services. This also meant that the kind of inpatient client they were working with was also different in certain respects from the kind of client today's inpatient service typically face. To begin with, the problem of the dual diagnosis client was not anywhere near so widespread in the late 1970s and early 1980s as it is today.

As Tables 6.1 and 6.2 illustrate, the overall picture is one in which, compared to the caseload of modern UK Assertive Outreach teams, Stein and Hoult worked with a somewhat younger client group, who were less frequently diagnosed as psychotic, and who had substantially less experience of hospitalization. In the Stein and Test (1980) client group, the average age was 31, with around half having a diagnosis of schizophrenia.

Table 6.1 Demographic characteristics of clients in classic studies (based on Stein and Test 1980, Hoult et al 1983)

Demographic characteristics of clients	Stein and Test	Hoult et al
Average age	31 years	Two-thirds aged under 40 years
Diagnosis of schizophrenia/ functional psychosis	50%	75%
Mean total duration of illness	14.5 months over five hospitalizations	?
Proportion without previous admission to hospital	17%	25%

Table 6.2   Demographic characteristics of clients in three recent UK studies

Demographic characteristics of clients	Thornicroft (1998)	Burns and Firn (2002)	Ryan et al (1999)
Average age	42 years	39 years	46 years
Diagnosis of schizophrenia/ functional psychosis	95%	87%	85%
Mean total duration of illness	184 months	120 months	264 months
Proportion without previous admission to hospital	0%	0%	0%

Seventeen per cent of Stein and Test's sample, and 25% of Hoult's, had never been in hospital before. By contrast, in three recent UK studies (see Table 6.2) the average age of the clients was at or over 40 years, and a higher proportion suffered from schizophrenia.

All clients in these studies had previously been hospitalized, and they had a far longer total period of contact with psychiatric services. In essence, this comparison would seem to suggest that the clients the modern UK studies were working with were an older, more disabled group. In comparison, the early classic studies, which established the reputation of Assertive Outreach as an effective intervention, would seem in retrospect to have been working with a younger, less disabled group, with far less experience of inpatient care. As an example there is no way that current UK Assertive Outreach teams would be working with clients with no prior hospital admissions, whilst 17% of Stein and Test's sample, and 25% of Hoult's, fell into that category.

The 'typical' client of Assertive Outreach teams cannot be easily described, as all people are individuals with their own stories and specific needs and wishes. The following two case profiles, in Boxes 6.1 and 6.2, give detailed accounts of the type of complex circumstances that many Assertive Outreach workers will be expected to work with on a daily basis.

Implications for mental health services as a whole

The policy requirements spelt out for Assertive Outreach clearly locate it in a particular position with respect to UK mental health services as a whole. To use a sporting analogy, one way to view this would be to say that Assertive Outreach has become the back-stop or sweeper for mental health services. The function of Assertive Outreach is to engage and work with clients whose difficulties are so severe that other parts of the service have simply failed to connect with them. Whilst all mental health services have increasingly focused on the severely mentally ill, Assertive Outreach focuses on the most problematic and difficult to engage clients of all.

Community mental health teams (CMHTs) in particular have a potentially problematic relationship with Assertive Outreach. Assertive Outreach teams are also, paradoxically, in a privileged position compared to other parts of the service. Whilst it is true that they work with

Box 6.1   Case profile 1: Margaret

Personal history

Margaret is a 49-year-old woman. She was born in London, an only child. She lost contact with her parents many years ago, whilst she was a hospital inpatient, and now believes they are deceased. She was married in her early 30s, to another patient she met in hospital, but her husband died five years ago. Margaret receives occasional visits from her sister-in-law but no other family or friends.

A poor achiever at school, Margaret was thought to be experiencing learning difficulties but no further investigations or support were pursued. As a result, she has been unable to gain any employment experience of any kind.

Her apparent disturbed behaviour through her teenage years, with profound social difficulties through volatile interpersonal contacts, resulted in social isolation, with no significant friendships developed. Her parents tended to increasingly restrict her access outside the family home. Margaret's only significant social and sexual relationships have developed through her many years as an inpatient at an old psychiatric hospital.

Psychiatric history

Margaret was admitted into institutional care at the age of 18 (in 1970). She had been diagnosed with schizophrenia following contact with the family doctor and a specialist psychiatric assessment. She experienced five long hospital admissions, totalling 13 of the next 15 years. These were interspersed with brief stays in hostel accommodation, and one tenancy of a council flat. The placements inevitably ended with relapse of her psychotic condition, and are reported to be the result of poor levels of support outside of the hospital environment.

In 1985, Margaret was discharged to a housing association flat with her husband, another longterm inpatient of the hospital, whom she had recently married. She has had only two hospital admissions since this time.

The first was for a month in 1990, on Section 2 of the 1983 Mental Health Act. This followed police intervention to a disturbance in a local supermarket, when Margaret was physically assaulting her husband. The second admission followed a prolonged period of severe self-neglect during the months immediately after her husband's death (from natural causes).

Physical health

Margaret is currently suffering a range of physical health problems, some of which are considered longstanding. Thyrotoxicosis has resulted from an overactive thyroid gland, with accompanying speeding up of her metabolism, abnormal protrusion of the eyes (exophthalmos), excessive growth of facial hair and a possible increasing of her extrapyramidal tremor.

The exophthalmos has also played a part in the development of a progressive infection and ulceration of her eyes, which is frequently aggravated by occasional periods of heavy smoking. In recent years, Margaret has developed a prolapsed bowel. Despite these complex and distressing physical complaints, Margaret continues to be distrustful of primary care and mental health services. She reluctantly accepted a brief hospital admission on a specialist eye conditions ward of a general hospital but generally prefers the persistent discomfort and occasional pain rather than fall for her perception that she will once again be held in hospital for several years.

Medication

Adherence to prescribed medication has presented unusual problems. Margaret has a general level of understanding that she needs to take medication to remain out of hospital. However, on occasions she has proved forgetful in her use of dosett boxes for oral medication, sometimes taking more and sometimes less than the prescribed doses (including prescribed steroids).

box continues

She only feels comfortable receiving depot psychiatric medication at the surgery. She visits the practice nurse, and she wishes to minimize the amount of access others have to her own personal space. She will not consider the psychiatric clinic at the hospital for similar reasons to her rejection of hospital services in general. She also does not wish to be in close proximity to other people for even short periods of time (a feeling that is reciprocated by most people who encounter her). Whilst Margaret became noncompliant with depot medication during the period of grieving and neglect immediately after her husband's death, she has not held issue against the 75 mg Piportil Depot prescribed for her every three weeks, as long as someone else reminds her when it is due.

Community support

Margaret is concerned that service providers wish to gain access to her flat to find reason for taking her tenancy, and thus her independence, away. At the point of her last admission (approximately four years ago), the flat had deteriorated into such a state of neglect, filth and dilapidation that urgent intervention was required to offset threats of eviction. Careful consideration needed to be given to the subsequent attempts at engaging some sort of relationship, in order to support Margaret's continuation of tenancy with the Housing Association.

The situation is made more complicated by the following issues:

- Margaret has an attention span of some 30 seconds before she feels compelled to end contact (verbally aggressively, if necessary).
- Many years of psychotropic medication have rendered Margaret subject to severe tardive dyskinesia.
- Her husband used to manage their joint finances (social security benefits) and the payment of bills.
- It is uncertain just how much Margaret is able to understand from the daily assortment of post she receives.
- Margaret does not accept that she has a problem with appearance and hygiene, despite wearing the same clothes in excessively soiled conditions (made worse by the prolapsed bowel) and her refusal to use the bath for anything other than for dumping soiled clothing.
- A number of professionals and nonprofessionals have expressed the view that Margaret may be better off in supported accommodation with other people. She is adamant about remaining in her current flat; contact with other people has shown a marked impact on the increase of psychotic symptoms, e.g. responding to auditory hallucinations, physical agitation and verbal aggression.

Current situation

Margaret continues to accept very brief daily access to the District Nurse, and even briefer doorstep contact with a community mental health worker. She states that everything is OK in the flat but she wishes the services would allow her husband out of the hospital so he could be with her at home (although she will occasionally acknowledge that he is dead). The District Nurse confirms that the condition of the living room is in a deteriorating state of neglect, but not to cause current concern about the environmental health hazard, as has previously been the case.

The Housing Association officer suggests that Margaret has been able to keep the rent account in substantial credit, but the new upstairs neighbour has phoned on several occasions to complain. Essentially, they are kept awake at night by the sound of Margaret holding strange conversations, sometimes in a loud and aggressive voice. They are not aware of anyone else living with her or visiting her. The neighbour is concerned that a strange and dirty woman is living in the same property without receiving any help.

Margaret has confirmed that she is awake at night and hears her husband's voice, with which she has conversations and arguments, but this does not cause her any concerns.

Box 6.2   Case profile 2: Wesley

Personal and family history

Wesley is a 34-year-old man of Antiguan origin, who moved to the UK with his mother and step-father when he was seven years old. He has two younger brothers, who were both born in the UK. He left school at the age of 16, with three O levels, and studied to be a book-keeper whilst working in the accounts department of a large national organization.

Wesley describes being a popular person in school, with a number of girlfriends during his teenage years. He was married at 21, and they had a daughter the following year. The marriage deteriorated rapidly at this point, coinciding with Wesley's deterioration in health and social circumstances. He is now divorced, with his ex-wife holding an injunction against him seeing her or their daughter.

He has little contact with his step-brothers and has had a very turbulent relationship with his step-father over the past 12 years.

Psychiatric history

Three hospital admissions are recorded between the ages of 23 and 27. On each occasion Wesley appears to have been referred by the Magistrates' Court for assessment and treatment, following charges of shoplifting, possession of marijuana and carrying an offensive weapon. On each occasion he was admitted for approximately one month, diagnosed with paranoid schizophrenia and/or drug-induced psychosis, commenced on anti-psychotic medication and subsequently discharged to community follow-up.

Wesley always denied having a mental health problem and the need for medication. His persistent refusal of injections or oral medication, and frequent failure to answer the door, resulted in his discharge from community psychiatric nurse caseloads.

Referral to Assertive Outreach

The persistent non-engagement with services, combined with a deterioration of social circumstances and criminal activity, caused Wesley's consultant psychiatrist to prioritize him as a candidate for the newly emerging community service. The diagnoses are felt to be accurate but in need of further assessment through more constructive contact between Wesley and the services.

Social history (from his mother)

A sad account is given of a son who was always helpful at home and achieving at school. He appears to have become involved in drugs and drinking alcohol through other people he was working with, but now he has lost all those contacts as well as his own family. He is now believed to drift about areas of the city, generally in contact with people involved in drugs. His mother says she has 'lost her son' but cannot simply ignore him or send him away, despite his volatile behaviour and dishevelled appearance.

Housing

On initial contacts, Wesley has refused to answer the door or to respond to written messages left for him. On the sixth call, racist graffiti is observed daubed on his front door, and a boarded-up window at the front of the flat. He lives on the ground floor of an inner city tenement block of flats, on a large council estate with a reputation for racial harassment and crime. The workers leave a message about wishing to help him with a housing transfer, possibly on the grounds of harassment.

Wesley appears at the door very dishevelled, with broken shoes, torn and dirty clothing, extremely long fingernails and long matted hair. He welcomes you by name and invites you in. The flat is sparsely furnished, generally broken items, and a mattress on the floor. It is covered with rubbish, cigarette lighters, penknives, and overflowing ashtrays. The kitchen is in the same condition, with empty alcohol bottles (wine and spirits) and cans (strong lagers).

box continues

When asked about how he is managing with his housing he smiles but appears distracted, then eventually answers: "It's a big problem, what with the underground well disturbing the energy forces...". He suggests he needs to get out of the flat but insists he copes quite independently, though his mother and step-father interfere "... by coming around tidying and cleaning, and generally rearranging the whole place...".

Criminal justice

Wesley does not deny the incidents when arrested by the police. However, he suggests that the police harass him, particularly when they keep him overnight in the cells, insisting that he should see a psychiatrist.

Health

He denies any mental health problem (without being asking), and suggests that the marijuana helps him to feel better within himself. He accepts that it costs him most of his money, and that the Social Security office requires him to turn up every week for over-the-counter payments, because he keeps losing his payment book.

Wesley claims his chesty cough is bronchitis, resulting from the damp conditions caused by the underground well and streams. He claims to go regularly to his doctor when the need arises. He suggests he would like to move from this flat, re-establish his book-keeping skills and visit Central and South America for a holiday.

He remains distracted throughout the discussion, with the above conversation taking a very disjointed course. He locks the front door from the inside, claiming personal security on a dangerous estate, and puts the key in his pocket. On returning from a couple of minutes in the kitchen, he has an angry expression on his face and begins shouting abusively. He paces the room threatening violence, without looking directly at the workers. He turns and smiles at them, and asks their names.

particularly complex and challenging clients, they also have a protected caseload, which a CMHT member, with a caseload of over 30, may well envy. Whilst CMHTs may well have referred on to Assertive Outreach some of their most challenging clients, in all likelihood they will still have on their books many clients who are equally difficult – but having to respond to them with a caseload two or three times as large as that of Assertive Outreach. It can also easily happen that Assertive Outreach teams fill up their caseload allocations quite rapidly, and when new equally complex and challenging cases are referred on to them they are put on a waiting list, which essentially means that CMHTs will be handling by default clients who really should be on the books of Assertive Outreach.

There is an important structural paradox here. As mental health services become more proficient at identifying the complex, challenging clients Assertive Outreach has been tasked to manage, 'overflow' can easily happen, resulting in other parts of the mental health system having to cope with clients they are in fact not equipped to manage. These clients are by definition more disorganized, with poorer coping skills, lower levels of motivation and at greater risk to themselves or others than the majority of clients with which local services operate.

Once Assertive Outreach engages with such clients, one of its tasks is to reconnect these highly vulnerable clients with complex needs to the services they need. The paradox is that, by consequence of the severity of their need and levels of disability, local services are often poorly equipped to offer services to this particularly disadvantaged group. Assertive Outreach, precisely because of its success in engaging with more complex and difficult clients than the rest of the service can deal with, then finds the rest of the service unwilling or unable to help – or both. Once engaged, Assertive Outreach clients often do not fit the eligibility criteria of the residential or day-care parts of the local system. Once engaged, both the clients and the Assertive Outreach team itself can be functionally excluded from local systems of care. This in turn places the team under constant pressure, often without sufficiently responsive local residential or day-care resources.

Assertive Outreach field workers are sometimes placed in a position where they feel forced to 'sell' their clients to other local services, persuading reluctant services to take a risk with clients they really do not want to take risks with themselves. The Assertive Outreach worker is often therefore in a situation where he or she has to give 'optimistic' accounts of the coping skills of their clients, and find ways to convince local services they fit criteria, which the worker knows they actually don't. The risk is that, if a local service takes on an Assertive Outreach client, it can find itself struggling to cope with a client who is actually more disabled than it has the capacity to manage, and the care arrangement can easily break down.

It is a small step from that to a downward spiral of mutual recrimination. The Assertive Outreach team can criticize unresponsive local services, whilst local services can criticize Assertive Outreach for being 'misled' concerning the actual capabilities of the client. If a local service loses confidence in Assertive Outreach in this way, it might itself withdraw from co-operation, not only with the client concerned but also with the Assertive Outreach service itself.

A SERVICE USER PERSPECTIVE: WHO WANTS TO BE A TARGET ANYWAY?

How are service users likely to respond to the targeting policy on Assertive Outreach? Viewed from a service user perspective, being contacted by an Assertive Outreach team might well appear very intimidating. A service user might be forgiven for thinking:

> "The team clearly think that I am one of the worst cases on the patch since all the other services must have given up on me. I must be a high-risk case and they think I am very likely to:
>
> - be involved in criminal activity like robbery or theft
> - taking drugs and alcohol
> - commit suicide, assault or murder people
> - be incapable of looking after myself
> - incapable of keeping a place to stay in the community
> - totally reject all approaches services make to me."

This is clearly a caricature but it is vital that services appreciate that targeting can, under certain circumstances, come very close to stigmatizing.

Given that Assertive Outreach is clearly aimed at 'the most problematic and potentially troublesome' client group amongst the severely mentally ill, this is a particularly high risk for Assertive Outreach services. How can this risk best be avoided?

'User-friendly' referral criteria: selecting clients for Assertive Outreach services

Drawing up selection criteria that do not inadvertently either 'medicalize' or stigmatize clients is a difficult undertaking. The following are based upon selection criteria of a number of Assertive Outreach teams the authors have worked with. Criteria for defining who is, and who is not, worked with can never clarify every set of circumstances. Assessments of eligibility will be taken on an individual basis but the following lists should broadly help prospective referrers and the Assertive Outreach service to make these decisions. Assertive Outreach services should be working with people presenting some of the most complex range of needs, so it is unlikely that only one or two of the following will be applicable to any one person being accepted into the service.

- Most usually, people will be subject to enhanced level of the CPA, Section 117, Section 25 or Guardianship.
- Individuals between the ages of 18 and 65. No new referrals will be accepted of people already 65 or over. However, the team is committed to continue working with people passing 65 years of age who are already in the service, and whose needs have not substantially changed through organic deterioration or the physical frailty of ageing.
- Ongoing severe and enduring mental health difficulties, most usually of a psychotic nature, that substantially affect the service user's ability to function in the demands of daily living and maintaining relationships, e.g. diagnoses of schizophrenia, affective psychosis or bipolar disorder.
- A history where other community mental health services have been unsuccessful in engaging the individual, either because services were unable to meet their needs or through the individual's choice.
- A history of repeated admissions to inpatient units following recurring crises.
- Where there is a reasoned belief that the person will benefit from intensive input (at least weekly, and potentially daily, contact).
- A history of violence, persistent offending or frequent involvement with the police because of the experience of mental health problems.
- At risk of neglect, or neglect of significant others.
- At risk from exploitation, i.e. financial or sexual, or harm from others.
- At times may present significant risk to their own safety or to the safety of others.
- Extreme isolation.
- Homelessness or difficulty maintaining a tenancy.
- Where the person's support network becomes unable to sustain the individual as a direct result of the experience of severe and enduring mental health problems.
- Severe and enduring mental health problems combined with a secondary diagnosis of substance misuse.

Exclusion criteria: who should not be selected for Assertive Outreach?

The following are determined on the basis that other services are, or should be, more skilled to meet the identified needs:

- Substance misuse as a primary diagnosis.
- Personality disorder as a primary diagnosis.
- Organic condition.
- Moderate to severe learning disability.
- Coping independently with existing levels of support.
- Living in high-support residential or institutional settings, and likely to stay there for the foreseeable future.
- Living outside the catchment area.

THE CLIENT WITH PERSONALITY DISORDER

It is often the case that local services refer personality disordered clients on to Assertive Outreach services. The rationale for this is usually that other services have failed to manage such clients successfully, and therefore Assertive Outreach is the last port of call. However, personality disordered clients often engage very intensively with services – indeed too intensively and chaotically for them to manage. This is *not* a criterion for referral to Assertive Outreach. Assertive Outreach is not, and must not become, a receptacle for clients whom other services generally find too difficult.

There is a case for accepting a client who may have a diagnosis of personality disorder, but also meets other criteria such as being difficult to engage or is a danger to self and others. However, Assertive Outreach teams who have accepted clients with personality disorder often report that such clients consume a disproportionate amount of time and resources. Most mental health services find personality disordered clients very problematic and difficult to manage, and it is tempting to refer them to a service which, because of its low caseload, may seem in an advantageous position to deal with them. Moreover, the emerging clinical impression is that Assertive Outreach is no more successful than other services in improving the clinical condition of these clients, and may serve no other purpose than keeping tabs on troublesome clients.

CONCLUSIONS

Assertive Outreach services have been tasked by government social policy with engaging with highly disabled service users, with a severe and enduring mental illness, who engage poorly with services, and who may be at high risk to self or others. It is clear from the pending legislation (Sainsbury Centre for Mental Health 2002) that mental health services will be given additional powers through the new community treatment orders to further protect public safety (or the safety of the client) by removing clients from the community back into hospital. Inevitably, Assertive Outreach teams will be at the forefront of implementing these new powers where public or personal safety is judged to be urgently at risk. It is likely therefore that the success or failure of Assertive Outreach will be largely determined by its success, or perceived success, in this specific area. This is a cause for concern, in that it is arguable that the research evidence would suggest that Assertive Outreach will be at its most effective with a younger, less problematic client group than that to which government social policy is now assigning it.

In any case, however successful Assertive Outreach may be in reducing risk levels for this client group, the elimination altogether of risk is arguably impossible. Inevitably therefore there will continue to be incidents in the community of self-harm or of violence towards others. Whenever such incidents do occur, albeit hopefully with decreased frequency, it seems almost inevitable that Assertive Outreach will be perceived by an irate public, and government, as having failed in its duty.

References

Appleby L 1997 National Confidential Enquiry into Suicide and Homicide by People with Mental Illness: Progress Report. HMSO, London

Burns T, Firn M 2002 Assertive Outreach in Mental Health: A Manual for Practitioners. Oxford University Press, Oxford

Department of Health 1990 The Care Programme Approach for People with a Mental Illness Referred to the Specialist Psychiatric Services. HC(90)23, LASSL(90)11. HMSO, London

Department of Health 1999a Effective Care Co-ordination in Mental Health Services: Modernising the Care Programme Approach. HMSO, London

Department of Health 1999b The National Service Framework for Mental Health: Modern Standards and Service Models. HMSO, London

Department of Health 2001 The Mental Health Policy Implementation Guide. HMSO, London

Hoult J, Reynolds I, Charbonneau-Powis M et al 1983 Hospital versus community treatment: the results of a randomised controlled trial. Australian and New Zealand Journal of Psychiatry 17: 160–167

Mueser K T, Bond G R, Drake R E et al 1998 Models of community care for severe mental illness: a review of research on case management. Schizophrenia Bulletin 24 (1): 37–73

NHS Executive 1994 Introduction of Supervision Registers for Mentally Ill People from 1st April 1994. HSG(94)5. Department of Health, London

Ryan P, Ford R, Beadsmoore A et al 1999 The enduring relevance of case management. British Journal of Social Work 29: 97–125

Sainsbury Centre for Mental Health 1998 Keys to Engagement: A Review of Care for People with Severe Mental Illness Who Are Hard to Engage with Services. Sainsbury Centre for Mental Health, London

Sainsbury Centre for Mental Health 2002 Briefing 18: An Executive Briefing on the Draft Mental Health Bill. Sainsbury Centre for Mental Health, London

Stein L, Test A 1980 Alternative to mental hospital treatment. I. conceptual model, treatment program, and clinical evaluation. Archives of General Psychiatry 37: 392–397

Thornicroft G 1998 The PRiSM Psychosis Study Articles 1–10. British Journal of Psychiatry 173: 363–431

Chapter **7**

Developing trusting working relationships

Steve Morgan and Peter Ryan

Without meaningful engagement we have nothing

INTRODUCTION

The strengths model of case management (Rapp 1988, 1998) clearly identifies 'engagement' of the relationship as a separate and distinct function of the helping process (Marty et al 2001, Morgan 1996). Burns and Firn (2002), however, conclude: "Engagement is not a separate function in itself but permeates everything that we do in this work." Both viewpoints describe a similar approach in practice but vary distinctly on the need to pay specific attention to how we engage the relationship. More frequently the starting point of the process is seen to be 'assessment' – the gathering of information to identify the problems and needs. There is an unspoken assumption that people will automatically engage with a service, on a basis of their need. Attention to the quality of the relationship is not so much forgotten as taken for granted.

Mental health services are provided to a large number of people, for a wide range of reasons or conditions. Most are satisfied with the service or simply accept what happens to them because of their need in distress. Assertive Outreach services are set up primarily to gain the trust and re-engage people who choose either not to become actively involved with, or to actively resist, mental health services. All too often, services negatively stereotype service users, and essentially blame the patient for the difficulties the service may be encountering with them. They are frequently thought to have 'slipped through the net of care' or to be 'treatment resistant', 'too disturbed' or 'unreachable'.

RESISTANCE TO SERVICES

The target group for Assertive Outreach services comprises people for whom a 'take it or leave it' philosophy of service provision simply does not work. Offering a few office-based appointments to such users and then discharging them for repeated non-attendance is not a satisfactory option. We at least owe it to people to explore the real and potential reasons why they disengage, rather than quickly attributing blame to them for non-attendance whilst conveniently avoiding any scrutiny of our own service provider shortcomings, which may be contributing to disaffection with what we are offering. Box 7.1 lists some of the reasons why people have become mistrusting of mental health services, and seek to avoid further contact.

This is not an exhaustive list of reasons, as different individuals have their own experiences and interpretations of information and events. It is important that practitioners recognize and validate the reasons for individual resistance to contact, at least as the commencement for developing a mutually trusting relationship in the longer term. Without such trust, other case management interventions may not follow, or will at best be delivered in a context of conflict. Service users can be engaged on levels other than 'illness', and this may need to be the most effective starting point for discussing different interpretations of experiences and behaviours (James 2002).

Box 7.1   Reasons for resistance to services

- Traumatic experiences of hospitalization, including actual physical, emotional and sexual abuse by other patients and by staff.
- Bad experiences of detention under mental health legislation.
- Bad experiences of the side-effects of medication, with little or no constructive reactions by the services when they have been reported.
- Rejecting the labels of psychiatric diagnoses, and the social and economic stigma associated with them.
- Not believing the concept of mental illness.
- Experiences of prejudicial treatment, e.g. racism and sexism.
- A feeling that services are dehumanizing and controlling.
- A feeling that personal experiences and opinions are not listened to.
- Dynamics of conflict within a family (with mental health service contact seen as an agenda, or validation, for one view over another).
- Having had a child taken away by social services.
- Having been in local authority care as a child.
- Bewildering experiences and contacts with the legal system during a mental health crisis.
- Frustrating experiences with government departments: housing; police; social services.

The 'hard-to-engage' service

Attributing the difficulties of developing trusting relationships solely to the service user is a premature assumption to make in many instances. In any analysis of the process of engagement, or resistance to services, we must firstly acknowledge the place the service may hold in creating barriers to trust. Services occasionally have an ability to present themselves in an inflexible way, often with an overlay of an authoritarian attitude, and an exaggerated belief in their own ability to determine what is best for other people.

A service's reliance on an appointment-based system may well suit many people referred to it, but for others it simply does not connect with their own view of their needs or how to meet them. Blaming the service user for not fitting in to the system only achieves further disconnection in these instances. There are many good reasons why a service establishes itself around a system of appointments, but to inflexibly hold on to them is more a fault of the service than the service user. There are equally as many good reasons why a service user cannot or does not want to fit into an appointment system, and these need to be recognized and respected.

In this chapter we will be focusing on engagement of the individual service user, rather than on changing the attitudes of narrow-sighted services.

Engagement is...

The 'therapeutic relationship' should be a priority for service users and service providers alike, as it is of central importance for enabling effective communication of information regarding needs and wishes on both sides (Box 7.2). The service user should rightfully be able to state their own needs and wants in a way that is respectfully heard, and practitioners should be able to state their observations and needs for further information in order to determine what they might be able to provide.

It is a two-way process of communication, with service users and practitioners getting to know each other as 'people'. It is about people 'connecting' with each other in a socially meaningful way, with a specific focus to the interactions based around experiences and alleviation of

---

Box 7.2   Proposed definition

" 'Engagement' is a separate and distinct function, the foundation for all aspects of the helping process. It is an attempt to build an on-going constructive partnership, and will most usually be facilitated by a series of unstructured, informal and shared encounters, that take place at the beginning of the process of relationship-building. It is a therapeutic activity within its own right, needing to be positively monitored and sustained throughout the duration of the helping process."

(Based on Morgan 1996)

[A mutual awareness that trust and respect on both sides of a relationship will help the things we want to happen]

mental distress. Burns and Firn (2002) remind us: "It is very often the intention of the activity that classifies it as 'engagement'." For example, working on increasing a person's income through maximizing their benefits entitlements is not usually set as a goal for achieving engagement, but the result of the personal interactions required to achieve more money often brings about more trust and respect for the working relationship.

Wolf (2002) suggests: "Good mental health work at ground level is chiefly about relationships. True relationships rely on the opening up and deployment of self in a state of disciplined and skilful emotional vulnerability...[*For service users it is*] that sense of linking with someone who's really there for you, who's working from the heart and not from the book." It is not to be assumed to be happening within the relationship where the professional tells the service user what has been assessed and what will be the prescribed interventions!

Rapp (1998) suggests that the essential characteristics of this new partnership are to be purposeful, reciprocal, friendly, trusting and empowering. It is a 'personal' skill, which can be taught, but is most commonly developed through life experience and common sense. No single profession can lay claim to monopolizing the skills of engagement. Indeed, it is not to be seen exclusively as a professional skill at all as quite often the person who mistrusts the motives of professionals will sometimes confide more information to the hospital cleaner, or the unqualified member of staff in a voluntary agency.

A theoretical framework for engagement

Motivational interviewing (Miller and Rollnick 1991) and the cycle of change (Prochaska and DiClemente 1982) provide a useful conceptualization of engagement from work more frequently associated with the substance misuse field. If we consider a disengaged and resistant individual as someone in a state of ambivalence regarding their mental health needs, then we need to direct our energies to the individual personal motivators that can support positive change. In this model, motivation is seen as a dynamic and cyclical process, rather than linear. It is characterized by a state of readiness, where this readiness can often change. The changes are captured by a six-stage wheel or cycle:

1. Pre-contemplation – where the person does not yet acknowledge the existence of a difficulty. We need to raise doubts by helping their increased awareness of the risks and problems with their current behaviour or stance.
2. Contemplation – a phase of tipping the balance to where the person begins to see reasons for change, and the risks of not changing their stance on an issue.
3. Determination – helping the person to determine their own best course of action for seeking to bring about their desired change.
4. Action – helping the person to take steps towards a desired change.
5. Maintenance – helping the person to identify strategies that will protect against the potential for relapse.

6. Relapse – still is a part of the cycle, a learning phase from which to renew contemplation from a different baseline of knowledge and experience.

In the ongoing process of engagement it is important to see that at a point in time an individual may be anywhere on this cycle, though active disengagement and resistance is clearly in the precontemplation phase. They may follow a logical path through to maintenance; they may go around the cycle several times before identifying a strong enough anchor for trusting engagement. The practitioner style of therapeutic approach will be a powerful determinant of the person's resistance or willingness to change. We need to recognize that ambivalence is normal, not pathological, and that facilitating a readiness for change and overcoming ambivalence is a key focus of our interventions with people.

Motivational interviewing (Miller and Rollnick 1991) is a therapeutic technique particularly useful as a means of considering engaging and working with people in the primary stages of change, notably precontemplation, contemplation, determination and action. It adopts the tenet that motivation is not something that an individual *has* but rather as something that an individual *does*. It aims to speed up movement around the cycle from the initial phases of precontemplation and contemplation by allowing the individual space and time to come up with their own list of positive and negative aspects of behaviour, which generates underlying discrepancies and helps the individual to come to their own conclusions about the benefits of engaging with a service. The predominant strategies within a motivational interviewing framework are summarized as:

- giving **A**DVICE
- removing **B**ARRIERS
- providing **C**HOICE
- decreasing **D**ESIRABILITY (of unhelpful choices)
- practising **E**MPATHY
- providing **F**EEDBACK
- clarifying **G**OALS
- active **H**ELPING.

Through the skills of supportive counselling, the practitioners are aiming to establish an appropriate sense of cognitive dissonance or discrepancy between the individual's current situation and the goals they personally wish to achieve. In this way, it provides a useful tool, which is highly compatible with the underlying philosophy and aims of the strengths practitioner.

MESSAGES FROM THE RESEARCH

Marty et al (2001) describe a study of responses from 96 *experts* in an attempt to identify the critical ingredients of a strengths model of case management. Their findings are organized into four categories: engagement; strengths assessment; personal plan; and resource acquisition. The following summary of 11 items (in rank order of agreement) were identified as critical ingredients of 'engagement':

- When a service user describes him or herself or their experiences, the practitioner assists them with identifying any achievement, interest or aspiration embedded in the event.
- Practitioners use every opportunity to identify the service user's interests, talents, abilities and resources.
- Practitioners discuss roles, responsibilities and mutual expectations of the working relationship.
- Once a service is requested, the practitioner does whatever it takes to meet with the new service user.
- The practitioner arranges meetings at a time that is most comfortable for the service user.
- The majority of contacts happen away from the office.
- The practitioner and service user are involved in an activity that is enjoyable to the service user as a backdrop for getting to know each other, e.g. over a cup of coffee, walking or listen to music.
- Practitioners inform service users of their rights as clients.
- If attempts to meet with the service user are unsuccessful, the practitioner discusses barriers in supervision.
- The practitioner and service user can feel able to discuss the interests and experiences they have in common.
- Practitioners can use purposeful self-disclosing statements to advance the engagement process.

PRACTICAL CONSIDERATIONS

Translating the messages from research into routine practice is never an easy exercise, but it is made all the more difficult when we are talking about concepts such as developing trust through empathic understanding and 'being with' someone. The indicators from the above list have been specifically developed from a practice standpoint, and so offer a starting point for considering the day-to-day practicalities of engagement. The following are a set of broad considerations in the practitioner–service user relationship:

- The social aspects of human interaction are skills needing attention to the detail of preparation in order to be most effective.
- We are dealing with complex human relationships, often at vulnerable and critical points in time, so we need to be clear in what we are saying, offering and doing with service users.
- Human services require humane consideration of how they are presented and delivered.
- Whether or not a person believes in the concept of mental illness, they will have their own ideas, interpretation and understanding of their own experiences. We need to hear and assimilate these messages.
- We need to be flexible and creative, but above all else responsive to the needs and wishes expressed by service users.

Detailed guidelines for developing the above considerations in routine practice are set out below. Box 7.3 describes the value base necessary for engagement to be effective, and Box 7.4 describes a three-stage process of engagement.

Box 7.3   The value base for engagement

1. Respect

- Whatever the person has done, or may do, they are worthy of respect, acceptance, attention and support.
- Respect a sense of self, dignity and integrity of all parties.
- Give plenty of time for people to talk and express their problems.
- Watch and listen for clues in what is said and how it is said.
- Acknowledge and address differences – of opinion and culture.
- Value the individual's experiences (including not dismissing them as 'mad').
- Honour people's views, rather than patronizing them.
- Develop co-operative rather than coercive approaches.
- Respect the need for privacy, confidentiality and rights to refuse a service.
- Relationships take time to develop – change may be slow and the person may not be able to acknowledge the relationship or the changes.
- Listen without judging or labelling.
- Do not talk about people in front of them or talk down to them.
- Do not use technical language, and be prepared to answer questions and explain things.

2. Reliability

- Trust is built by demonstrating commitment and ability to deliver the goods (from the other's point of view).
- Appropriate interdependence can be promoted more easily if there is a trust that an effective response can be offered when required.
- Often simply 'being available' is all that is required.

Box 7.4   Guidelines for engagement

1. Prepare thoroughly

- The importance of planning for the first meeting. 'You don't get a second chance to make first impressions.'
- Make yourself a real person who has come from somewhere – encourage the service user to experience you as a real person rather than a role or an office.
- Identify possible successful and meaningful ways of approaching the individual, e.g. asking the referrer if they know what may be the best form of approach.
- Consider the need for direct and/or indirect early contacts.
- A telephone call or a letter, prior to the first meeting, can set the context – stating who you are, where you are from and how you come to be making the approach; we should not assume that because a

box continues

person has been referred to Assertive Outreach that they are aware of this fact or know why.

- Introduce yourself properly (by name rather than designation) and reinforce information by describing why you are visiting at this particular time.
- Use people's names – ask them what they want to be called.
- Keep administration separate from engagement; structure and formality should only be introduced if and when necessary.
- Do not rush into the formal administrative needs of the service; exclude all but absolutely essential data gathering from first meetings.
- Establish links with individuals known and trusted by the service user.
- Consider how you are able to demonstrate trust and openness about yourself in relation to others.
- Place the emphasis on getting to know each other at the start.
- Consider how you may be able to get alongside the service user – problem-solve on issues that the service user is presenting there and then.
- Persist where appropriate, or try another tack where initial approaches have been rejected or failed.
- Plan to avoid early disagreements wherever possible.

2. Communicate clearly

- Communicate effectively, starting as you mean to go on; avoid jargon as it often serves to mystify and creates a barrier.
- Establish a two-way process of interaction – keep it as informal and conversational as possible.
- Monitor your use of language and encourage the person to check ambiguities with you.
- Be honest but tactful (careful and considerate use of the truth); there are circumstances where blunt delivery of the truth may be very counterproductive to developing a working relationship.
- Education and information sharing can help service users to understand how the process leads them to achieve their wants and needs.
- Identify the difference between real and pretend collaboration – whilst acting in the service user's best interests, the case manager may occasionally have to act against the service user's stated wishes (our clients' wishes deserve our respect but not always our support).
- State the possible limits of your powers and access to resources – do not be tempted to raise unrealistic expectations as a means of making quick gains in developing the relationship; the longterm nature of the relationship makes deception unhelpful and unlikely to succeed.
- Avoid allowing ambiguity about your role which may lead to disappointment and distrust later; the relationship will need clear boundaries and limitations on roles for both sides.
- Have an idea of what may be on offer (including your own support) and how to be clear in explaining it.
- Avoid confusion over personal boundaries – being a friend and delivering a service in a more friendly manner are very different things.

- Diagrams and flowcharts can be a useful way of explaining complex issues or ideas (but they are not a usual method of *ordinary* interaction so can be a barrier if handled in a clumsy way).

3. Proactive collaboration: invitation to partnership

- Be assertive in asking the service user's opinion.
- Maximize information – leaving power with a person means giving them choice.
- Wherever possible, arrange to see people where, when and for what duration of time they prefer in order to help them feel more comfortable with what is primarily a service-led process.
- Be flexible and involve the person in the pace and pattern of work done.
- Give permission for the person to rely on you.
- Be aware of actions that could easily be interpreted as overstepping boundaries or 'abandoning' people.
- The focus of interactions should address topics of interest to the service user (not just an assessment of medical and social problems).
- Identify common ground, e.g. agreed areas to work on or similar interests for discussion.
- Understanding other's views helps to create patience and constructive relationships.
- Use of appropriate self-disclosure challenges traditional professional training, but can help to promote more equality in the working relationship.
- The sharing of practical tasks can enhance a service user's trust in the case manager to work 'with' them (it's very much a 'doing with' rather than a 'doing for' approach, with the aim of supporting the service user to do it themselves).
- Appropriate use of humour can lighten an otherwise difficult series of interactions; it can also help to make the service appear less formal and more natural.
- Understand that actions that seem like resistance or unreliability can be an inevitable 'testing' part of many engagement processes.

The above lists are based on Onyett (1992), Morgan (1996) and Bleach (1997).

A WORKING EXAMPLE OF ENGAGEMENT IN PRACTICE

The following (Box 7.5) is a case profile of a person in contact with Kettering Assertive Outreach team, to illustrate the process of 'engagement' in practice.

How do we know if we have engaged successfully?

The efforts made by case managers/practitioners to focus on the need to effectively engage trusting working relationships have not gone unnoticed by the users of specific services prioritizing such an approach. Box 7.6 sets out responses from service users in one USA and two UK studies, which aimed to identify what characteristics attracted them to

Box 7.5   Case profile: Robin

Robin is a 40-year-old man who has lived in the local town all his life. He has a diagnosis of paranoid schizophrenia and experiences alcohol-related problems. He has experienced numerous admissions to hospital under sections of the Mental Health Act, including secure and intensive care beds, following deterioration of his mental state and presenting as threatening and a risk to others. He was referred to the Assertive Outreach team by the community mental health team (CMHT) following concerns expressed by neighbours, and a prolonged time of refusing access to CMHT staff or contact with his GP. At this point, little was known about Robin's lifestyle or social circumstances; despite his history he remained reluctant to engage with services.

The team employs a 'team approach' (five staff), setting an immediate challenge in the work with Robin, to enable all the team to get to know him, and for him to get to meet the whole team. The early contacts with new referrals are made by the team in pairs, not just for safety reasons but to also enable the service user to experience the different personalities making up the team.

Engagement

The initial contact was by a personalized letter, also enclosing a team information leaflet. The first couple of visits, on the same day, by two team members, failed to achieve any contact due to the locked entrance to the flats (with buzzer/intercom communication). The team made some contact with the concerned neighbours, who provided a code for accessing the building to gain access to Robin's front door. Regular visits to knock at his door usually resulted in staff being sworn at and told to go away, through a closed door. On one occasion, Robin told them: "You can't help me. I know what I want and you social workers will not be able to help me." This was a chance for the staff members to explain that they were not social workers, and that they would try to work in a different way to what he had been used to, if he would let them try.

With some gentle persuasion, he opened the door and expressed his anger at their earlier use of his buzzer, as he believed it allowed people to infiltrate into his flat. The workers apologized, and asked if there was another way of letting him know of their arrival. Robin told them to use their car horns, and he would let them in. This the team agreed to; it had taken approximately six weeks from the time of the first visit.

The flat was in a considerable state of neglect, and Robin expressed views of being persecuted by God, and delusional ideas that were clearly distressing to him. He was drinking alcohol 'to help him sleep', and the flat was extremely littered with empty cans. He asked what the team would do, and they asked him what he wanted. Robin's reply was more adamant about what he did not want – no hospital admission, no doctors and no eviction. His one expressed wish was for his family to visit his flat for a meal (they lived locally but had never visited him).

Two-person visits continued, occasionally on a daily basis, and the team gradually built up a picture of Robin's likes, dislikes and interests, as they spent time working alongside him to clear, clean and paint his flat. It transpired that Robin felt his family would not visit because of the dirty and dilapidated state of his flat. He chose items of furniture he wanted, as a result of the team helping him to claim £3500 in backdated benefits owed to him (as a result of him not opening his post over a long period). Gradually his debts were all cleared and the flat was completely redecorated and refurnished. Robin began to suggest he looked forward to the team's visits, while continuing to express his beliefs about being persecuted, that people were infiltrating his flat, that God thought he was bad, and occasionally listening to and reciting from biblical tapes. He now knew the first names of all the team and enquired how people were that he had not seen for a short time.

Sustaining the engagement

Whilst continuing the help in the flat towards Robin's goal of inviting his family for a meal, it became clear that his Christian faith was extremely important to him, and he wanted to be confirmed. One team member pursued this idea with Robin, and over a period of 20 weeks they attended confirmation classes together, one evening a week between 7.00 and 9.00 pm. They were confirmed together, with all the team attending and celebrating the occasion.

Once the decorating was completed the team members visited local country pubs and restaurants with Robin, to browse menus for ideas for the family meal. Whilst on these visits, open discussion of his alcohol intake was made possible, and Robin's drinking reduced. It also enabled discussion of the potential for medication to replace the alcohol as the source of sleep, and its potential for tackling some of his distressing thoughts. The team were able to use the trust they had achieved to be open about the difficult topics of conversation. Initially they were able to take medication to his flat on a daily basis, and to openly discuss with Robin his concerns about possible side-effects. This reassured him that if he had any reactions to the medication the team would address them immediately. They also backed up discussions with written information. On the basis of these discussions, Robin chose to visit his GP for a physical examination and a liver function test, with team members attending in support.

Robin chose a four-course menu, despite only having cooked convenience food previously.

Team members practised cooking items on his chosen menu with him, and Robin set a date for the family meal. On the afternoon before the evening meal, two team members helped Robin to prepare, stayed with him until the family members arrived and sat down for the main course, then left him with his family. The following day team members visited to help Robin with the washing-up. This event enabled Robin's family to make a connection with the team, and to express their own anxieties and concerns. With the support of team members Robin was able to answer most of the family enquiries himself.

Outcomes

To date, Robin has had no further hospital admissions. He accepts twice-weekly visits by the Assertive Outreach team but this can be increased at Robin's request in line with a collab-oratively developed crisis plan. He regularly takes prescribed medication and attends psychiatric outpatients supported by team members.

A further interest has rekindled new ambitions – developing a social life through attending 'soul nights'. Robin now wants to be a DJ. He has achieved a half-hour slot, and is hoping to DJ a whole soul night completely arranged by himself, raising money for people experiencing mental health problems as a result.

Robin works on a voluntary basis in a local sports club, attends church twice a week, a gym to improve his physical condition, and sees his family twice a week. His flat is main-tained in a reasonable condition, he has more control of his alcohol intake and enjoys a more settled sleep pattern.

make more use of the service. A common theme seems to be that the user felt that the worker had 'got through' to them, that there was a basis of trust, help and support. In a sense, the worker was seen as a vital ally in collaborating with the life projects which were important to the user.

Sustaining trusting relationships

Engagement is not a function that can be achieved then assumed to always be in place. As with other aspects of the mental health process, e.g. assessment, it is something that requires continual attention. It is not

Box 7.6   Illustrative examples of what service users said influenced them to work with specific services

Kisthardt (1992)

- "Really cared for me as a person."
- "Was always there for me."
- "Respected what I had to say."
- "Asked me what I wanted, where I wanted to meet, what I wanted to do."
- "Didn't force me to do things, went at my pace."
- "Took it slow and easy, had a calm manner with a soft soothing voice."
- "Did fun things with me, like go for a coffee or just drive me in their car."
- "Didn't try to be a snoopervisor, didn't try to analyze everything I said."
- "Shared something about their own life, was more like a friend."
- "Had a great sense of humour. We laughed together, that made me feel good."
- "Was real honest with me.... Was a real person."
- "I could tell she was really listening to me."
- "Told me she was going to focus on what I can do."
- "Said that she had a lot to learn from me."
- "We talked about a lot of things we have in common."
- "The big thing was how she was with my son, he took to her right away."
- "We talked about right now, not 20 years ago."
- "Didn't judge what I was saying."

Beeforth et al (1994)

- "I can't talk to him about everything, but most things."
- "The case manager is my friend, but I can't tell her everything."
- "She doesn't let me get away with anything – she's not too soft."
- "My case manager backs me up in what I want to do."
- "The case manager mended my front door, which was really good."
- "She helps me with benefits. I now have more money and I can pay my bills."

Graley-Wetherell and Morgan (2001)

- "They asked what I needed, just let me talk, I wasn't keen at first but they went at my pace, they waited to see what it was that I needed."
- "We just chat – if I have an important issue then I just tell them."
- "If there is something concrete they have to raise they just say it, but they are gentle with me and go at my pace."
- "They ask how I am, I tell them, I ask questions and things, I usually lead it."
- "We just natter about what's happening, unless something important has occurred."
- "They treat me as a person not a number."

> - "They are like friends, if I don't keep in touch they send little notes and cards. I get trapped in my environment but they stop me from being alienated. They are not intrusive; they talk about everyday problems not just mental health. They also help with the practical stuff like washing, and when I almost lost all my possessions they tried to stop that happening."
> - "They are professionally different, they do normal things."
> - "Hospitals treat you like you are not normal, I feel like I am looked down on. Julian Housing treat you as a person should be treated, they make a conscious effort to do that. I feel like I do when I am with friends."
> - "They give me help, but they do it with dignity, I don't feel patronised."
> - "They have helped me with my correspondence and forms, also with my language difficulties."
> - "They believe what I tell them, they really listen and don't dismiss what I say."
> - "They were the only visitors that I had when I was in hospital."

a linear process with a defined start and completion point; it is an essential function of human interaction, which will necessarily fluctuate and adopt a path of its own in response to interactions, moods and behaviours. Practitioners need to feel comfortable with occasionally checking out with the person how they perceive the relationship aspect of the work to be. Initial degrees of trust can be hard gained, and easily undermined by a careless statement or change of working priorities without the expected degree of consultation.

'Degrees' of engagement

The idea that engagement is the first function of the care process, and that assessment comes later, can be taken too literally with the effect of paralysing the current ability to offer support. We are assessing the situation from the outset, but not fully and accurately with confidence until the trusting relationship feels engaged. It would be wrong to assume that our assessment is comprehensive when the service user continues to actively question the reasons why they should be meeting you. Similarly, it would be wrong to just assume that a trusting relationship is engaged when the person is speaking with you under the legal requirements of being sectioned under mental health legislation.

What constitutes actual engagement in practice will necessarily vary from person to person, and situation to situation (Box 7.7). In some instances, openly explicit connections through kept meeting times and a sense of open and honest discussion will offer a strong sense of engagement being achieved. This should not cloud our judgement through establishing predetermined ideas of what constitutes defined standards or preconditions for engagement to be taking place. The most important issue is that the practitioner is actively monitoring the quality and nature of the relationship, to ensure that they are making considerable efforts to involve the service user in all aspects of care and support.

> **Box 7.7   A case example of engagement by degrees**
>
> **Case profile: Margaret**
> The case profile of Margaret (in Chapter 5) is a good illustration of how we may consider engagement by degrees. For the first 18 months of case management contact, the meetings constituted little more than 30 seconds on the doorstep to her property. She was frequently verbally abusive and quick to curtail the conversation. However, on team reflection the content of what was relayed to her, verbally and through written notes, was achieving some of the intentions of gaining her views about aspects of her care. It was also time used creatively to remind her of ongoing health care needs, e.g. reminders to attend her surgery for her depot medication (which she did not appear to question either on the doorstep or with the practice nurse administering the regular injection). For Margaret there was an element of responding to reminders for something at a three-weekly interval rather than trying to remember herself.
>
> With time she reduced her verbal aggression, and felt more able to express her concerns that services were simply out to remove her from her home. Practical help in the interim with letters in the post enabled her to eventually see that the case management team were there to help her achieve her wishes, specifically retention of her tenancy. Duration of contact on the doorstep increased, the focus of the conversations was able to be planned more around engaging her ideas and wishes, and occasional invites into the flat were completely in her control (and respected by the case managers). This is not to say that assessment was not happening within the first 18 months, or that there was not at least some tenuous degree of engagement for the case managers to hang on to and work with from the early stages.

Whether formally or informally, we need to adopt a flexible template in our minds for checking out the quality of engagement. In its simplest form, such a template needs to be constantly evaluating the timing, location and intensity of contacts and content of what we are collaboratively working on. Whilst the service user is a vitally important person to be evaluating these decisions with, it can also be of benefit to check out your assessment of the engagement function in other arenas, e.g. individual supervision or team meetings, as a training and/or team development tool.

Strategies for enhancing engagement

At a service level, the Julian Housing Active Outreach team recognizes these needs by focusing continuing attention and energy into 'engagement'. The team believes it requires chameleon-like qualities in its outreach workers to respond to rapidly changing circumstances respectfully, and a constant desire to bring a feel-good factor into the working relationships whenever possible, e.g. sharing a sense of humour. The following are some examples of creative approaches they have employed to engage, and sustain engagement of, individuals (there can never be an exhaustive list of approaches to engagement as all circumstances are different and fluctuating):

- a focus on pets, e.g. talking about service users' pets, walking the dog, ongoing correspondence with the office dog, caring for a parakeet, taking animals to the vet and visiting rescue centres
- talking about art
- washing up and cleaning, with the service user
- painting and decorating
- use of the office washing machine
- use of the office shower
- attending horse racing and football matches
- giving Italian lessons
- donations of food
- facials and washing hair
- forming a rock band (due to record a CD!), linked to the local community not solely a mental health venture
- going to church
- accessing community resources.

POSITIVE DISENGAGEMENT AS A STEPPING-STONE TOWARDS RECOVERY

What is it about Assertive Outreach teams that promotes good levels of engagement, and sometimes generates reluctance in people to return to the service of the community mental health teams? The intensity of contact cannot be the answer, as most people involved have previously been reluctant to engage with the lesser intensity of CMHTs. Within a strengths approach it is more likely to be the flexibility and creativity engendered from a different service value base, which promotes a greater appreciation of real service user involvement and genuine working with needs and wants. The challenge for other parts of the system would be to assimilate these principles into their different methods of practice.

Helping people to move on should be initiated from the same value base that informs the approaches to initial engagement and progressive work. Moving on should be seen as integral with the whole process of 'recovery' (Box 7.8). In the strengths approach it is closely associated with the principle of 'the person as director of the helping process' (see Chapter 3). Moving on should aim to demonstrate the following characteristics:

- gradual disengagement guided by the pace of the person themselves
- not using the concept of 'discharge'
- seeing the process as function led rather than time limited
- accepting fluctuations in the intensity of contact over the period of positive disengagement
- linking to other resources as appropriate to the needs of the individual, considering the CMHT as only one potential option (not necessarily the first)
- considering outpatients, primary care, voluntary and independent sector, and non-mental health services as equally valid options

- maintaining a 'dormant' contact list with the Assertive Outreach team, whereby former active cases can re-access the service without having to jump through the more usual service hoops.

The most frequent concerns expressed in relation to 'dormant' lists by other service providers is that they continue to foster the sense of dependency referred to earlier; and by Assertive Outreach services themselves, that many people on a dormant list going into crisis at the same time would be unmanageable. With regard to the former criticism, the strengths approach promotes the reality of a healthy interdependence, as opposed to a fear of dependency that more frequently ends in discharge and subsequent later relapse. In respect of managing multiple crises, the possibility is always real but unlikely if the gradual process of 'positive disengagement' has been afforded careful attention, with real connections established in the person's social network, and longer-term crisis and contingency plans put into place.

Box 7.8   A case example of positive disengagement

Case profile: Molly

Molly is 26, and experienced a chaotic childhood largely in social services care. She has had seven years' contact with mental health services and is generally considered to be experiencing psychotic relapses most probably aggravated by drug misuse. The first four years of contact were largely characterized by repeated hospital admissions, with short periods of time in the community disengaging from CMHT attempts to monitor her follow-up treatment. Consequently, Molly was referred to the locally developing Assertive Outreach service approximately three years ago.

The initial attempts at engagement were slow to develop, with Molly seeing the Assertive Outreach service as just another part of the community mental health team. The first year of engaging included three shorter than previous admissions to the inpatient unit, with the Assertive Outreach workers gradually making more inroads to engagement through regular visits to the unit. The more flexible approach to home visits and being open to meet with Molly at other locations began to connect with her as a different way of working as the first year progressed.

Through a focus on a 'strengths' assessment a childhood talent and interest in music emerged, and the team spent significant amounts of contact time discussing this aspect of Molly's life with her. Ultimately, these discussions led to helping her to find other like-minded musicians in the local area, and she began playing saxophone for the first time in nearly 10 years. Molly proved to be a fast learner, and also became more involved in jamming sessions.

Some of the Assertive Outreach workers felt able to continue involvement in these developments for Molly, without it looking like a mental health service keeping an eye on her. She continued to lead a chaotic social life but felt able to confide much more personal information through the trust she was developing with the Assertive Outreach team.

In the last two years there have been no hospital admissions. Molly has recently decided to cut down the level of contact with the team through her own decision, taking more control of contacts related to her needs. She has come to understand her seven years of psychotic experiences more through her discussions with team members, and become more aware of triggers and early warning signs. Just recently she has had a stormy episode in a personal relationship but she instigated more contact with the team to help her through the distress.

With her current emotional stability being supported by a new relationship she has felt able to recommence her earlier plan of reducing contact with the team. She feels that her new girlfriend also has a good connection with the team that she can trust as a bridge to support her. Molly has talked of not wanting to lose the support she has found in the Assertive Outreach team, but also having a desire to feel strong in herself. She is talking of taking full control of the contacts with the team in the near future, and the plan for the next two contacts are to be through the informal setting of Assertive Outreach workers dropping in on a jamming session and a local gig that has been arranged for a few weeks' time. (The staff are clear about the boundaries they maintain in these social settings, and the workers who become involved in these contacts are the ones with a specific interest in jazz and the local scene.)

These changes to practice call for major cultural changes, both within the longterm planning priorities of Assertive Outreach teams themselves, and for the host organizations of the teams. It challenges the more usual service management short-term economic considerations – driving for a point of discharge in order to take on new referrals at a consistent pace. The impact of working to service-oriented needs, through responding to the existing pressures, is most likely one of creating further revolving doors but at a slower speed of rotation. This would be an area ripe for longterm research into the health, social and economic effectiveness.

CONCLUSIONS

We are working with people who have lost, or never had, the opportunity to establish their trust in mental health services. This will be for a wide variety of reasons, which require our respect without attribution of blame. It is incumbent on practitioners to go further than the extra mile in order to attempt to establish that trust in the potential of the working relationship. The quality of all subsequent aspects of our work will be strongly influenced by the quality of that trusting relationship.

Repper et al (1994) found that: "… developing and maintaining the client–case manager relationship was the central vehicle through which the needs of service users were assessed, direct care delivered, and the necessary service co-ordinated." The positive philosophical framework of many practitioners in this UK case management study was informed by a strengths approach to their work, founded on principles of realism, taking a longterm perspective, positive empathic understanding and client-centred flexibility. Specific attention to engaging a trusting working relationship was the foundation.

Similarly, we need to be thinking differently about how we disengage people from services at the time and in the way that is appropriate to individual circumstances. Previous experiences of contact followed by discharge to situations of coping without support is a good enough reason why some service users become disenchanted with the services being offered. We need to be as creative in our thinking and actions at the later parts of our contact as we are at the commencement of contact. Reliance on a rigid number of disengagement options only sets up a creative service with an inflexible end point. Timescales and types of continuing contact are equally open to flexibility.

References

Beeforth M, Conlan E, Graley R 1994 Have We Got Views For You: User evaluation of case management. Sainsbury Centre for Mental Health, London

Bleach A 1997 The Process of Engagement. Acetates prepared for workshop presentations (unpublished)

Burns T, Firn M 2002 Assertive Outreach in Mental Health: A Manual for Practitioners. Oxford University Press, Oxford

Graley-Wetherell R, Morgan S 2001 Active Outreach: An independent service user evaluation of a model of assertive outreach practice. Sainsbury Centre for Mental Health, London

James A 2002 Douglas Turkington: a profile of a psychiatrist prepared to go the extra mile. Openmind 118: 7

Kisthardt W 1992 A strengths model of case management: the principles and functioning of helping partnerships with persons with persistent mental illness. In: Saleeby D (ed) The Strengths Perspective in Social Work. Longman, New York, p 59–83

Marty D, Rapp C A, Carlson L 2001 The experts speak: the critical ingredients of strengths model case management. Psychiatric Rehabilitation Journal 24 (3): 214–221

Miller W R, Rollnick S 1991 Motivational Interviewing. Guilford Press, New York

Morgan S 1996 Helping Relationships in Mental Health. Chapman & Hall, London

Onyett S 1992 Case Management in Mental Health. Chapman & Hall, London

Prochaska J O, DiClemente C C 1982 Transtheoretical therapy: toward a more integrative model of change. Psychotherapy Theory, Research and Practice 19: 276–288

Rapp C A 1988 The Strengths Perspective of Case Management with Persons Suffering from Severe Mental Illness. University of Kansas and NIMH, Lawrence

Rapp CA 1998 The Strengths Model: Case Management with People Suffering from Severe and Persistent Mental Illness. Oxford University Press, New York

Repper J, Ford R, Cooke A 1994 How can nurses build trusting relationships with people who have severe and long-term mental health problems? Experiences of case managers and their clients. Journal of Advanced Nursing 19: 1096–1104

Wolf R 2002 From the heart. Openmind 118: 9

Chapter 8

Strengths assessment

Peter Ryan and Steve Morgan

Does doing a strengths assessment mean you forget about the client's problems?

INTRODUCTION

Assessment is a complex issue, not least because it covers a multiplicity of tasks and functions. Often, it is driven by the underlying assumption that it is primarily about defining a problem, to which a service offers its best approximation to a solution. There are also medical assumptions that assessment is best addressed at least in part through arriving at a medical diagnosis of dysfunction or disability.

This chapter commences by attempting to clarify and tease out some of the separate tasks and functions often lumped together by the term 'assessment'. It then goes on to explore some of the underlying assumptions that characterize 'problem definition–problem solution' approaches to assessment. The chapter then proceeds to make the case for a 'strengths approach' to assessment, which is outlined in some detail. Some 'frequently asked questions' about strengths assessment are addressed.

TASKS AND FUNCTIONS IN ASSESSMENT

One of the difficulties in discussing assessment is that the term is often used to describe a variety of different tasks. These complexities are well addressed by Onyett (1992): "The object of assessment is to gain a developing picture of the needs and strengths of the user and their social and physical environment. However, definition of need is a difficult issue. A need can be considered as a problem, or deficit, a desire, a demand or a solution. Services tend to define need in terms of services available. Thus assessment becomes an exercise in determining the user's eligibility for services. Clearly assessment of this kind provides no information on needs that are not already addressed by existing services."

Medical diagnosis and its links to assessment

Obtaining a medical diagnosis is useful for the information it can contain concerning the signs, symptoms and indications of mental illness which a service user may be experiencing. It is typically arrived at through a careful process of systematically assessing the mood, thought processes, perceptions, appearance, speech and behaviour of the service user (Craig 2000). When well conducted and presented, it contains a wealth of information concerning cognitive and emotional functioning. It is a skilled and specialized application of assessment. However, useful as it is, a medical diagnosis per se gives little information concerning the broader psychosocial adjustment of the service user, and offers few clues, apart from implications for medication, as to what should be included in a care plan or package of care. On the other hand, diagnosis may and indeed often is used as an indicator of severity of illness, and therefore of eligibility for services. Medical diagnosis is often part of the screening criteria for Assertive Outreach, and therefore can be a crucial determinant as to whether a given user receives an Assertive Outreach service at all.

Information gathering, referral and screening for service eligibility

As the chapter on targeting made clear (see Chapter 6), Assertive Outreach is a very carefully restricted service. It is not designed to be applicable to everybody. A vital preliminary process in Assertive Outreach, therefore, is determining eligibility. This in part is an information gathering process, in which as much referral information as possible is gathered from referrers. Some basic information (date of birth; family members; GPs; primary language; educational and work history; diagnosis; history of use of psychiatric services) obviously needs collation at this stage, or checking from previous files.

In addition, the Assertive Outreach team may well carry out a series of screening interviews in order to assess for themselves whether a referred service user actually meets the team's criteria for acceptance as an Assertive Outreach client. Some of this information, such as number and length of previous admissions, can be difficult to get but is relatively 'hard evidence'. It can be much more difficult to come to a firm judgement concerning other criteria, such as 'difficulties in engaging with services'. This is essentially a subjective judgement on which opinions can legitimately differ.

For Assertive Outreach services in particular, screening for eligibility is a crucial function, and one which can be locally highly controversial, where an Assertive Outreach team rejects a referral from its local community mental health team. Screening for eligibility is a highly specialized and important function, which clearly requires highly developed assessment skills. It can also be an important part of an engagement process with an Assertive Outreach client. It can be distinguished from a comprehensive assessment process or a strengths assessment mainly in terms of its objectives. The focus for a screening assessment is necessarily on gathering such information about the client as to enable the team to come to an informed judgement as to whether the client concerned is excluded or included in the team's caseload.

ASSESSMENT: SOME UNDERLYING ISSUES

Once a given service user has passed through a screening for eligibility threshold, and has been accepted onto the team's caseload, a more complete and comprehensive assessment process can be initiated. The nature of that assessment and its usefulness in giving a comprehensive picture of the service user's needs are clearly crucial. It is important therefore to consider very carefully the nature of the assessment undertaken and its implications for the client.

Service-led assessment

It can happen that services draw little distinction between the individual needs of a particular service user, and what services are available to meet those needs. This would mean that what were called assessments simply consisted of checking the suitability for a particular service which happened to be available, and in which a 'service slot' was located, rather than genuinely addressing the unique concerns and aspirations of individual users, and coming up with a uniquely specific response to that particular expressed need. Hence, a service-led response might ask: 'Is there a place available in the day centre, group home or hostel?' rather than attempting to create a specific and unique response. Often assessment is prompted by the identification of problems for which services are available. This leads to the assessment of those problems from the perspective of what services can respond to, resulting in what services can most conveniently offer rather than what the service user necessarily most wants or can optimally respond to.

Confusions of language and definition

An additional area of concern in service-led assessment is the confusion of terms and definitions, in that the concepts of problems and needs are generally used in such an unclear way that they become confounded. For example, a service user who is deemed to be socially isolated may be assessed as having 'problems socializing' and therefore *needing* a social skills training group. This is a service-led response in that a problem the client is perceived as experiencing is defined as best being met by what the service has available to offer, whether or not it is actually what the user themselves really wants, and regardless of the actual aspirations the user may have in terms of social contact.

A strengths assessment might reveal that the user lives a long way from friends, and what the user themselves wants is to move house in order to be closer to them. If needs and problems are mixed up in this way, then it becomes effectively impossible for the service user to 'own' a service response that may be only vaguely and indirectly related to what actually keys in to their own aspirations. If, in addition, the availability of services and resources become the controlling factor in what the user is offered, then the assessment of 'need' becomes functionally defined purely by what the service has to offer. The term 'need' therefore can become detached and divorced from any real engagement with what the user wants, and becomes a euphemism for what the service provides irrespective of the user's actual aspirations.

The language of problems and strengths contrasts strongly (Morgan 1997) as shown in Table 8.1.

A problems approach tends to describe people in a way that promotes categorization into groups, offering little or no sense of the individual person, for example:

- poor motivation
- low self-esteem
- poor personal hygiene
- self-neglect
- social isolation.

In contrast, a strengths approach helps to draw out the individuality of the person, for example:

- watching the local football league team on Saturdays
- reading suspense and drama novels
- writing poetry
- eating Chinese food.

The problem with a problems orientation

Rapp (1998) summarizes the problems of a 'problems focus' as follows: "Attention to people's inability to cope is a central expression of the prevailing perspectives on helping. Approaches differ in the way the 'problem' is defined, but virtually all schools of therapeutic thought rest on the assumption that people need help because they have a problem – a problem that in some way sets them apart ... The terminology

Table 8.1   Contrast between the language of problems and strengths

Problems	Strengths
Needs based	Wants based
Service centred	Person centred
Prescription	Choice
Intervention	Collaboration
Professional jargon	Shared language
Generating artificial motivations	Tapping intrinsic motivations
Daily occupation supplementary to medicine	Medicine supplementary to daily occupation

'having a problem' suggests that problems belong to, or inhere in people, and in some way, express an important and limiting fact about who they are." In other words, a problems approach to working with clients may inadvertently add to rather than remove from service users' stigmatic assumptions about disablement and disability.

Hall (1981) argues that the purpose of problems-based assessment includes:

- judging the individual's level of disability
- planning a programme of care and observing progress over time
- planning service provision.

To invite, as a point of departure, a person to talk about their problems, difficulties, dysfunctions and disabilities is to invite possibly painful memories of failures, conflicts and difficulties inherent in their career as a 'mental patient.' However indirectly, it is a reminder of the social status and stigma attached to being a mental patient. A problems-based approach (Fox and Conroy 2000) is further operationalized through what is traditionally called the five Ws:

- **What** do you see as your main problem?
- **When** is the problem worse/better?
- **Where** is the problem worse/better?
- **With** whom is the problem worse/better?
- **Why?** – What do you think causes or maintains your problems?

From a strengths perspective this of course creates an intrinsic difficulty. Rappaport (1990) makes this point well:

> "To work with an empowering ideology requires us to identify (for our-selves, for others and for the people with whom we work) the abilities which they possess which may not be obvious, even to themselves... It is always easier to see what is wrong, and what people lack. [*An empower-ment agenda*] seeks to identify what is right about people, and what resources are already available, so as to encourage their use and expansion under the control of the people of concern."

An empowerment approach promotes the recognition and development of the strengths, resources and skills that an individual possesses. It attempts to facilitate the further development of those resources whilst taking on board all the constraints and limitations of circumstance and personal difficulty, which an individual may be faced with. Strengths assessment challenges a problems-oriented model by developing an approach to assessment – and care planning – that is empowering and which enhances a service user's ability to make choices.

CARRYING OUT A STRENGTHS ASSESSMENT: CORE QUESTIONS

There are three main areas of focus in a strengths assessment. These core questions are:

> **Box 8.1   The service user's situation**
>
> For example, the service user is finding the bed-sit accommodation where he is living stressful, and he is being pressured by the landlord through non-payment of rent. He is not currently taking medication, is hearing voices and is increasingly worried about having to go back to hospital. The neighbours are also complaining and the physical standard of the bed-sit is very poor, the cooker is not working and the service user is not keeping up with tidying and cleaning. His parents used to come round to help with tidying up but their own physical health is deteriorating and they can no longer keep up (Bleach and Ryan 1995).

1. What is the situation for the service user at the moment?

This focus area tries to be as clear as possible about what is currently going on in the life of the service user in the domains covered by the assessment: housing; financial/legal; health; leisure; occupation; daily living; social support; and spiritual/cultural. What specifically are the issues the service user is dealing with in this current situation (Box 8.1)?

2. What does the service user want in relation to this situation?

Given this situation, what does the service user want? What are their own aspirations and aims? How do these translate in terms of what the user needs to meet these aims (Box 8.2)?

> **Box 8.2   What the service user wants**
>
> For example, the service user wants to stay living where he is but needs to get the landlord and neighbours off his back. *This might entail working out fixed rental repayments with the landlord, and working with the neighbours to help them understand the situation.*
>
> He wants to keep out of hospital but is fed up with the medication and hates the side-effects. *This might entail working out, with the service user and the team's psychiatrist, a more acceptable medication regime with reduced side-effects.*
>
> He does feel lonely and isolated in the bed-sit and would like to have more social contact. *This might entail working with interests and hobbies the service user used to have and finding ways to re-establish them, and through this having a more active social life.*
>
> He wants the bed-sit to be neat and tidy, and would like his parents to visit – but not just to tidy up. *This might entail working with social services to supply a home help, and working with the parents to arrange transport so that they can come over for an afternoon.*

3. What resources are available to respond to this?

What past and present physical skills, experience and achievements could the user themselves, with encouragement and support, draw upon to help address the current situation? Are there any resources available in the user's friends or family? What do local mental health services have to offer which could be tailored to specifically meet these needs? Are there any resources in the community itself which the user could key into (Box 8.3)?

THE LIFE DOMAINS COVERED BY STRENGTHS ASSESSMENT

According to Rapp (1998) strengths assessment is a process by which a client's personal and environmental assets are identified. These assets are organized into life domains.

These domains can be outlined as follows:

Housing

This includes the user's accommodation and other pertinent details including availability of informal/formal support, location, quality of furnishing, method of payment and level of tidiness.

Financial/Legal

This focuses on the sources and amounts of income, debts and loans, financial management skills, any financial assets and savings, etc.

Health

This means the whole domain of physical and mental health, including needs for dental care, physical health problems, level of physical fitness (diet and exercise) as well as mental illness (medications taken, major side-effects, attitude towards medication, early warning signs where known, level of contact with and support by the psychiatrist, etc.).

Leisure

This focuses on any interests, hobbies or other recreational activities – how they spend (or would like to spend) their spare time, including where, with whom, etc.

Occupation

This addresses paid, unpaid or voluntary work activities, any meaningful and structured day-time activities, any training or education undertaken, etc.

Box 8.3   The service user's progress

For example, the service user used to have interests in sport and going to the cinema but these have dropped off over the last few years. When he is well he is able to take care of himself adequately, and did cope quite well for the first six months he lived in the bed-sit. Again, over this period, he got on quite well with the landlord and with one of the neighbours. His parents still wish to visit and support him, if they could be helped over transport.

Daily living

This focuses on how the service user manages the challenges of daily living such as cooking, cleaning, self-care and transport as well as such characteristics as punctuality and time keeping.

Social support

This includes the service user's network of support defined in its broadest sense as including links to family, friends, neighbours, as well as such specific social support as is provided by the mental health service itself. This may include the role of the Assertive Outreach worker in supporting the service user.

Spiritual/Cultural

This includes the service user's moral, ethical and religious beliefs about the world around them, as well as their feeling of connection to specific groups of people based on race, ethnicity, gender, sexuality, organization, etc.

Rapp (1998) summarizes the life domains as corresponding "to those life domains that clients are most concerned about. They also reflect the major niches that people occupy. The focus is on actual life activities that reflect successful community functioning of the person, and the resources, personal and environmental, that are and have been employed."

STYLE OF APPROACH IN STRENGTHS ASSESSMENT

It is important to remember that this is intended to be part of a continuous process. At the start, it will be more of engagement: a gentle process of 'getting to know each other', which will probably suggest some urgent work, which will itself help to establish trust, and assist in further exploration and understanding. To a large extent, once priorities are established, plans set and work begins, further needs and aims will become identified as work proceeds. The assessment and planning processes are ongoing and cyclical in nature, and it is not necessary or realistic to identify all possible future steps before initial plans are implemented. Strengths assessment is based on some underlying principles of practice (Rapp 1998, Bleach and Ryan 1995), and as an ongoing process rapidly become part of everyday working practice (Box 8.4).

The use of questions in strengths assessment

Questioning should be carried out in the informal, friendly style outlined in Chapter 7. Assessment should not suddenly set another, more formal note. Good strengths assessment is seamlessly interwoven with the engagement process and should be congruent with it in terms of how it is approached. Having said that, guidelines for questioning are essentially good practice that is common to many different approaches. The following points are suggested as general guidelines:

- Start by using open-ended questions as this approach is less threatening and has the potential for yielding richer and more detailed information, which gives the service user a better opportunity for defining their own agenda in their own most natural form of expression.

Box 8.4 The underlying principles of practice of strengths assessment

- Strengths assessment is best carried out using a brief, specific, detailed narrative or descriptive statements. Statements that are interpretive or analytical in nature are to be avoided. For example, a statement saying that the user likes sport is very general and globalized. A statement saying that the service user used to enjoy playing Sunday morning football in the local park with a neighbourhood team gives far more precise information.
- The assessment is focused on gathering information relevant to each individual's current circumstances, and what they aspire to or want to achieve in the 'life domains' in which they have expressed interest; and what resources are available to help achieve these.
- The process is flexible, ongoing and continuous: circumstances change, as may the service user's aspirations. The assessment is not therefore fixed and new facets of a person continuously emerge. The gathering of information, assessment, care planning and implementation operate as a continuous process.
- Urgent issues are worked on immediately to help build up the trusting relationship between the Assertive Outreach worker and the service user. For example, Mr F's longterm plan was to broaden his social contacts and to keep more active during the day through pursuing his interests in sport, but the immediate priority agreed on was tidying up the flat and getting the cooker to work.
- The assessment is best conducted in an informal, conversational manner, rather than a structured interview. It is best conducted so far as is possible on the client's own 'territory' and in places where the user feels comfortable, rather than in formal service or institutional settings. The user's own home is usually where they feel most able to relax. For example, in the day hospital Mr F displayed a lot of defensiveness and antisocial behaviours but when at home on his own territory he was much more open and forthcoming. However, there are exceptions (Onyett 1992). The user might be in an abusive or highly conflict-ridden family relationship, in which case the assessment might well be better undertaken on neutral territory. Sometimes a user may feel that being seen at home is an invasion of privacy and may wish to be seen elsewhere. The golden rule is to be flexible and imaginative as to where the assessment is carried out, and to be guided by the user's own preferences.
- The assessment develops at each user's pace and comfort level, and adapts to change. For example, as soon as Mr F's flat was tidied up, his antisocial behaviour decreased but he was still worried that 'getting better' might mean saying goodbye to the help and support he was beginning to value.
- The assessment is made as detailed and specific as possible. It should, as clearly and accurately as possible, describe, where possible using the

box continues

service user's own words, their aspirations, circumstances, options and choices. Each strengths assessment should therefore be unique and so pre-packing it to fit into service requirements should always be avoided.

- The assessment should be a positive, hopeful and constructive process – the act of looking at strengths, possibilities and motivations is in itself constructive. For example, discovering that Mr F used to be good at playing the piano helped him to remember the respect with which he was treated and the simple act of remembering his achievement helped him to reconnect with a sense of potential development.
- The assessment should paint a holistic picture of a user's life. Strengths and motivations noted in one life domain may be useful in promoting positive improvement in another. For example, remembering the hard work involved in learning to play the piano was helpful in encouraging Mr F to feel more relaxed and comfortable in considering broadening his social horizons by going out to meet new people.
- Wants, aims and aspirations are important anchors to drive plans forward, to clarify what resources are needed from whom in order to achieve them, and to identify what barriers or difficulties may need to be overcome. For example, the untidiness and messiness in his flat was not initially a problem for Mr F but, when he realized that he wanted to invite potential new friends round, Mr F was sufficiently motivated to work at keeping his flat tidier.
- The assessment makes clear, thought-through connections between the specific care plans that are worked on. For example, Mr F's assessment and care plan made clear connections between his situation of isolation, his need to change aspects of his behaviour to enhance his chances of making new friends, and his longer term aspiration of living independently of institutional and service support.

- Focus in (from more general open-ended questions) on more specific questions. The five Ws can be helpful ways to generate more specific information:
  - **What** are your main aims and aspirations?
  - **When?** What kind of timescales do you have for them?
  - **Where** is the location or whereabouts?
  - **With** whom would you like to be involved?
  - **Why?** What is your motivation and 'driver' for this?
- Go where the client takes you. Rapp (1998) states: "Since the strengths assessment is to be done conversationally, adhering to a row or column on the form is contraindicated." For example, if the client spontaneously mentions that he or she went to the cinema with two friends from church, this would suggest focusing and further exploring the leisure and social support domains.
- Reflection and self-disclosure. As a client shares information about themselves, the practitioner should share and self-disclose appropriately, so as to illustrate that they have things in common. It can be

helpful in facilitating a trusting relationship in which the service user will begin to feel confident in sharing information about themselves, if they begin to feel that there are things in common between them, and that having a severe mental illness does not make them utterly different. For example, 'Yes, I too sometimes get nervous if I am meeting new people for the first time.'

- Use active listening to tune in to the underlying moods or feelings that the user may be beginning to communicate.
- Help the user see, accept and value their positive strengths and achievements. A client's life and the experience with the mental health system is such that many clients have difficulty in seeing their lives as one of strengths, talents and achievements. A client who says 'I only completed one year in college and then I had to drop out' is conveying that self-identity as a failure. The case manager might respond 'So you have a high school diploma and one year in college under your belt.' Case managers should use every opportunity to feed back to clients that, while their life contains pain and disappointment, like others it also contains a history of achievement. As one client reflected: "I remember her doing the strengths assessment. I think she saw a lot more in me than I saw in myself. It felt better talking about me as a person rather than as a manic-depressive."

The following gives an overview of some of the starter questions that may be useful in the various strengths assessment life domains:

General
- What do you most want to do in your life right now?
- What do you enjoy doing most?
- What do you like most about yourself?
- What do others most like about you?
- What do you still want to achieve in your life?

Housing
- What do you most like about where you are living right now?
- What could make where you are living right now more satisfying or enjoyable?
- Is there anything you would like to change about the way it looks?
- Do you know any of the neighbours? How do you get on with them?
- Where would you most like to live?
- Where else have you lived?

Financial/Legal
- Where does your income come from?
- How well do you manage on it?
- Is there anything you need legal advice on?

Health
- How is your physical health right now?
- Mentally, how do you feel at the moment?
- When do you feel strongest physically?
- What can you do to feel better physically?
- Who do you contact if you are not feeling well?

- Are there any ways in which you think you could be stronger and/or healthier?

Leisure
- What do (did) you especially enjoy doing in terms of hobbies and pastimes?
- Have you or do you belong to any clubs or organizations?
- What do (did) you enjoy doing on your holidays?
- How do (did) you like passing your free time?
- Anyone in particular you enjoy(ed) doing these things with?
- Are there any hobbies or activities which you would like to take up?

Occupation
- Have you had any work/voluntary work which you particularly enjoyed doing?
- What do you enjoy most about your work?
- What were you best at in your work?
- How long were you employed for?
- Is there any work in particular you would like to go for?
- What kind of work would you like to do? Part-time or full-time? Paid or voluntary?
- Is there any training you would like to have?

Daily living
- What daily chores are you able to do?
- What kind of work around the house do you most like doing?
- How do you manage with getting chores around the house done?
- What would make things easier for you round the house?
- How do you get on with shopping?
- How about transport?

Social support
- Who of your family/friends do you spend most time with? Whose company do you most enjoy?
- Are there any family members or friends you can rely on to help you?
- What kinds of things do you do/like to do with family and friends?
- Who of your family/friends would you like to see or hear more from?
- What kinds of things would you like to do when you meet up with family/friends?

Spiritual/Cultural
- What spiritual beliefs are important to you?
- How important is your faith to you?
- What (cultural) groups of people do you feel most closely associated with?
- How would you like to express the things that feel important to you?

When interviewing for service user strengths, De Jong and Miller (1995) acknowledge that the person may not always respond to straight-forward questions about positive attributes and achievements. Experiences of severe depression or of frequently being referred to as a failure are not conducive to thinking in the positive. If more creative lines of questioning are called for, they suggest trying some of the following techniques:

Exception-finding questions

- Are there times, in the present or past, when you noticed a significant change to the way you feel now?
- In what ways would your life be different if the current difficulty were resolved?
- When these changes would be noticeable, what is it that you would be doing differently on these days?

Scaling questions

- On a scale of 1 to 10, with 1 being the difficulty at its most intense, where would you place yourself at present?
- What is different in your life that has contributed to the higher score?

Coping questions

- How do you feel you best manage to cope when things are not going so well for you?
- What sorts of things help you to get out of bed to face another day?

'What's better' questions

- What is happening in your life that is better than before?
- When was the last time you noticed this type of positive change?
- What will increase the chances of this positive change continuing?

FREQUENTLY ASKED QUESTIONS

Q. Does a strengths assessment simply mean an unquestioning acceptance of 'whatever the user wants the user gets'?

A. Taking a strengths approach does not mean that the user's views or preferences should not be questioned. What is required, however, is that the user's views, preferences and aspirations are acknowledged and dealt with through negotiation, in which the user is supported and empowered, not controlled, by the assessor. It is advisable, indeed essential, that the strengths practitioner takes an independent view as to the desirability/reality/justifiability of the user's view. This does not mean that a user's views should simply be summarily dismissed even if they seem to be extreme, unrealistic or potentially harmful. The role of the practitioner under these circumstances is to understand 'where the user is coming from' as clearly as possible, and identify and negotiate ways forward which the user ultimately accepts, even though the action taken may be very different from what was initially expressed. This is still best achieved in a collaborative and co-operative manner in which collusion and coercion are equally avoided.

It is useful to remember that the role of the practitioner is to listen carefully to and acknowledge the user's views as expressed, and to work collaboratively with the user to achieve the 'negotiated compromise'. It is not necessary or desirable for a practitioner to compromise on their view as to what is really needed. If the practitioner feels that the user's view is odd, unrealistic or unwise, it is not necessary to humour or collude with them, only to respect and include them, whilst also presenting to the user the realities and constraints of the user's situation.

Q. Is a strengths approach to assessment simply a naïve reframing into the positive, which overlooks or ignores the difficulties, disabilities or dysfunctions which a service user may be experiencing?

A. Both philosophically and technically, strengths assessment is a great deal more than this. Philosophically, strengths assessment can be a very powerful way to destigmatize the self-definitions which the service user may be holding about themselves. Many of their experiences within the mental health services may well have reinforced a deep sense of worthlessness and helplessness, that having a severe mental illness is effectively a life sentence without remission. By assisting the service user to identify some continuities in their lives, in which they too had achievements and accomplishments, can over time powerfully affect their self-esteem and transform a sense of profound hopelessness into the possibility of growth and development.

Technically, also, there are some quite sophisticated skills underlying strengths assessment. An important component of cognitive behavioural therapy is addressing and systematically working with the negative, distorted or dysfunctional belief systems that a service user may have, both with respect to their 'voices' and more generally (Fowler et al 1995, Chadwick et al 1996). There is an important sense in which strengths assessment is also involved in challenging predominantly negative self-attributions, which the service user is likely to hold about themselves.

Q. How does strengths assessment link up with systematic assessments required by my Trust, and through the CPA?

A. There is indeed a whole series of assessments, particularly in the enhanced CPA, where the majority of Assertive Outreach clients are likely to be located. The designated care co-ordinator under the enhanced CPA is required to undertake a comprehensive assessment in the following areas:

- psychiatric, psychological and social functioning
- risk to the individual and others, including previous violence and criminal record
- needs arising from co-morbidity
- personal circumstances including family or other carers
- housing, financial and occupational status
- physical health needs
- user and carer views.

On that basis they are required to develop a care plan which should include:

- arrangements for mental health care including medication
- an assessment of the nature of any risk posed and the arrangements for the management of this risk, including the circumstances in which contingency action should be taken
- arrangements for physical health care
- action needed to secure accommodation appropriate to the user's needs
- arrangements to provide domestic support
- action needed for employment, education or training
- arrangements needed for an adequate income

- action to provide for cultural and faith needs
- arrangements to promote independence and sustain social contact
- date of next planned review.

Given this somewhat intimidating array of assessments and required paperwork, is there really a place for strengths assessment? Perhaps the main point to make is that the required enhanced CPA care plan does cover all the life domain areas covered in strengths assessment. Therefore undertaking a strengths assessment is an excellent, user-friendly 'road map', which in fact provides in a simple yet comprehensive fashion much of the information required by care planning under the enhanced CPA. It has the additional advantage from a user perspective of doing so in a way that emphasizes the user's own point of view and which is based on working collaboratively with the user to achieve their own aims and aspirations. The main area that is not covered is risk assessment, which it would be relatively easy to carry out in parallel with the strengths assessment.

Q. How does the process of strengths assessment happen in practice?

A. The formalized approach of so many mental health procedures needs to be substantially discarded, if we are to create the right environmental conditions for a strengths assessment to happen. As practitioners, we need to refrain from working to the unrealistic expectations of completing an assessment within the confines of a short space of time. The service user will be acclimatized to a more traditional set of assessment procedures, e.g. the formal interview. Many will be exhausted by the experiences of repeatedly having to answer the same questions about their history to each new practitioner they have to see. The promise of a different experience is unlikely to garner much favour, at least until proved different.

Essentially, the strengths assessment is a continuous process that develops over time. It may be completed in one session on very rare occasions. But such a success should be treated with caution, and regularly reviewed in the light of new information. People have the right to change their minds about their future aspirations and priorities. So, strengths assessments share the need equally with all other forms of assessment to be reviewed and revised at regular intervals.

The ultimate aim is for the assessment to be completed collaboratively, with or without an example of the form being introduced into the conversations. It is not something that is done to someone but rather an outcome of mutual dialogue (Rapp 1998). Paperwork in meetings does have a habit of formalizing the situation and thus getting in the way of the intended purpose. In rare instances, the whole process has been described to the service user, and the form left with them to ponder and complete in their own time. This has then successfully formed a basis for the service user to lead a subsequent discussion of their strengths and aspirations with the practitioner. On equally rare occasions, where the service user has expressed a particular disregard for any process or positive procedure the practitioner wishes to explain, the strengths assessment has been gradually documented by the practitioner in the office, following each occasion where strengths have been identified through ongoing conversations.

There is no single way of doing it or documenting it. The outcome still becomes a positive inventory of achievements, resources and aspirations individualized to the experience of the person themselves (Morgan 1997) (Fig. 8.1). More frequently than any other type of assessment, service users have come to accept or request a copy of their strengths assessment, largely because of the unusually positive and constructive record it unearths. It becomes an easier task to explore a person's motivations, where the starting point is positively agreed.

Its flexibility has also been demonstrated through one known example of using it with a tragic situation of a person with mental health problems dying from cancer in a general hospital ward. The practitioner was able to adapt the approach to help the person express unfulfilled aspirations, and their wishes for loved ones being left behind.

Figure 8.1   A completed strengths assessment form

STRENGTHS ASSESSMENT		Date: 24/2/03
Service User's Name: MEHMET		Worker: S. MORGAN
What has worked for me in the past? (How have I coped?)	What is going on for me today? (What is available?)	What are my aims for the future? (What do I want?)
HOUSING		
Living in council tenancies, and living with different members of the family	Recently moved into a new one-bedroom housing association flat, on the 4th floor of a block of flats	A larger flat on a better estate
FINANCIAL/LEGAL		
Wages from employment, and social security benefits. One judge in the court had a good understanding of my mental illness, and gave me good advice	Social security benefits: Income Support, Disability Living Allowance and Housing Benefit	Eventually to return to a job. But to keep my current benefits until I am ready. To stay out of trouble with the police

HEALTH		
People taking me into hospital when I was not realizing I was unwell. High doses of the injection have helped me when I have been ill and getting violent towards other people	Regular contact with my community mental health worker, GP and psychiatrist. Low doses of the injections, and taking my tablets	No more hospital admissions. To understand my illness better. To keep on the lowest dose of injection for a few years, then just stay on the tablets
LEISURE		
Drinking in local pubs	Started driving lessons. Going to English classes to improve my speaking and reading. Playing with our young son	Pass the driving test, and get a car. To read and write better, by catching up on my education. Help my son get a good education
OCCUPATION		
Labouring jobs	Trying to make good use of my time towards getting a job in the future	Get back into work, when I am ready
DAILY LIVING		
Using cafes and take-aways. My step-mother's cooking	I like cooking some Turkish foods. Shopping at a Turkish super-market	Share looking after the flat and our son with my girlfriend. Do more of the cooking at home
SOCIAL SUPPORT		
People in the cafes. Going to a local gym	My girlfriend and our young son	Maybe get married. New friends through English classes and a different gym I go to with my girlfriend. Maybe meet the community mental health worker outside of his work, if it would be okay
SPIRITUAL/CULTURAL		
No particular beliefs. Feeling part of Turkish communities in London	Now that I have a new life with my girlfriend and son, I think more about being proud to be Turkish	Help my son to understand his Turkish roots. To visit Turkey and Cyprus

STRENGTHS ASSESSMENT: A WORKING EXAMPLE

My chief priorities are:
- staying well, and out of hospital
- getting a bigger flat for the family
- to improve my reading and writing
- to understand my illness and the medication better.

Signed: Service user
Signed: Worker

[The above case example of a strengths assessment is further developed in Chapter 9: Care planning and care co-ordination.]

CONCLUSIONS

The dominant assessment procedures in mental health focus directly on the negative: problems; deficits; deficiencies; and failings. This inevitably leads the service user to feel negative about themselves, reinforced by the external view perpetuated and documented by every practitioner gathering information on them (Morgan 1996, Rapp 1998). Essentially the strengths approach requires us to accept the more challenging focus on identifying the strengths, passed achievements and interests, capabilities and future aspirations of the individual. Most people in service provision make a claim to be doing this already but in reality are just paying lip service to the concept.

Rapp (1998) reminds us that practitioners will find it difficult to shift from their more natural interrogative approach to a more conversational approach, and also the more fluid approach moving away from the need to complete one area of investigation before moving on to the next. It is difficult to hold the attention on identifying positives for someone who can more easily identify and articulate the negative experiences. We easily become distracted ourselves by self-evident problems. Moreover, the person receiving the service will have become acclimatized to talking about their weaknesses and problems through their history of previous contact with the services.

However, the benefits of persisting with the practice of strengths assessment make a significant gain towards engagement of a trusting working relationship. Ultimately, both parties learn to strike up more rewarding conversations, and create realistic and achievable action plans. The approach itself is positively compatible with the intentions underpinning the CPA, thus offering a light for what is widely regarded as an over-bureaucratic aspect of contemporary mental health practice.

References

Bleach A, Ryan P 1995 Community Support for Mental Health. Pavilion, Brighton

Chadwick P, Birchwood M, Trower P 1996 Cognitive Therapy. Wiley, London

Craig T 2000 Severe mental illness: signs, symptoms and diagnosis. In: Gamble C, Brennan G (eds) Working with Serious Mental Illness: A Manual for Clinical Practice. Baillière Tindall, London, p 41–64

De Jong P, Miller S 1995 How to interview for client strengths. Social Work 40 (6): 729–736

Fowler D, Garety P, Kuipers E 1995 Cognitive Behaviour Therapy for Psychosis for Delusions, Voices and Paranoia. Wiley, London

Fox A, Conroy P 2000 Assessing clients' needs: the semi-structured interview. In: Gamble C, Brennan G (eds) Working with Serious Mental Illness: A Manual for Clinical Practice. Baillière Tindall, London, p 85–97

Hall N 1981 Psychological assessment. In: Wing J K, Morris B (eds) Handbook of Psychiatric Rehabilitation Practice. Oxford University Press, Oxford

Morgan S 1996 Helping Relationships in Mental Health. Chapman & Hall, London

Morgan S 1997 Assessing personal strengths. Materia Prima (Argentinian Journal of Occupational Therapy) 1 (2): 5–6

Onyett S 1992 Case Management in Mental Health. Chapman & Hall, London

Rapp C A 1998 The Strengths Model: Case Management with People Suffering from Severe and Persistent Mental Illness. Oxford University Press, New York

Rappaport J 1990 Research methods and the empowerment agenda. In: Tolan P, Keys C, Chertak F et al (eds) Researching Community Psychology. American Psychological Association, Washington DC

Chapter **9**

Care planning and care co-ordination

Peter Ryan and Steve Morgan

"Humans are purposeful; we do things for a reason"

(Rapp 1998)

INTRODUCTION

Morgan and Akbar-Khan (2000) suggest that, in its simplest form, care planning is the process of translating identified needs and wants into real actions. These may cover a complex range of health and social care issues, including housing, finances and personally meaningful occupation and activity. It is a dynamic, cyclical process in the here and now – stating the achievable tasks, responsibilities and timescales for practical action to take place. It sets the agreed goals for the future, as well as reviewing the achievement of those set in the past. In this way, it should not be so much of a bureaucratic exercise but rather a regular checkpoint for the service user and service providers to be aware of the progress of the work they are doing together. The emphasis is very much on the service user as an active partner at the centre of the care planning process, not just as a passive recipient of care determined by professional judgement.

Direct work with the service user is explicitly based on strengths assessment, and ensures that whatever direct work is done is directly linked to user aspirations, and based on care plans worked on and negotiated with the service user (Kisthardt 1992). However, many user aspirations (e.g. accommodation and their living situation) clearly require linkage into and co-ordination of care with a potentially vast range of voluntary, private sector and statutory agencies. This chapter follows on from Chapter 8 on strengths assessment to consider strengths care planning. In this respect, it is particularly important to ensure that the goal setting involved in care planning is user directed; this is discussed in some detail. The chapter continues with an exploration of care co-ordination. It is in this arena that the practitioner has to liaise with the other agencies in the 'patch' in order to deliver the agreed care plan. The section on care co-ordination describes some of the conflicts and difficulties this can create, and then goes on to propose some practical solutions.

However, before we establish a false sense of the dynamic process in action, it is important to reflect that many service users and carers remain unclear about the whole process of care planning and care co-ordination (Allen 1998, Phillips 1998). This raises the important question of whether we as practitioners often get carried away with a rose-tinted perception of how well we are implementing what is primarily a service-centred function. Do we really attend sufficiently to the information and explanations to service users and carers about the processes we attempt to engage them in? Are we really just meeting the administrative requirements of organizational audit, by processing and filing the paper-work? Does a service user's signature on a piece of paper represent real service user involvement in their process of care?

THE IMPORTANCE OF USER–LED GOAL SETTING

Viewed from the perspective of empowerment, goal setting is perhaps the most crucial part of the whole strengths approach in that it is where the user and the practitioner come together to find ways of optimizing user choice. In the chapter on ethics (see Chapter 4), reference was made to the work of Dworkin, particularly the concept of 'decisional privacy', denoting that we are free to direct our own lives. Clearly, from a strengths perspective, this value of decisional privacy is central to the whole approach, and has clear civil liberty implications, in terms of freedom of choice and hence the right to choose.

Burns and Firn (2002) rightly make the point that: "Issues of free will and personal autonomy are at the heart of all mental health practice." There will be occasions, as we have discussed in the ethics chapter, when issues of compulsion cannot be avoided. However, whenever and wherever possible, the primary commitment of mental health practitioners is to optimize user choice so as to enable them to exercise optimal control over their own decisions, and hence over their lives.

Through the progressive exercising of choice, service users can, over time, develop a sense of significance, meaning and purpose in their lives, which we believe to be an important staging post on the road to recovery. Victor Frankl (2000) has written movingly about the importance of personal meaning as the vehicle through which individuals can creatively live through the most traumatic, painful and difficult of personal circumstances. Himself a Holocaust survivor, Frankl writes: "Usually, in his everyday life, man lives and moves in a dimension whose positive pole is success and whose negative pole is failure. This is the dimension of the competent man … but the *homo pasiens,* the suffering man who is capable of rising above, and taking a stand to, his suffering, moves in a dimension whose positive pole is fulfilment and whose negative pole is despair. A human being strives for success but, if need be, does not depend upon his fate, which does or does not *allow* for success. A human being, by the very attitude he chooses, is capable of finding and fulfilling meaning even in a hopeless situation." Somebody who has experienced longterm severe mental illness is highly likely to have experienced their fare share of suffering. Frankl (1988) reminds us that there still remains as a matter of choice the stance taken with respect to the suffering experienced. It is crucial therefore that as much choice as possible remains with the service user. By so doing, a service user can build in a personal meaning to their lives, by building upon the personal choices they are able to make.

Rapp (1998) suggests that: "Participation leads to more ambitious goals, increased commitment, and acceptance of goals. The importance of using client-directed goals lies not only with the improved performance that results, but also in potential long-term benefits." He goes on to support the claim of Moore-Kirkland (1981) that collaborative goal setting is intrinsically justified: "By being involved in the setting of goals, the client sees them as coming largely from themselves and more easily incorporates them. As a result, chances for success are enhanced since the problem is one he or she has helped define rather than one that has been thrust upon him. Equally important is the feeling of competence resulting from satisfaction demonstrating to the client that change is possible and rewarding, and it lays the groundwork for subsequent success instilling hope."

There is an emerging body of research which supports the importance of user choice through optimizing the opportunities for participation, defined by Fitzsimmons and Fuller (2002) as referring to the level of influence which people can exercise over events in their life, and with the following operational outcomes:

- A sense of control or self-determination over goals or circumstances that are important to the individual.
- A sense of self-efficacy or self-confidence in one's ability to achieve desired outcomes.
- Increased levels of self-acceptance and self-worth.
- A sense of being valued and respected by others.
- A sense of purpose, and of actively advancing one's own interests.
- A hopeful and motivated stance.

There is some evidence that lack of influence or control can lead to poor health outcomes. Conversely, the ability to exercise control and influence, even where high stress is present, can act as a protective factor against levels of risk against cardiovascular disease (Theorell et al 1984). Also compatible with these findings is the literature on learned helplessness, which suggests that absence of influence or control can lead to the onset of depression (Garber and Seligman 1980). Powerlessness has therefore emerged as a key risk factor in the aetiology of disease. The corollary is that there is now a good deal of evidence from a number of different fields which suggests that empowerment is not just a set of values but that it leads to positive outcomes in care. These include increased emotional well-being, independence, motivation to participate and more effective coping strategies (Prilleltensky and Laurendeau 1994, Ryan and Deci 2000, Thompson and Spacapan 1991, Macleod and Nelson 2000).

Barham (1994) has described how "…loss of confidence in the viability and value of their life projects and the reconstruction of themselves as useless are as much as anything powerful determinants in the transformation of a potentially manageable disability into a permanent social disablement." Trainor and Tremblay (1992) found that active participation in self-help and mutual aid schemes was associated with lower rates of psychiatric admission, and reduced use of community mental health services. In a qualitative approach that generated service user narratives, Nelson et al (2001) found that several strategies were cited by users as facilitating their recovery, all of which are key components of the strengths approach to Assertive Outreach:

- Choosing which services to receive.
- Designing their own care plan.
- A sense of meaningful involvement and participation in the services received.

Lecomte et al (1999) found an increase in active coping strategies for users in outpatient services who were involved in an empowerment-based self-esteem group. A strengths approach can also enhance outcomes in the area of housing and independent living: Ware (1999) found that service users in an innovative housing project, which emphasized a strengths approach, made significant progress towards independent living. The intervention emphasized group self-management, access to financial resources and reducing staffing levels.

Rappaport (1990) expresses the importance of choice in user empowerment well: "To be committed to an empowerment agenda is to be committed to identify, facilitate or create contexts in which heretofore silent and isolated people, those who are outsiders in various settings, organisations and communities, gain understanding, voice and influence over decisions that affect their lives… leading to the development of a personal sense of being able to effect important life aims, to acquire psychological or material resources necessary to accomplish them and to make progress towards achieving personal goals."

PRINCIPLES OF STRENGTHS CARE PLANNING

Care planning 'carries on the good work' commenced in strengths assessment. In strengths care planning the purpose is to establish through a process of discussion and negotiation a 'joint-working agenda' focusing on achieving the goals the user has set. Morgan and Akbar-Khan (2000) suggest that these discussions are often an amalgamation of conversations, formal assessments, disagreements, negotiations and decisions, made in the dynamic interactions of service user and Assertive Outreach workers, and between the Assertive Outreach team and other service providers. This leads them to a common agreement on the longterm goal, any short-term goals along the way, and all the operationally specified, measurable action steps needed to get there. For each action step, there is clear agreement as to who will do what and by when. This 'technology' is by no means unique to strengths care planning. Indeed, it is an essential underpinning of behavioural psychotherapy and cognitive behavioural therapy (Chadwick et al 1996, Fowler et al 1995). What we do here is to interpret some of the elements of these approaches in the context of a strengths philosophical framework.

The service user is aided to set their own goals and in their own words

It is crucial that no compromises are made in terms of setting the longterm goal. This should be set by the service user, in their own words as far as is possible. Even if they appear 'thought disordered' or bizarre, these goals should not be rejected out of hand. Rather, through discussion and exploration over time, they can be worked with empathically and creatively. The client who wanted to be Queen illustrates this process (Box 9.1).

Box 9.1   The client who wanted to be Queen

Mrs J was due to be discharged into the community after a long stay of hospital residence. When faced with discussing the care programme approach discharge plan, she was considerably upset. She stated her wants in terms of residence in a nursing home with no responsibility plus daily care activities. Everyone agreed that her likely self-care skills and anxiety levels seemed to indicate that this would be the best plan. Once a trusting relationship had been established, Mrs J divulged that she hated the idea of going into a home, and going to day-centres, and that she really wanted to be the Queen. She challenged the practitioner to work towards that aim. Without promising that, the practitioner did however begin to work out with Mrs J what she felt the Queen did that was worth aiming for. It emerged that Mrs J believed that the Queen did not have financial or administrative worries, she always knew where she was going to live, people respected her because she helped them and, most importantly, she had 'companions' and 'ladies in waiting' who helped her and kept her company.

The subsequent assessment stated that Mrs J needed a strong sense of financial security and the guarantee of help with day-to-day organization, she needed to move to one location and be promised that she need never move again, she needed to feel that she was helping people and feel respected for it, and she needed some 'old-fashioned' companionship. Mrs J eventually began considering sharing a long-stay group home with another person being discharged who was already a firm friend, and an effective organizer of both good works and daily living (Bleach and Ryan 1995).

Goals are prioritized by the service user not by the service

It is important to optimize assigning client responsibility for goal completion. It is better to assign a 'microtask', however small, which can be completed by the client, rather than assigning more ambitious targets which, in practice, are undertaken not by the client but by the practitioner. The more a client can achieve independently or in a normally interdependent way, the greater the sense of achievement and empowerment, and the greater the likelihood of subsequent goal-directed efforts being exerted.

The first port of call for many a care programme approach (CPA) discharge plan might for example be *monitoring mental state* twinned with the need for *medication compliance* (adherence or concordance in an increasingly politically correct world!). This not-so-unexpected view can easily be linked to the notion that any person experiencing severe and enduring problems would require the symptoms of mental illness to be reasonably stabilized before dealing with the social and environmental concerns. However, this more usual approach may be seen as overpaternalistic, and certainly as a failure to connect with the individual's view of their world and their personal priorities within it. It is a truth universally acknowledged that service users do not like medication and resent its side-effects. They are highly unlikely, if left to their own devices, to have 'medication adherence' prominent in their care plans. This raises a very simple question: whose goal is 'medication adherence' likely to be? Very frequently, a goal in the care plan is in fact the service's not the service user's.

This simple adherence to traditional expectations of service delivery might well be a significant contribution to the reasons why many people

---

Box 9.2   Medication adherence

Mr A was referred whilst in imminent danger of losing his hostel place and becoming homeless, or being admitted to hospital because of his lack of compliance to his medication regime. Initially he would not accept taking his medication as part of his care plan since he clearly hated taking it. He was adamant that he did not wish to stay in a hostel where the rules insisted that he should take his medication. He was unwilling to accept that homelessness was a worse option than staying in the hostel. However, one of his aims was eventually to get a flat of his own, and in the short term he expressed a preference for not being admitted to hospital. Initially his primary aim in his care plan was recorded as wanting to find his own flat. When he was assisted in exploring this, he came to the conclusion that he would be unlikely to be accepted into any of the potential options unless he could demonstrate a greater stability and stay out of hospital for longer than he had in the past. He and his practitioner then agreed that a priority was to demonstrate this stability through a very public return to a limited but acceptable level of medication, which would enable him to gain the endorsement of his psychiatrist and the manager of the hostel (Bleach and Ryan 1995).

in the so-called Assertive Outreach client group disengage from the services prescribed to them. The case study in Box 9.2 illustrates a situation in which medication adherence did in fact become part of the user's care plan although very much on his own terms, and linked very clearly to his own longer-term aspirations.

Goals are stated in terms of positive attainment

Goals should be stated positively. The goal should specify what the user has agreed to do positively rather than what they should avoid trying not to do. For example, rather than 'Bob will not stay in bed until midday' it is preferable to state the same goal positively as 'Bob will get up every day by 11 am.' De Jong and Miller (1995) make the useful point that: "Practice outcomes are improved when clients are helped to express their goals as the presence of something – for example, 'taking walks', rather than the absence of something."

Longer-term goals are analysed into smaller achievable pieces

It is useful to go for 'quick wins'. Goals are broken down into small manageable 'chunks', in each of which the probability of success is optimized. For each goal or task, a target date for achieving it should be set. This further structures and directs the goal-directed process and enhances the likelihood of completion. As a rule of thumb, it is desirable to set target dates that can be achieved between the current visit and the next one. This clearly also implies that the size and complexity of the task is realistically achievable in the given time-frame.

It is important to help the service user in specifiying neither too many goals at any given time nor too few – pacing at a level that the client can manage. Having too many tasks assigned at any given time can be counterproductive. It can lead to the client experiencing confusion, diffusion of effort and to a feeling of being overwhelmed. Where a client comes up with too many tasks, Rapp (1998) recommends feedback along the lines of: "This seems like a lot. I know that when this happens to me, I am less likely to accomplish anything. Do you ever feel like that? How about just focusing on one priority for the moment?"

Goals are concrete, specific and operationally defined

Goals should be tangible and observable in such a way that it should be clear and unambiguous whether or not they have been achieved. Global and vague descriptive terms such as 'appropriately' or 'regularly' should be avoided. Goals need to be precisely stated wherever possible, with respect to:

- **what** behavioural target is specified
- the **location(s)** under which the behaviour is to be performed (e.g. transport, the particular setting, etc.)
- **frequency** and **duration**.

For example, perhaps the practitioner is working with the service user's stated aim to develop greater independence and self-care. A concrete, specific and measurable goal could be:

Shopping alone, twice a week, by getting a bus to the local supermarket.

In this instance, the goal components are:

- the behaviour – shopping alone
- the location(s) – getting a bus to the local supermarket
- the frequency – twice a week
- the duration – for one hour.

Goals are specified separately

Each goal statement should be stated separately. To have two or more goals mixed up together in the same goal statement confuses the measurability of what has been achieved, or not achieved.

Goals should be measurable and lead to a definable outcome

If the preceding guidelines have been followed, then any goal specified should in principle be measurable. Measuring the success with which goals have been achieved is an intrinsic element of strengths goal planning; it provides a useful framework in which the achievements of the service user can be praised, encouraged and reinforced. Where goals have not been achieved or only partially, this may provide much useful information for discussion between the service user and the practitioner. In addition, measuring goal achievement provides useful information for the team, and beyond that for the clinical governance procedures of the Trust itself. Progress towards goal achievement is monitored openly and discussed by both the service user and the practitioner. Figure 9.1 illustrates a useful format.

Figure 9.1   Rating goal attainment

Service User Goal Attainment Rating					
Goal Specified: Shopping alone, at a busy time, twice a week, to the local supermarket.					
My progress towards this goal is:					
Indicate here	0	2	4	6	8
	0% no luck so far	25% made a start	50% substantial	75% very considerable	100% complete success
Practitioner Goal Attainment Rating					
Service user's progress towards goal specified above:					
Indicate here	0	2	4	6	8
	0% no luck so far	25% made a start	50% substantial	75% very considerable	100% complete success
Any comments (Service User)					
Any comments (Practitioner)					

STRENGTHS CARE PLAN: A WORKING EXAMPLE

From the strengths assessment in Chapter 8, Mehmet had expressed the following priorities:

- staying well and out of hospital
- getting a bigger flat for the family
- improve my reading and writing
- understand my illness and the medication better.

In subsequent discussions with members of the Assertive Outreach team, he developed care plans for each of the priority areas he personally identified. In relation to his first priority, the plans identified focused on building up a picture of early warning signs of emerging problems, through set times for Mehmet, his partner and one specific Assertive Outreach worker to discuss the precipitants of many previous hospital admissions. A crisis plan was to be agreed for actions that may prevent getting to the point of needing an admission in the future. It was recognized that these discussions would become linked to the educational proposals developed for meeting his fourth priority and that these issues were necessarily longterm initiatives for all people involved. The plan concerning housing turned out to be the most immediate in terms of specific practical tasks, and is outlined in Fig. 9.2.

Figure 9.2

CARE PLAN		Date: 24/2/03			
Service User: MEHMET		Worker: S. MORGAN			
Planned frequency of contact: 3×/week					
Life Domain focused on:	**Housing** Financial/Legal Health Occupation	Leisure Daily Living Social Support Spiritual/Cultural			
Service User's own longterm goal (expressed in own words):					
To move into a two bedroom flat on a better housing estate, on the ground floor with a small garden					
What user is aiming to achieve towards longterm goal	Who has to do it?	Date to be done by	Date achieved	Comments (what happened?)	
Keep current housing benefit application updated	Mehmet and AO worker	March 03			
Set up a housing transfer interview	AO worker	February 03			
Attend the housing department for interview	Mehmet and partner	When invited			
Maintain current tenancy in good condition	Mehmet and partner	Ongoing			
Discuss a supporting letter for transfer	AO worker, Mehmet and his partner	March 03			

FROM CARE PLANNING TO CARE CO-ORDINATION

Once a care plan is articulated, it translates into work the practitioner undertakes directly with the service user (see Chapter 10), and care co-ordination with whatever agencies are indicated by the care plan. The complexity of the needs of people most frequently referred to Assertive Outreach makes it highly unlikely that the team will be able to meet them all solely from its own resources, e.g. housing and financial issues require a great deal of input from the specialist services responsible for providing accommodation and welfare benefits, respectively. Hence, service delivery requires multidisciplinary and multi-agency involvement, with a demanding role for care co-ordination.

In UK mental health services, the policy context for care co-ordination has been set through the introduction of the CPA (Department of Health 1990) being implemented from April 1991, and modernized and reaffirmed as a part of the more recent review of service provision (Department of Health 1999). It is important to be reminded that the broad principles are positive in their construction:

- systematic arrangements for assessing the health and social needs of people accepted into specialist mental health services
- the formation of a care plan, which identifies the health and social care required from a variety of providers
- the appointment of a key worker (care co-ordinator) to keep in close touch with the service user, and to monitor and co-ordinate care
- regular review and, where necessary, agreed changes to the care plan.

Morgan and Akbar-Khan (2000) state: "The key to effective care planning requires collaborative joint working between all agencies involved in the delivery of care with the individual service user. This requires clear lines of communication, whilst also respecting the principle of client confidentiality; and the acceptance of responsibility by individual workers to coordinate the various inputs to the total care plan." This sounds positive in principle, but may not be so easy to deliver in practice. Complex care co-ordination primarily requires a large administrative input to be made by practitioners. It also assumes that communication will be taking place between receptive people and agencies, which is not always the case.

It is highly likely that the service users the team has engaged with present an even greater challenge to local agencies than they do to the Assertive Outreach team itself. Local services are not necessarily geared up to working with service users with the range of risk and difficulties of Assertive Outreach clients. This can create difficulties both for local services, and for the Assertive Outreach team itself. Ryan and Green (2001) explored the problems involved in care co-ordination, through tracking in detail the experience of one rural and one inner city team. Both teams had established a strengths approach to their practice. Neither team had an in-house psychiatrist who had dedicated session time with the team. Particularly with respect to co-ordinating care around hospitalization, this lack of dedicated specialist psychiatric input proved to be a major disadvantage (Boxes 9.3 and 9.4).

There were different obstacles to overcome when it came to liaison and co-ordination of care with community services. Many of the local

---

Box 9.3   Care co-ordination with hospital admission and discharge

The teams felt disempowered from having a genuine influence in decisions to admit or discharge from hospital. The teams reported having to 'sell' the user to the inpatient team for admission, whether a compulsory or voluntary admission was concerned. This was mainly due to the hospitals concerned being unsure about the team and not believing that an acute crisis could be managed in the community. When it came down to it, it was the consultants who made the critical decisions with respect to admission and discharge, and the Assertive Outreach teams were somewhat left outside decision making for these critical issues. For example, care co-ordinators were not able to admit informally.

What militated against a 'good' admission was having to use the liaison psychiatrist in the A & E department, since teams experienced that this created needless delays and added to the bureaucracy. So far as discharge was concerned, the team tried to optimize its influence by putting a lot of work on developing a very detailed discharge plan, which could demonstrate to the hospital that the requisite community supports were in fact in place. A 'good' discharge from the care co-ordinators' point of view consisted of working intensively with the ward and doing a great deal of liaison there to educate the ward about what could be achieved in the community. Good 'in reach' to the inpatient unit was also useful for a smooth discharge (Ryan and Green 2001).

---

services had fixed referral criteria, which were aimed at a considerably less disadvantaged and generally 'difficult' and risky client group than those the Assertive Outreach teams were working with. Consequently, many local services either excluded or rapidly ejected, once admitted, the clients referred on to them by the Assertive Outreach teams.

Box 9.4   Care co-ordination with community services

Both teams stated that they felt they were pushed into having to plan from a service-led point of view. They reported substantial difficulties in terms of shifting local services from service-led perspectives. The most common barrier mentioned was that most services in the catchment area operated a limited hours, 9 am–5 pm, opening policy, and therefore were often not available when clients needed to use them. Also, services were not set up in a way to meet the needs of the Assertive Outreach target client group. The housing benefit department created a lot of work for the teams, as a constant threat hanging over many clients was that of eviction. One care co-ordinator stated: "We have been waiting for one client to have their housing benefit processed for over two years.

box continues

This creates such problems with eviction, courts, etc., which could be prevented if we had a better working relationship with them."

Often local services refused to accept Assertive Outreach clients because they did not meet their referral criteria. These local services were looking to work with clients with far higher levels of motivation, organization and psychosocial functioning than that typically demonstrated by Assertive Outreach clients. Also, the levels of risk of harm to self or others demonstrated by Assertive Outreach clients were too high to be acceptable to local services.

All team members reported difficulties in placing users into suitable accommodation. One major factor was simply the lack of suitable accommodation, including council housing and voluntary sector supported accommodation. There were often disagreements between the housing department and the user concerning what was, and what was not, suitable accommodation; also, for a variety of reasons the user might be unwilling to move to improved housing. Also, neighbours were often a source of difficulty in placing users, and would object to a mental health service user being placed nearby. Most team members reported that finding and maintaining users in appropriate accommodation was an ongoing difficulty. Locally, there was a vulnerability panel set up as a problem-solving group between the Trust and the housing department, as one of the only ways of stating the needs or unmet needs of the client group.

Both teams stated that it was difficult to maintain users in their existing accommodation. This was for several reasons. Chief amongst them was the lack of stimulating or meaningful daytime activities appropriate for the needs of this highly vulnerable and disabled group. Also, there were constant problems with housing benefit, which were difficult and time-consuming to resolve. Many users had ongoing battles with the local estate office over non-payment of rent, or neglect of the property.

Potentially, it was a small step to a downward spiral of mutual recrimination. The Assertive Outreach team can criticize unresponsive local services, whilst local services can criticize Assertive Outreach for being 'misled' concerning the actual capabilities of the client. If a local service loses confidence in Assertive Outreach in this way, it might itself withdraw from co-operation, not only with the client concerned but also with the Assertive Outreach service itself.

One of the team leaders despairingly commented: "Residential providers don't want to know because our clients are too much trouble, but the problem for us is trying to fit people into systems that we know aren't appropriate, and knowing that things will fail and fall apart sooner or later. Either the system is failing our clients or our clients are failing the system. And the system places the blame on us if our clients fail. We have to live with a constant sense of failure... Sometimes our clients have to fail in order to prove that the system is. It's so frustrating knowing what you know and knowing that you can't deliver." Another team member said: "You can't win really, the system becomes fragmented and it's just a battleground between teams" (Ryan and Green 2001).

It is important to remember that Assertive Outreach teams actually are targeted to meet the needs of the most disadvantaged, problematic and risky of clients. Inevitably, therefore, it can be a considerable 'shock to the system' when local services are forced by referrals from Assertive Outreach teams to examine their referral criteria, and be prepared to work with substantially more disadvantaged clients than they are used to. This can be very frustrating and alienating for the Assertive Outreach teams, who can themselves feel isolated and distanced from non-responsive local services.

For this reason, we feel it is very important that Assertive Outreach teams develop a strengths approach, not only to engage their service users but just as importantly to engage their local services. Local services can be even more difficult to engage than the service users!

TOWARDS A STRENGTHS APPROACH TO CARE CO-ORDINATION

Essentially, this approach would aim to take all the strengths principles and practices associated with good service user engagement, and apply them to other service providers. It becomes a serious selling game if we are to change minds and attitudes in order to open up the needed opportunities for service users to participate fully and achieve greater social inclusion. At a more practical level, strengths-based Assertive Outreach can play a significant role in redefining how the functions of care co-ordination can be delivered.

Traditionally, the CPA has been seen by many practitioners as becoming a bureaucratic and administrative process that essentially takes time away from the real work of direct contact with service users. The individual care co-ordinator carries an identified caseload of people for whom they are charged with particular responsibility 'to co-ordinate the delivery of the care plan' (Department of Health 1999). This usually entails the time-consuming demands of setting up the 'review meeting' in order to complete the CPA form. Telephone calls to co-ordinate different people's diaries can seem to take more time than is spent delivering the decisions agreed in the previous care plan. Pressure of time, and a consultant psychiatrist-oriented process in many local services, can lead to an unrepresentative use of time – where mental state and medication reviews are often the primary achievement of the meeting. It is highly unlikely that this really represents a review of complex needs in a service user-involving way. Service users and Assertive Outreach practitioners may both feel dissatisfied by the process in these circumstances.

Potential considerations for positive change

1. Establish a system for prioritizing the service users who require a complex meeting attended by multidisciplinary and multi-agency personnel, with or without the service user or carer present.
2. Identify the service users for whom 'the meeting' is not necessarily the best mode of care plan review.
3. Ensure that the regular service user contacts and interventions involve a user-led review of care.

4. Ensure that Assertive Outreach contacts with other service providers can enable a review of care, in place of the wider meeting, where appropriate.
5. Tie in the contact reviews with close proximity to supported attendance at outpatient appointments.
6. Check if realistic expectations are being placed on the individuals, the team and the process itself, within the available resources and priorities.
7. Set up routine systems for good communication within the team, and with other agencies – additional to reliance on the CPA form as the main method of communication.
8. Consider how the team approach method of care planning, review and co-ordination can achieve the principles set out in national guidance and local policy, i.e. the 'Assertive Outreach team' *is* the care co-ordinator if it fulfils all the functions.
9. Target team training and practice development resources to prioritize the skills of effective communication and co-ordination, including chairing meetings with authority and confidence.

CONCLUSIONS

Care planning is the method for articulating the service user's identified needs into coherent actions. By linking short-term goals to the bigger picture of longterm personal aspirations, Kisthardt (1992) reminds us that the process helps people to see how small-scale immediate achievements provide the stepping-stones toward greater positive change. It operationalizes a number of the underlying principles of the strengths approach: with the person directing the helping process through their articulation of priority needs and wants; the ability to learn, grow and change, through developing short-term goals with positive expectations of success; and linking in all the available community and professional resources in their own defined neighbourhood.

Service users occupy a very complex place, with statutory sector services provided by health and social care agencies, housing and welfare rights administered through entirely different agencies, and the voluntary sector and local neighbourhood made up of a patchwork of flexible and creative resources. No single Assertive Outreach team is able to deliver on the complex range of needs from its resources alone, so systems of co-ordination are required in order for the care plans to be effectively implemented. Active listening to the service user, and attention to strengths and abilities, will offer greater opportunities for involving people at the centre of their care, and engage people more fully with the process.

Care planning and care co-ordination is frequently seen as the aspect of work concerned with the paperwork representation of an office-based administrative process (Morgan 2001). It needs to be seen in a more positive light, responsive to the recording of practical and dynamic interrelationships between all the people involved in the care and support of service users (Sanderson et al 1997).

References

Allen C 1998 The Care Programme Approach: the experiences and views of carers. Mental Health Care 1 (5): 160–162

Barham P 1994 Schizophrenia and Human Value. Routledge, London

Bleach A, Ryan P 1995 Community Support for Mental Health. Pavilion, Brighton

Burns T, Firn M 2002 Assertive outreach in mental health: a manual for practitioners. Oxford University Press, Oxford

Chadwick P, Birchwood M, Trower P 1996 Cognitive Therapy for Delusions, Voices and Paranoia. Wiley, Chichester

De Jong P, Miller S 1995 How to interview for client strengths. Social Work 40 (6): 729–736

Department of Health 1990 The Care Programme Approach for People with a Mental Illness Referred to the Specialist Psychiatric Services. HC(90)23/LASSL(90)11. HMSO, London

Department of Health 1999 Effective Care Co-ordination in Mental Health Services: Modernising the Care Programme Approach. HMSO, London

Fitzsimmons S, Fuller R 2002 Empowerment and its implications for clinical practice in mental health: a review. Journal of Mental Health 11 (5): 481–499

Fowler D, Garety P, Kuipers L 1995 Cognitive Behaviour Therapy for Psychosis: Theory and Practice. Wiley, Chichester

Frankl V 1988 The Will to Meaning. Meridian, New York

Frankl V 2000 Man's Search for Ultimate Meaning. Perseus, Cambridge (Mass.)

Garber J, Seligman M 1980 Human Helplessness: Theory and Applications. Academic Press, New York

Kisthardt W E 1992 The strengths model of case management: the principles and functions of a helping partnership with persons with persistent mental illness. In: Saleeby D (ed) A Strengths Perspective for Social Work Practice. Longman, New York, p 59–83

Lecomte T, Cyr M, Lesage A et al 1999 Efficacy of a self-esteem module in the empowerment of individuals with chronic schizophrenia. Journal of Nervous and Mental Disease 187: 406–413

Macleod J, Nelson G 2000 Programs for the promotion of family wellness and the prevention of child maltreatment: a meta-analytic review. Child Abuse and Neglect 24: 1127–1149

Moore-Kirkland J 1981 Mobilising motivation: from theory to practice. In: Maluccio A (ed) Promoting Competence in Clients. New York Free Press, New York

Morgan S 2001 Scaling paper mountains. Openmind 107 (1): 20–21

Morgan S, Akbar-Khan S 2000 Individual care planning in the UK. In: Basset T (ed) Looking to the Future: Key Issues for Contemporary Mental Health Services. Pavilion/Mental Health Foundation, Brighton, p 77–86

Nelson G, Lord J, Ochocka J 2001 Empowerment and mental health in the community: narratives of psychiatric survivors. Journal of Community and Applied Social Psychology 11: 125–142

Phillips P 1998 The Care Programme Approach: the views and experiences of service users. Mental Health Care 1 (5): 166–168

Prilleltensky J, Laurendeau M 1994 Introduction, prevention and the public good. Canadian Journal of Community Mental Health 13: 5–9

Rapp C A 1998 The Strengths Model: Case Management with People Suffering from Severe and Persistent Mental Illness. Oxford University Press, New York

Rappaport J 1990 Research methods and the empowerment agenda. In: Tolan P, Keys C, Chertak F et al (eds) Researching Community Psychology. American Psychological Association, Washington DC

Ryan M, Deci E 2000 Self-determination theory and the facilitation of intrinsic motivation, social development and well-being. American Psychologist 55: 68–78

Ryan P, Green D 2001 Implementing Assertive Outreach: A Pilot Study. Internal Report, Middlesex University

Sanderson H, Kennedy J, Ritchie P et al 1997 People, Plans and Possibilities: Exploring person centred planning. SHS, Edinburgh

Theorell T, Alfredsson L, Knox S et al 1984 On the interplay between socio-economic factors, personality and work environment in the pathogenesis of cardiovascular disease. Scandinavian Journal of Work, Environment and Health 10: 373–380

Thompson S, Spacapan S 1991 Perceptions of control in vulnerable populations. Journal of Social Issues 47: 1–21

Trainor J, Tremblay J 1992 Consumer/survivor businesses in Ontario: challenging the rehabilitation model. Canadian Journal of Community Mental Health 11: 65–71

Ware N 1999 Evolving consumer households: an experiment in community living for people with people with severe psychiatric disorders. Psychiatric Rehabilitation Journal 23: 3–10

Chapter 10

Using psychosocial interventions with the service user

Steve Morgan and Peter Ryan

Don't do things to me, do things for me, but preferably do things with me

INTRODUCTION

Theories and research evidence play an important role in the development and evolution of mental health services. Without them we would most likely find a very ad hoc loosely defined patchwork of services developed largely on individual whim and initiative, with little coherent rationale for doing what is provided locally: a 'postcode lottery' of health care. Over the last 20 years there have been some very exciting developments in the community treatment of people with severe, longterm mental illness. Mueser et al (2001) define psychosocial intervention as meaning: "nonpharmacological interventions designed to decrease symptom severity or distress, avoid hospitalisations, improve psychosocial functioning (e.g. work and social relationships) or improve satisfaction with life." The psychosocial interventions to be discussed in this chapter are:

- relapse prevention – early signs, relapse signatures and relapse drills
- medication adherence
- cognitive behavioural interventions – working with service user cognitive appraisals
- behavioural family intervention.

Many of these new developments have been extensively evaluated, on the whole with encouraging results. The best single overview of the psychosocial interventions is by Gamble and Brennan (2000). The research evidence has also been well summarized by Mueser et al (2001), Brooker (2001) and Bustillo et al (2001). The advent of the new 'evidence-based interventions' present an exciting challenge to Assertive Outreach as to many other areas of mental health care. There is however also quite a lot of evidence (Fadden 1997) to suggest that these new evidence-based interventions, certainly with respect to family intervention, fail to be implemented satisfactorily. Creative, flexible adaptation to real-life requirements (practice-based evidence) is necessary therefore to enable effective implementation of these approaches to occur. This involves a lot more than training. The challenge is how the psychosocial interventions can best be integrated within existing modalities of service delivery so as to give 'added value' to mental health service users. A process of practice development needs to be established, which leads to a seamless process of embedding them into practice (see Chapter 12 for our views as to how this can best be achieved).

It is important to recognize that for many if not all service users the benefits and attractions of Assertive Outreach lie in its flexibility, and responsiveness to priorities and agendas set by service users themselves. Usually, these priorities are extremely practical: fix my cooker; sort out my welfare benefits; get me better housing. It may be humbling for professionals but the availability of psychosocial intervention per se is likely to be a matter of indifference to service users: it is only if they can make a practical contribution to the achievement of service user goals that they become relevant.

This chapter will adopt the framework of one complex case study to provide continuity of a theme in presenting the many challenges for the effective implementation of psychosocial interventions within Assertive Outreach. The chapter commences quite deliberately with 'prioritizing the practical', as a reminder to us that this is the touchstone for effective delivery. The chapter then briefly outlines the major elements of these new interventions and summarizes the evidence base underpinning them. It then explores the underlying principles as to how the main psychosocial interventions discussed here can best be integrated within Assertive Outreach. The implications of crisis and crisis response are then discussed. The chapter then gives a series of practice examples of integration into practice and illustrates the implementation difficulties of doing so.

PRIORITIZING THE PRACTICAL

The predominant focus of the relationship between service users and service practitioners is the provision and delivery of care, support, treatment and interventions. At the crux of the matter is how much practitioners do this work *with* people, or whether it is something done *to* or *for* people. Strengths Assertive Outreach (or strengths applied to any other part of the mental health system) promotes the notion of working with people in a very real way. This is not just an academic debate, it lies at the very heart of the differences of approach to practice that will greatly influence how an individual service user perceives and ultimately engages with a service – or not.

Engagement should never be considered simply as a first and entirely discrete function that can be ticked off as completed before progressing to the important business of delivering mental health interventions. It is not 'sleight of hand' possessed by the discerning Assertive Outreach worker alone. The flexible and creative approaches necessary for developing some degree of engagement are likely to set up expectations in the service user (and some carers). Having demonstrated a service with a difference, the difficult challenge then becomes one of sustaining the difference throughout all aspects of the work. The strengths approach will only come to be seen as a valid vehicle for positive change where such expectations are sustained.

The baseline for developing the strengths approach to the individuality of people is established through strengths assessments and care planning (see Chapters 8 and 9). The potential range of activities that may be used as part of working with service users is never-ending but some of the more frequent areas of work are as follows:

- creative, meaningful engagement on the service user's terms
- assessment (including mental state, risk, needs and strengths)
- symptom management
- psychosocial interventions, e.g. cognitive behavioural therapy and behavioural family interventions
- care planning, implementation, evaluation and review (to include relapse prevention, crisis resolution/contingency planning)
- medication management, including education, promoting informed choice, assessment, monitoring side-effects and collaborative review
- meeting and maintaining accommodation needs within local resources
- ensuring rightful entitlement to welfare benefits
- financial management
- practical assistance and supporting activities of daily living, with the aim of promoting a level of independence in shopping, cooking, laundry, housekeeping and self-care
- accessing and supporting appropriate resources for physical health
- promotion of meaningful daytime occupations, including social, leisure, education, employment and vocation
- consideration for cultural and spiritual well-being
- working with substance misuse
- working with the criminal justice system
- working towards social inclusion, through accessing the ordinary resources available to the local neighbourhood
- advocacy, for accessing rights and entitlements
- interagency and multidisciplinary liaison
- carer/family work
- working to reduce stigma and discriminatory practices towards persons with mental health problems.

This list illustrates one of the core components of effective Assertive Outreach practice – that service practitioners will need to be flexible and creative in the ways they are able to deliver a broad range of working options and interventions in their practice. At the root of this ability will be a further core component of a team approach, enabling access to the full range of knowledge, skills and personalities of a team. More often, it is the simple practical tasks that people are finding difficulty with that may offer an insight to personal priorities, help to establish a sense of trust in the difference offered by the service, and subsequently provide the basis for the more challenging conversations around experiences and management of mental distress.

Assertive Outreach is charged with finding ways of re-engaging and motivating people who have clearly become disenchanted or even dis- enfranchised by the more traditional and restrictive methods of service delivery. The challenge becomes one of adapting rather than adopting formal models, in ways that connect with the experiences and aspira- tions of the service user, with due regard and attention paid to risks, crises and the positive potentials of risk taking.

Application to practice

The principles of a strengths approach to Assertive Outreach (see Chapter 3) clearly identify 'working on the person's own territory' as an essential core component of effective practice, and as an important shift for providing service delivery with a difference. The delivery of an Assertive Outreach service requires creativity and flexibility if it is to meet the needs of people previously mistrustful of the services offered. These qualities will be demonstrated in many ways but most simply in the places where workers are prepared to deliver the service. It requires a substantial shift away from relying on service-based locations, though these will be relevant for some people at certain times, e.g. assertive 'inreach' during inpatient admissions.

Within a necessary context of personal safety, the list of places where Assertive Outreach workers could be expected to work is endless. The issue is about responding to the service user's expression of where they feel most comfortable to meet, and work on the identified needs. The all- important change is one of getting away from thinking about service venues as a first option.

The challenge presented to practitioners working within the strengths approach is to suspend our natural tendency as people to make judge- ments of others based on our own codes or standards. This automat- ically leads us to interpret things we see as different in the environment to be a likely consequence of a relapsing mental state, and as a problem needing to be fixed. In Gavin's example (Boxes 10.1–10.7), it is important to establish an understanding of how he perceives and lives in his world. Is it necessarily a problem for him? If it is not, we could spend a great deal of wasted time and energy trying to change something by working against a natural wall of resistance. Is he unaware of a clear causal link between the way he chooses to live, and the abuse or threats he receives from others? Is it ultimately more beneficial to support taking the risk of him continuing with his current choices, or hope that he will change his ways by gentle persuasion of the alternative ways? There are no simple answers to these complex individual questions but they are the questions that mental health workers need to be more open to debating, amongst themselves and with service users.

Box 10.1   Case scenario: basic background

Gavin is 41 years old and lives alone in a first-floor one-bedroom council maisonette in a block of flats on a large inner-city estate. He has lived in his current accommodation for 14 years. He has been diagnosed with paranoid schizophrenia and personality disorder since his late teenage years. He has had four lengthy stays in hospital, all by compulsory admission following concerns expressed by his family who live locally, or from neighbours contacting the police.

He is believed to be very suspicious of specific people on the estate, and rarely ventures out of his home. He is generally described as being very neglectful of his appearance and environment. He appears to order much of his shopping through home delivery services, paying by credit card, or through contacts with family members. He always converses with delivery people through a closed door, and asks for the goods to be left outside the front door. Neighbours new and old are generally disturbed by his rare appearances – regardless of weather conditions he wears a lot of old and dishevelled clothing, and keeps his head and face covered by a balaclava and scarf drawn up over his nose.

Referral (from the community mental health team consultant psychiatrist to the Assertive Outreach team)

Referral was triggered by concerns expressed by Gavin's mother that he is becoming increasingly concerned about threats from other people living on the estate. She feels he is probably concealing weapons for protection against intruders. Community mental health team staff have recently written several appointment letters and made weekly brief visits, but have still managed no further contact with Gavin – he was last seen by services at hospital discharge two years ago.

Initial Assertive Outreach contacts

A letter from the team introduces who they are, who will be visiting and at what time, clearly stating they wish to hear about his concerns for his safety on the estate. Prior contact is made with Gavin's mother, as the person expressing concerns for him currently, and to enquire if there is anything that will help their approach to him to be more successful. The two named workers arrive as scheduled. It is suggested that they remain at the doorstep for some considerable time, as he will understandably be suspicious of strangers and will watch them through the spy-hole.

After 10 minutes of silence from within the flat Gavin opens the front door, and states the names of the two workers. They acknowledge his obvious reading of the letter of introduction and wait to be invited in. They do not make presumptions about his behaviour and aim to do things at his pace. Dressed in worn and soiled clothing, shoes and coat, he stares silently at the two workers from between hat and scarf for some further time, before furtively checking the surrounding estate from his doorstep. Before entering the workers enquire whether Gavin feels suspicious of

box continues

them – he replies that he is suspicious of all strangers but he does not think they are there to do him any harm. On entry to the maisonette they find the stairs covered in piles of newspapers, magazines, post and carrier-bags of unidentified items. On closer examination, these are carefully placed and stacked, with a cleared space for walking up the stairs. Gavin locks the front door in an apparent routine method of checking its security, and watches out of the spy-hole for a further few minutes.

The whole maisonette appears to be similarly arranged with carefully placed and stacked items, with cleared narrow pathways for walking from room to room. Furniture is sparse, and Gavin appears to spend most of his time on a mattress on the living-room floor facing the television in the corner of the room. After a somewhat bizarre and drawn out conversation, with many pauses and repetitions of phrases, Gavin states that he has been beaten up several times outside the flat by people on the estate waiting for him to come out, and on one occasion they broke open his old front door and threatened him inside his home. He produces a jagged piece of wood, which he proclaims to be his only souvenir of his old door. He also suggests that he frequently gets objects and abuse through the letterbox.

The two workers engage in conversation led by him about his way of coping with the practicalities of daily living in the maisonette. He shops by phone, and has social security benefits paid into a bank account, which he manages from home. They ask him if they can be of any help with any of these matters. Only on the fourth visit, when Gavin has also met a third team member, does he begin to negotiate help to check some of his post to see if he is receiving his full benefits entitlement. He also suggests that some of the older items stored around his flat are now rubbish, and need taking to the main bins and bottle bank across the estate. But, he gives no permission for anything to be cleared that he has not first checked himself. The workers remain cautious of the potential risks of a man who is deeply suspicious of a number of local people; Gavin assures them that he does keep a kitchen knife about his person but as a means of self-defence if he were to be attacked again. No overt discussion of mental state, symptoms or history of illness, or issues of medication are yet discussed with Gavin. The workers begin to ask him about his views and aspirations for accommodation, and most importantly continue to get to see him on a regular basis.

[More of Gavin's story follows in Boxes 10.2–10.7.]

RELAPSE PREVENTION

Psychotic relapse may be more predictable than we have traditionally believed, particularly if we subscribe to its close relationship to stress levels in the environment, i.e. a stress–vulnerability model (Nuechterlein and Dawson 1984). Cognitive, perceptual and behavioural processes indicative of an increased risk of relapse may precede the point of relapse. The frequency of relapse is associated with increased vulnerability to further episodes, as well as increased incidence of social difficulties and deficits in daily functioning. Therefore, it is important to address the potential for relapse at an early stage, to prevent its progression if possible.

In a review of recent literature, French and Walford (2001) highlight the confusion in using the term 'early intervention' as there are three distinct areas of practical application:

1. Primary – pre-onset of the first episode of psychosis.
2. Secondary – post-onset of the first episode of psychosis.
3. Tertiary – relapse prevention in established psychoses.

In this chapter, we are particularly concerned with tertiary early intervention as the client group most closely associated with Assertive Outreach services is likely to contain established histories of psychosis. The aim of developing greater knowledge and application of the techniques will be to promote early detection to reduce the length of duration that developing psychotic experiences remain untreated, with the goal of improving longer-term outcomes for reduced frequency of relapse and improved levels of functioning.

Each person may have a unique set of early signs: the 'relapse signature' (Birchwood 1996). Close monitoring of this can lead to early identification and potential intervention to minimize the severity of an episode of illness. The total elimination of the risk of relapse is not possible but targeted medical and psychosocial interventions are believed to support the aim of relapse prevention. Birchwood et al (1989) developed four categories associated with the prodromal lead-up to psychotic relapse:

1. Anxiety/agitation (sleep disturbance; tense; afraid; anxious; irritable; quick tempered).
2. Depression/withdrawal (quiet; withdrawn; depressed; low; poor appetite).
3. Disinhibition (aggression; restless; stubborn).
4. Incipient psychosis (behaves as if hallucinated; behaves as if being laughed at/talked about; behaves 'oddly').

A significant key to this area of work is that the earliest signs may not always be the usual medical symptoms of psychotic relapse but behavioural changes often recognizable to the service user and close carer or relative. French and Walford (2001) give examples of the early changes as:

- listening to a certain piece of music over and over
- wearing a piece of clothing that the person does not normally wear
- spending time in church, out of character with their normal beliefs or patterns of attendance.

Figure 10.1 gives an example of a service user's relapse signature, with the accompanying relapse drill, is based on a format developed by Plaistow and Birchwood (1996). The relapse drill is an important part of relapse prevention in that it enables the service user to keep in charge, and guide what happens at a stage when their signs and symptoms may be becoming very troublesome, and which if not acted upon could lead to relapse.

Figure 10.1   Relapse prevention sheet

Relapse signature	Relapse drill
Low mood/lack of motivation Greenhouse feeling (trapped, not achieving) Feeling increasingly sensitive and irritable Listening to the same music over and over Not eating very well Wake up early (4 am) and can't get back to sleep Frightened I am 'losing it' Stop taking medication Voices from the radio telling me to cut myself and end it all Assertive Outreach worker: Tel: Email:	**Step 1** • Get up by 11 am • Keep on going out (table tennis, snooker) • Contact my Assertive Outreach worker to set small achievable daily targets **Step 2** • See my Assertive Outreach worker to help me challenge my voices telling me to cut myself • Agree to depot medication **Step 3** • Arrange respite care • Refer myself to home treatment if my Assertive Outreach worker and I still feel I am losing it

The supporting evidence

One of the problems in the research literature is that the research does not give equal weight to French and Walford's (2001) useful distinction between primary, secondary and tertiary early intervention. Most of the evidence focuses mainly on secondary early intervention (post-onset of first-episode psychosis). With respect to secondary early intervention, Crow et al (1986) found that first-admission patients with schizophrenia who had been treated with medication during the first year of the onset of their condition were less likely to relapse at follow-up compared to patients who had been untreated during this first year. Crow concluded that failure to initiate early treatment may heighten the risk of relapse.

McGlashan et al (2001) report how by commencing to track patients with prodromal features of schizophrenia, and monitoring that through to the onset of a first psychotic episode, they are in fact able to reduce DUP (duration until psychosis) by timing their intervention to coincide with the onset of the psychotic episode. McGlashan et al (2001) report that for all patients so treated the outcome so far has been highly positive: no patient has required hospitalization; all but one patient has continued with scheduled daily activities at home or school; overall compliance with medication has been very high (93%); and all patients have retained their relationships with family and friends and maintained their social networks.

In the EPPIC model in Melbourne (McGorry et al 1996, McGorry and Jackson 1999), this early treatment consisted of short-term inpatient care, low-dose antipsychotic medication, outpatient case management, day care, vocational rehabilitation, family support and education, and cognitive therapy. This study compared a group of patients who had received the EPPIC approach with a matched group who had not. Patients receiving the EPPIC early treatment approach spent less time in hospital, and took lower doses of antipsychotic medication; however, at one-year follow-up there was no difference in symptomatology.

Warner (2001) suggests that a lengthy duration of untreated psychosis is likely to be associated with poor psychosocial adjustment, increased treatment costs, increased duration of the psychotic episode, and poorer course and outcome. He concludes that: "Although there is no conclusive evidence that early intervention in schizophrenia carries substantial benefits, the prevention of psycho-social decline secondary to prolonged illness is an attractive concept. The provision of optimal well-coordinated treatment as early as possible in the disorder could reduce relapse and maximise benefits for the patient and his or her family."

Relapse prevention: application into practice

Monitoring mental health, particularly its impact on day-to-day functioning and early signs of potential relapse, is a skill that all Assertive Outreach team members are able to provide. The team possesses a solid base of professional expertise from the diverse backgrounds of its members. The routine documentation of relapse signatures to better inform the team and wider network of early signs is an important aim, but as Gavin's experience highlights it is not something that can easily fit into a standard routine method of practice. The client group engaged with Assertive Outreach services is naturally a diverse range of people and personalities, and as such requires enormous flexibility in the application of theoretical models and approaches.

For some, the development of time-lines and full relapse signatures will flow from open discussions with the service user and others in their informal network. For others, it will be patchy and piecemeal, picked up from scraps of information observed rather than mutually agreed. There will also be many examples lying between these extremes. However, the application of tertiary early intervention practice into the Assertive Outreach team model of working will have a vitally important part to play.

As a response to identified warning signs, high-functioning Assertive Outreach teams are quick to discuss and implement practical strategies for closer monitoring of mental state, and rapid links to other specialist services, e.g. psychiatrists where cover is available. Accompanying people to appointments and monitoring medication adherence is seen to be a useful tool in relapse prevention, but the teams should also counterbalance this role by advocating for service user rights, sometimes for medication review and reduction, or occasional complaints about the service they are receiving from statutory agencies. Use of the team's supervision structures, and the development of risk management plans, are two strategies commonly used for working with early warning signs.

The two concepts of 'strengths working' and 'early intervention' share a great deal of harmony in their underlying principles. They both adopt a positive standpoint towards the service user's and carer's abilities, and they both prioritize the sharing of information to support informed choice within a context of service user decision making. The strengths principle of 'the service user as director of the helping process' (see Chapter 3) relies on good quality care plans, contingency plans and crisis plans being in place, based on attention to identifying the early warning signs as a method of protection against the damaging effects of repeated relapse.

The strengths practitioner will make every positive effort to introduce the ideas of early intervention and relapse prevention to service users and carers. The chosen approach will reflect individuals' reactions to the concept of relapse, recognizing that it can be an emotive subject to people who do not believe they experience a mental health problem. It should largely arise from a basis of open discussion, either to introduce the formal tools for a person's own use or, by reflecting back the observations made by the practitioners themselves, to check out possible validity in the service user's experience. The focus on strengths should potentially identify the person's abilities to work with the concepts of early signs monitoring. The focus on engaging the relationship should help to underpin the trust needed for disclosing early signs if they are recognized. Furthermore, the focus on strengths assessment may also help to uncover potential protective strategies from the individual's experiences and aspirations, extending the range of possible responses beyond a reliance on medication alone.

We cannot underestimate the importance of establishing alliances with the service user and other people in their informal network, as they generally have earlier opportunities to identify the early warning signs. Each episode needs to be seen as a further learning opportunity, and the service user and carers should be fully involved, informed and educated about changes to the pattern of the relapse signature resulting from new information. The overall approach is one of:

- developing the relapse signature through identifying the prodromal signs
- identifying the stress-related triggers and risk factors
- developing a relapse prevention plan with the service user and others
- monitoring for early signs
- responding rapidly when early signs are recognized by targeting responses to what you see rather than what it may become.

The first line of treatment will most often be through maintenance medication and increased compliance but associated with other appropriate interventions, e.g. family work, substance misuse treatment strategies, supportive counselling, 'hearing voices' groups and crisis intervention strategies. Continuous monitoring offers the opportunity of assessing the severity and potential timescales of relapse, as some people spiral down very quickly into a distressed and chaotic condition, while others can maintain their more usual levels of functioning for much longer periods.

The experience of relapse is not something that usually happens suddenly overnight, and the quicker it is picked up the greater is the chance of offering appropriate treatment and support to minimize the impact. The timescales between stages will vary between individuals, and even between episodes, and one tool for identifying and recording appropriate information will be a 'time-line' – plotting the significant events and changes in their chronological order.

Watkins (2001) reminds us: "A relapse prevention plan that includes early signs monitoring is essential for people who want to try living without long-term medication or who want to reduce it and avoid a further disruptive breakdown in their personal and social functioning...". However, Birchwood et al (1998) also indicate that despite a growing wealth of research in this area of emerging clinical practice continuous monitoring of early warning signs of relapse can be very detrimental for some people, causing them greater anxiety through the focus on the potential for relapse.

Box 10.2   Gavin's story (continued)

When the Assertive Outreach workers felt able to raise the subject of monitoring for early warning signs of relapse they felt the need to approach the subject very tactfully. Gavin had made his views known on several occasions that he did not necessarily agree with the diagnoses of schizophrenia and personality disorder. He had given an impression of being open to discuss what they meant and to consider their possible applicability to his circumstances. However, on occasions when the subject was reintroduced by the team he would frequently deny having experienced anything that could be given such labels, and claim to have no idea what reasons he presented to justify being taken into hospital on all the previous occasions.

Gavin consistently maintained that his problems all result from the actions of other people on the local estate. When the notion of 'early signs' was introduced, he quickly interpreted this as a mechanism for justifying his view of the world – the early signs were the actions of others threatening him! Discussion amongst the team, back in a specific team meeting, concluded that the discussion should be maintained at a low level with Gavin, not to risk him refusing contact. The team would accept his views but continually watch for any signs of changed behaviour or emotional reaction to his environment.

Discussion with Gavin's mother

Permission was asked from Gavin for the team to talk with his mother about her knowledge of the troubles he had experienced on the estate, and possible reasons for his previous hospital admissions. Gavin suggested that she had such little contact with him that she would not have much information to give them, but he raised no objections to such contact, stating that both she and the team were of some use to him.

box continues

His mother confirmed that she did not have regular close contact with Gavin to be able to provide the kind of detail that would describe what happens when things are not going so well. For her the main issue was Gavin's increased concern for the thoughts and actions of other people he perceived to be threatening him on the estate. She did think that he carried a kitchen knife with him, or kept it behind the front door at times when all he could talk about was 'them'. She was convinced that he was threatened by others, and had been assaulted on occasions by gangs of local youths. She admitted his behaviour, way of talking and living was 'extremely odd' but said he had been that way for many years, it was not something that she had thought of in terms of deteriorating as he became unwell.

The conclusion of this area of working was an agreement that Gavin's mother would try to think about the ideas of early warning signs and discuss her thoughts with the team. The Assertive Outreach team would continue to work with Gavin on practical issues, while also continuing to watch for potential early signs, and to keep raising questions of diagnosis, medication and lead up to hospital admissions with him in a low key and consistent manner that respected his views on the subject matter.

MEDICATION ADHERENCE

Since the first use of chlorpromazine for the treatment of psychiatric disturbance in 1951, medication has occupied a central role in the medical management of severe mental distress as services have progressively moved from an institutional base to a dispersed community focus. Medication is the most widely researched form of intervention available to mental health services. Johnstone (1989) suggests that medication offers no cure but may have some qualified success in suppressing distressing symptoms, helping people to live reasonable lives outside of hospital and helping the prevention of some relapses. Shepherd (1991) echoes these sentiments, suggesting that 'chronic' conditions, with persistent and sometimes intractable symptoms, cannot realistically expect to achieve anything more than degrees of symptom relief. The primary aim becomes one of trying to help people develop their functional abilities and, at the very least, enable them to function at an optimal level despite their symptoms. 'Symptoms' and 'functioning' must therefore be considered as potentially independent domains. Realistically, we are looking to support a person's ability to manage and cope with the experience of distress.

Working to reduce side-effects

When weighing up the value of medication we need to be equally aware of the potential side-effects and damaging impact on functioning (Diamond 1998), which can significantly reduce a person's ability to motivate themselves to engage in meaningful activity. The introduction of clozapine (Clozaril) and the atypical antipsychotics has greatly increased the options open in terms of optimizing medication levels whilst reducing

Table 10.1 Side-effects of antipsychotic drugs

Side-effects	Signs/Symptoms
Hypotension	Reduced blood pressure, dizziness
Dystonia	Muscle spasm (especially neck), fixed gaze
Akathisia	Restlessness, inability to sit or stand for long, shifting or tapping feet
Parkinsonism	Rigidity, tremor, 'masked face', shuffling gait
Tardive dyskinesia	Abnormal mouth or tongue movements, bodily tics or abnormal movements or grunting
Antipsychotic malignant syndrome	Muscle rigidity, rapid heart beat
Anticholinergic effects	Dry mouth, blurred vision, constipation, sexual dysfunction (erectile problems)

side-effects to a minimum. Table 10.1 summarizes some of the side-effects people suffering from schizophrenia can experience. Burns and Firn (2002) make the useful point that: "Simply having a range of possible treatments, with different profiles of effects and side-effects, means that negotiation is not simply a token but a meaningful and concrete component in the therapeutic relationship. It is no longer taking the medicine or not taking the medicine but choosing *which medicine*."

Working to increase adherence

Certainly in the context of a strengths approach to Assertive Outreach, it never makes sense to consider issues around adhering to medication outside the context of the user's own aspirations. Very rarely, if ever, is a user likely to put taking the tablets as a major life goal in its own right, although adhering to medication might well make sense in the context of an expressed wish, for example, to stay out of hospital or to seek paid employment. If taking medication fits within an aspiration the user themselves puts forward, and is seen as materially instrumental in achieving that aim, then adherence is a good deal more likely. Seen in this context, Kemp et al (1997) have developed a useful model of 'compliance therapy' (Table 10.2). The approach is based on a collaborative approach, which emphasizes client choice. It also references motivational interviewing approaches (Rollnick et al 1992), which again emphasize going at the service user's pace, and gentle encouragement rather than prescription.

The supporting evidence

Both Curson et al (1985) and Hirsch et al (1973) conducted randomized controlled trials in which they found that patients receiving (depot) medication stayed out of hospital for longer periods than those not taking medication. However, Curson et al also found that the patients receiving depot medication fared slightly worse than those not taking medication in terms of social and occupational adjustment. A number of studies have explored the impact of medication adherence programmes. Kemp et al (1997) undertook a randomized controlled trial based in an inpatient unit.

Table 10.2 Principles and phases of compliance therapy (adapted with permission from Kemp et al 1997)

Principles

- Framed in terms of contribution towards achieving user's own goals
- Emphasis on personal choice and responsibility
- Non-blaming
- Support self-monitoring and self-management

Phases

Phase 1 Explore user's attitude towards medication

- Review previous experience of medication
- Explore user's attitude towards taking medication
- Acknowledge negative experience
- Explore user's experience of mental health services and hospitalization in particular
- Explore any links between hospitalization and ceasing to take medication

Phase 2 Explore ambivalence to treatment

- Explore dislike of medication – side-effects, stigma, etc.
- Identify side-effects experienced by user
- Provide information and clarify any misunderstandings
- Explore advantages and disadvantages – what has helped or hindered?
- Clarify what the advantages of taking medication might be in the context of user's own expressed aspirations

Phase 3 Negotiate a rationale and plan for taking medication

- Confirm with user how medication fits into expressed aspiration/user goal
- Review with user and psychiatrist current medication as to how side-effects can be minimized – including change of medication where indicated
- Identify relapse signature and relapse drill if not done before

It compared brief (four to six) sessions of 'compliance therapy' against nonspecific counselling. The trial took under three weeks to complete and showed that the experimental group of patients did significantly better than the control group in increasing their levels of compliance. These were maintained over the ensuing 6, 12 and 18 months (Kemp et al 1998).

Cramer and Rosenheck (1999) found that behavioural tailoring produced good results. They developed a Medication Usage for Effectiveness (MUSE) programme, which consisted of a 15-minute initial orientation followed up by monthly checks. After six months they found that the clients receiving the MUSE programme did significantly better in maintaining improvements in adherence.

Medication adherence: application to practice

Onyett (1992) states that the closer and more intensive relationship established through case management (Assertive Outreach) could be beneficial for monitoring symptom changes and variable use of medication. This relationship can ensure more detailed and open discussion with people about their own views and experiences of using medication, with improved two-way communication of the essential information to support constructive negotiation or even adherence to prescribed medication regimes.

People have many personal reasons for objecting to the medication prescribed for them: experience of side-effects; experience of stigma; fear of being on it for life; objections to relying on chemical agents; and enjoyment or acceptance of some positive symptoms. Morgan (1993) suggests that, whatever the basis of the objections raised, it is important that they are acknowledged constructively. Refusal should not be dealt with in a punitive manner or be seen as a failure on the part of the practitioner(s). Even though there is much evidence that medication can have positive effects for people experiencing severe and enduring mental health problems, its prescription should always be approached on an individual case-by-case basis, acknowledging the potential negative consequences and the need for constant review and reduction. Above all else, there should be a clear acknowledgement and response to the person's right to make an informed choice.

Box 10.3   Gavin's story (continued)

The Assertive Outreach team were already aware from the details of the referral that Gavin had not been seen by anybody in the community mental health team during the last two years, so may not have been taking any prescribed medication during this time. He was not apparently enthusiastic about taking medication during his last admission on the inpatient unit.

No proactive discussion about medication was planned for the first few visits but on the fourth visit Gavin suddenly mentioned that he had been told previously that he was 'schizophrenic and a personality disorder.' One of the Assertive Outreach workers responded to the comment, encouraging Gavin to explain the situation in which this information arose. The subsequent discussion was relatively short, with Gavin suggesting that he did hear voices in his head but did not want medication to block them out. He suggested that the predominant voice was that of a woman, commenting on the people around the estate who troubled him. Occasionally other voices would make disparaging comments about him but Gavin claimed these did not trouble him.

The Assertive Outreach workers acknowledged Gavin's views and thanked him for sharing this personal information with them. They offered to discuss schizophrenia, personality disorder and the medication he was previously prescribed, without any pressure to rush such discussions.

Morgan (1993) suggests that greater adherence can only be genuinely advocated through workers assisting service users to see ways in which taking medication genuinely links into their own aspirations. The use of supportive counselling and the provision of additional information concerning the likely consequences of not taking medication in any given instance can play an important role in helping people to weigh up the positive and negative impact of decisions about the taking or ceasing of medication. Reliance on a strong trusting relationship can also provide the basis for negotiating medication reductions and drug-free periods, with the support and close monitoring of the service users themselves, their carers and the Assertive Outreach staff (Onyett 1992).

COGNITIVE BEHAVIOURAL THERAPY

Over the past decade there has been growing interest in applying cognitive behavioural therapy (CBT) techniques to clients with severe longterm mental illness, especially those who continue to experience psychotic symptoms despite taking the appropriate medication. The principal aims of CBT tend to be to reduce the intensity and the distress of the service user's delusional system, and to promote their active participation in reducing the risk of relapse and levels of disability. One formative influence in it has been Beck's (1976) analysis of how cognitions or inferences can be distorted or biased through the interaction with strong affective states or moods. Beck identified six such 'distortions':

- **Arbitrary inference** where a conclusion is drawn arbitrarily and at some distance from the facts available.
- **Selective abstraction** where a detail is taken out of context, other salient issues ignored and focused on to the exclusion of everything else.
- **Overgeneralization** where a conclusion or general rule is made on the basis of one or more isolated incidents, and is applied to virtually all situations.
- **Magnification and minimization** where errors of judgement are made either in exaggerating or in minimizing the significance or importance of a particular event.
- **Absolutistic, dichotomous or black-and-white thinking** where all judgements or statements are placed into one of two polarized and categorical opposites.

The rationale for CBT is that an individual's emotional response is mediated through their system of beliefs, cognitions and making inferences. A CBT intervention seeks to explore, challenge and dispute dysfunctional beliefs, leading to decreasing negative emotions and to developing more adaptive perceptions and beliefs. CBT typically consists of:

- development of a collaborative relationship with the client
- exploration of the symptoms and their meaning to the client
- assisting the client in checking the objective evidence supporting the stated assumptions
- encouraging the client to 'reality test' his or her assumptions.

The supporting evidence

Kuipers et al (1997) found that clients receiving CBT achieved a significant reduction in overall symptoms compared to standard treatment but did not experience reductions in specific psychotic symptoms. Tarrier et al (1998) did find significant reductions in psychotic symptoms compared to standard care, which were maintained over a 12-month follow-up period. This study included blind rating of symptoms. Working in an inpatient setting, Drury et al (1996) found that CBT plus antipsychotic medication led to significantly faster and more complete recovery from the psychotic episode. At nine-month follow-up, 95% of the CBT group reported no or only minor psychotic symptoms, compared to 44% of the control group. In this study, the CBT clinicians themselves carried out symptom ratings.

In summary, the relatively few randomized controlled trials of CBT do provide positive evidence for its efficacy in either reducing overall symptom levels, or in some cases having specific effects in reducing psychotic symptomatology in particular. It would seem to have applicability both in acute inpatient and in community settings, and to have effects that last over time. However, CBT does not appear to extend to other areas of functioning such as social adjustment. Neither is there currently evidence that it reduces relapse rates.

BEHAVIOURAL FAMILY INTERVENTION

The components of effective family intervention are:

- acceptance of a stress–vulnerability model of schizophrenia
- the service user maintained on medication
- commencing family intervention when the family motivation is at its highest, i.e. just after an acute episode of relapse
- developing a trusting working relationship between the practitioners and family members
- the service user and family being seen together, at least for some of the time
- family sessions generally conducted at home
- an emphasis on information and education to enhance understanding of the illness
- cognitive behavioural interventions focused on practical day-to-day issues
- enhancing family problem-solving skills
- a focus on the communication patterns used in the family, attempting to reduce the negative and critical exchanges
- realistic expectations held by all
- encouraging interests outside the family for all family members
- interventions provided with follow-up or embedded in the ongoing package of care.

(based with permission on Fadden 1998)

A number of formal tools have been designed to support the implementation of effective family interventions. Barrowclough and Tarrier (1992) include:

- relative assessment interview
- family questionnaire

- social functioning scale
- personal functioning scale
- knowledge about schizophrenia interview.

One danger lies in overformalizing the approach, to the extent of burdening the service user, relatives and practitioners with too much paperwork, and losing sight of the real needs of the individual and family members. The effectiveness of family interventions is also largely dependent on the availability and quality of training and supervision for the practitioners delivering the service. Brooker et al (1994) demonstrated the importance of highly skilled trainers and intense supervision as essential for successful implementation. However, even with attention to the need for skilled training and supervision Fadden (1997) reported that many practitioners struggled to implement these interventions in their routine work because of the lack of support within the service to resolve the competing tensions of other work responsibilities and creating sufficient time.

The supporting evidence

Since 1980, over a dozen randomized controlled trials have been carried out on behavioural family intervention, where the duration of treatment has been over nine months (Mueser et al 2001). There are clear indications that family intervention works best over relatively extended periods of time. All short-term family interventions of less than three months' duration except one (Goldstein et al 1978) have been ineffective. The primary outcomes for which behavioural family intervention has been evaluated are the prevention of psychotic relapse and the avoidance of hospitalization. In addition to family intervention, all clients in these studies have also received a programme of medication, case management, and other services such as day care where available. Typically, studies have compared behavioural family intervention and family psycho-educational approaches, to 'standard' outpatient care and/or individual psychotherapy. The impact of multiple family therapy has also been evaluated (McFarlane et al 1995).

Barrowclough and Tarrier (1992) summarized the findings from a number of international studies in the early 1980s through to the mid-1990s demonstrating the effectiveness of family interventions with people experiencing schizophrenia. They primarily focused on practical problems and coping skills within the family, with the services developing a specific emphasis on providing psycho-education for all family members. Fadden (1998) suggested that when these approaches were combined with psychopharmacological treatments there was a consistent drop in relapse rates. "The interventions have also been found to be culturally robust, applicable to routine clinical settings, and to result in reduced costs for the care of the people with schizophrenia. In spite of the evidence of their effectiveness, these approaches are not being applied routinely, and the majority of people with schizophrenia do not receive family intervention."

Dixon and Lehman (1995) raise the point that the evidence is more conclusive that family interventions delay rather than prevent relapse in people who have significant family contacts. However, Tarrier et al (1994) have produced evidence to indicate reduction in relapse rates being sustained across five- and eight-year follow-up periods, where the specific short-term interventions are carefully integrated into ongoing care packages. Fadden (1998) reports that for families identified as having high 'expressed emotion' the evidence suggests that effectiveness is closely associated to the use of individual family therapy where the service user is involved in most sessions, and that psychodynamic and multifamily approaches are far less effective. There is a danger in assuming that families with low expressed emotion are in less need of family intervention. Tarrier et al (1988) found that low 'EE' families had a potential to develop more critical or hostile responses over time where there was no psycho-educational input. Fadden (1998) also reviews the evidence that interventions provided in the home have a higher success rate, largely due to the non-attendance rates associated with clinic-based programmes.

Bustillo et al (2001) concluded: "On average, relapse rates amongst schizophrenic patients whose treatment involves family therapy are approximately 24% as compared to about 64% for those who receive routine treatment. In addition, the beneficial effects of long term intervention (i.e. greater than nine months) appear to be quite durable, and may be maintained for two years or longer." However, it is also important to note that two studies (Linszen et al 1996, Hogarty et al 1997) found low relapse rates for both control and experimental groups but with no advantage for the experimental group receiving family intervention. Mueser et al (2001) concluded: "Both single family and multiple family interventions… were associated with fewer relapses and rehospitalisations, with rates about half that of routine treatment. It might be expected that the profound effect of family intervention on reducing relapse and rehospitalisations would result in substantial cost savings. Two studies of family intervention (Cardin et al 1986, Tarrier et al 1991) conducted cost analysis. In both cases, family intervention resulted in significant cost savings, mainly through reduced use of inpatient treatment costs." For example, Cardin et al (1986) found that the total costs of family intervention were 19% less than those of individual treatment, with the overall benefits favouring the family intervention.

Family intervention: application in practice

Assertive Outreach services are frequently working with people who are socially isolated to the extent of having lost most or all contact with their families and friends. For some people, the rare fleeting contact with a neighbour, or people serving in local shops, or the practitioners in the mental health services, may be the sum total of their social connections with the world. This must not lead teams to assume limited contact for all people referred to them. It is important to draw a wide definition of carers and friends, as the application of the principles of family intervention may have benefit beyond the scope of blood relatives alone. However, in contemporary society the significance given to connections with people outside the family circle also has to be closely scrutinized, e.g. people whose main contacts happen to be the suppliers of their non-prescription illicit drugs. There may be some benefits in making contact with some drug-related acquaintances, in order to negotiate and educate regarding the potential difficulties and dangers that drug misuse may be having on the service user, but this approach carries significant dangers of violence and aggression generally associated with accessing and taking drugs.

The formality of the approach encapsulated in the research does not easily relate to the experiences of delivering Assertive Outreach services. A planned approach to family intervention may be of use in establishing the aims you feel are important to achieve, but the route for getting there is likely to be far more tortuous than the simple expectations of delivering

---

Box 10.4   Gavin's story (continued)

Gavin's mother has continued her regular contact over the years but his father and two older siblings (sister and brother) have long since lost contact. His sister married and has a family of her own and, though she is concerned about Gavin, her husband does not want their children meeting him, or even knowing much about his existence. His brother only sees Gavin as a complete embarrassment and tries to deny they are in any way related. His father believes that Gavin's mother should let go of the contact, suggesting that it is detrimental to their own marital relationship.

Attempts at family interventions are severely restricted by the family dynamics. However, the Assertive Outreach team maintain regular contact with Gavin's mother (with his knowledge) to offer advice, information and support. She has been able to talk for the first time about the son she feels she has lost, and that she still thinks of him as the little boy and teenager who once had prospects and a future. She understands why other family members wish to disown him but still feels angry with them for not supporting her to help him more. Attempts to meet Gavin and his mother together at the flat have been largely blocked by him stating he has little need for such formality. There has been one brief meeting by the Assertive Outreach workers with Gavin and his mother on his doorstep – with the workers taking the few minutes' opportunity just to review how the overall work was going, without intruding into any sense of formality.

The general view held by both of them is that the services have done very little to explain what his condition is, or what they could offer to help other than hospital admissions and medication. This has led Gavin and his mother to be more negative about mental health services. This knowledge has been important for the Assertive Outreach team to consider how it tailors its approach to the needs of both people. The emphasis on offering information without imposing formal meetings has helped the team's engagement with both people.

a set number of face-to-face sessions. The research talks of the applicability of the approach to clinical settings but the bizarre circumstances encountered by Assertive Outreach services may frequently require a major adaptation of the methods in practice. For example, psycho-education may be offered through numerous very brief discussions with a person on their doorstep, over protracted periods, or you could be working with the conflicting views of family members who do not even sit down in the same room to talk, e.g. conducting multiple conversations by moving back and forth to different people located in the kitchen and the living room.

In an attempt to identify the positive potentials of the individual, and their wider social network, a strengths approach will naturally focus on the knowledge, skills and abilities of all the people significantly involved with the service user. We need to respect the limited amount of contact and input we have as practitioners, even in so-called intensive work, whereas a close friend, relative or neighbour is likely to be a much more significant resource and potential influence in the person's daily functioning. The strengths perspective is one that attempts to strengthen the positive sources of support and influence, by valuing the naturally occurring resources of the individual's definition of their own local neighbourhood. Adapting the messages from family intervention research and literature will be one way of articulating this particular strengths principle in practice. The team often provides ongoing education to both clients and their families into the nature and management of longterm mental illness. Behavioural family interventions (Fadden 1998) are used in order to optimize communication and support in the family. Essentially it is a form of individually tailored psycho-educational programme, which seeks to preserve the family as an asset and resource to the patient. The programme attempts to facilitate a supportive but not overinvolved or destructive relationship with the patient and the family.

CRISIS RESPONSES

Assertive Outreach and crisis response teams are being seen as two specialist elements of a comprehensive and integrated local mental health system (Department of Health 1999, 2000). Even with the coexistence of a crisis team, the reasonable expectations are that the Assertive Outreach team has a strong and intensive working relationship with their service users, and should be in a position to identify and manage crises sooner. They should have in place, as a part of the CPA care plan, a detailed and individualized response to potential crises, which will be triggered and followed when the circumstances arise. In the rarer event that the Assertive Outreach team cannot respond effectively to the needs of a crisis, it would have developed good links with other crisis services in the local system, which will be in a position to negotiate more intensive out-of-hours support or joint working arrangements.

Watkins (2001) suggests: "Crises can occur for many reasons. They commonly occur at times of transition, either developmental, situational or both, when the challenges of living overwhelm or exhaust our resources. How well we cope with the challenges of living depends on three factors:

- The nature of the challenge. The meaning it has for us. The magnitude and predictability of it, and the amount of control we have.
- The resources we have to draw on. Our personal coping strategies and the support we have available.
- Our sense of personal agency, of being in control of our lives."

It is natural for a crisis to be seen as a negative, frightening and damaging experience for service users and their wider social connections – a point of failure to cope, with demoralizing consequences that frequently lead to reliance on hospital admissions and medication. Similarly, practitioners may feel a service user's crisis is a reflection on their inability to manage and support a person effectively, or to prevent the cycle of relapses and remissions through hospital admission. Caplan (1964) suggests an alternative view that underpins the philosophy of the more effective and responsive crisis services – that, however painful and disorganizing a crisis seems to be at the time of acute illness, it is a crucial point if the person is open to be learning something about themselves. It can become a turning point where some people emerge stronger and more integrated. However, there are also many people for whom the opportunity of learning is too much of a challenge – they remain fragile and susceptible to return to a state of crises, requiring a greater dependence on others.

The South Camden Crisis Resolution and Response Team (2001) defines a psychiatric crisis as: "The point where an individual experiences a sudden or gradual change in their mental health and well-being, and their more usual coping strategies and mechanisms are no longer adequate to address the emerging predicament. It is characterised by a reduction in the individual's normal functioning, indicating a need for an increase in the intensity of support, which cannot be delivered by the present arrangement of support structures. In the past such episodes might have necessitated in-patient care." During a subsequent team away day in 2003, the team summarized its approach as "... providing short-term, intensive and supportive interventions, that are task-oriented, problem-solving, information giving, and dealing with the wider social systems as well as issues of medication compliance. It aims to promote the maximum level of independence and integration into the individual's own system or community by empowering people to exercise choices, and by learning the valuable information arising from the experience of the crises."

What are the differences between 'crisis prevention', 'crisis intervention', and 'crisis response and resolution'? We may be able to distinguish the value of good early signs monitoring as a way of identifying the early onset of relapse, with the aim of intervening appropriately to prevent the otherwise downward spiral into a psychiatric emergency. Crisis intervention involves brief periods of intensive support aimed at helping people through periods of high levels of distress, which may prevent the full-blown crisis or help to minimize its impact if it has already developed (Watkins 2001). Minghella et al (1998) suggest it is the responsibility of mental health services to support people through these chaotic periods in the most sensitive and effective way possible, minimizing further distress, risk and loss of liberty. The effectiveness of the response to the individual circumstances will determine the rapidity of the resolution of the particular crisis. In summary, we should prioritize the prevention of the potential crisis; failing this we should intervene to support the person through the crisis to the most satisfactory means of resolution.

A further core component of effective Assertive Outreach service delivery is its ability to ensure cover for 24 hours a day, seven days a week, 365 days a year. The tradition of 'normal' working hours misses the point of the experience of mental health distress – people cannot limit their crises from nine to five, and most services record an over-representation of hospital admissions or A&E visits at the periods of time when the normal support systems are unavailable. This does not necessarily mean that the Assertive Outreach team stretches its limited resources to be directly available at all times but that it should make every effort to connect service users and carers with the necessary contacts at any point of the 24-hour period.

Crisis resolution: application in practice

Staff within a strengths approach adopt an attitude that crises are learning experiences, forming a basis for the principle that people can learn, grow and change (see Chapter 3). Watkins (2001) reminds us that staff and service users can see a point of crisis as an opportunity for learning ways of managing the difficulties of daily living more effectively. It contributes to the knowledge that informs the relapse signature, thus improving our chances of future relapse prevention. In this way, an otherwise debilitating crisis can be seen as something positive. The approach is also characterized by frequent enquiries into 'what has worked well for you in the past?'.

The intrinsic activity of a strengths approach is involved in identifying personal and wider social resources. Thus, when a crisis is developing it is hoped that the person, their informal networks and practitioners are better equipped to mobilize the necessary resources to manage the crisis in a more effective way. Furthermore, the strengths assessment has helped the person to identify their personal aspirations and abilities, giving anchor points to stabilize the natural tendency for spiralling into a chaotic and disorganized state when in crisis.

The strengths approach does not ignore difficulties, crises and risks. It develops a more positive standpoint from which to assess and work with the difficulties. The enormous ongoing investment in developing a trusting relationship can be used as a buffer at times of crisis, even occasionally where the situation still results in a hospital admission. At these times, the strengths approach maintains the intensity of contact, through 'assertive inreach' to the inpatient unit, continuing to provide a different orientation to the service user's previous experience of the services. It works at reinforcing the validity of the strengths portrait already built up, as a catalyst for a quicker and positively co-ordinated discharge from hospital. People do not lose their previous achievements, their current resources or their most valued aspirations just because they have to go into hospital. They will most likely need a trusted ally to help remind them of the positive aspects of themselves while they are in an acute condition, and also to use the time constructively by adding to the body of personal knowledge and resources as clues arise.

Box 10.5   Gavin's story (continued)

A previous absence of mental health service engagement with Gavin or his mother has resulted in four hospital admissions, in distressing situations involving compulsion and a police presence, because of the perceived high risks of assault by Gavin on others. These circumstances have only served to raise Gavin's profile as an outcast on the estate. Whilst this situation is considered unsatisfactory, it has been the only expectation that they have both held for some time.

The Assertive Outreach workers use every available opportunity to remind Gavin and his mother that they could possibly avoid a repeat of these events in the future if they felt able to trust the Assertive Outreach team enough to disclose any difficulties or repeat patterns of crises at an early stage. The discussions take the form of asking about details of the lead up time to the previous crises, and consideration of what might be done at the different stages to prevent it getting to the point of hospital admission. An important basis for continuing these discussions with Gavin is enquiring about and valuing what he wants for the future. His expressed wishes are to not go back into hospital.

The Assertive Outreach workers use this aspiration as the reason for continuing to engage him in discussions about future crisis prevention. More frequently than not Gavin will resort to blaming others on the estate, accepting little or no personal responsibility for the difficulties that have arisen. The workers refrain from judging him on this one-sided view of events, preferring to keep the lines of communication open rather than risk his refusal to discuss the matter again.

Both Gavin and his mother are encouraged repeatedly by the Assertive Outreach workers to accept a list of emergency contacts for the late evenings and nights when the team is not immediately available. The negotiations continue to revolve around Assertive Outreach being the first point of contact in a crisis, hopefully, at least picking up any early signs during their 8.00 am to 8.00 pm hours of availability, rather than waiting for the possibility of more acute concerns arising by the early hours of the morning because the early concerns remained unattended. In the event that a response is needed out of hours, the Assertive Outreach team plans to introduce a member of the crisis team on one of their routine visits, to discuss the service they offer locally outside the Assertive Outreach team's hours of working.

WORKING WITHIN A WIDER SYSTEM

Effective functioning of an Assertive Outreach service largely depends on integration and good communication with other statutory and non-statutory mental health services. Assertive Outreach teams may carry high expectations but they cannot be set up, or set themselves up, to meet all the needs of all the people referred to them. However, they are expected to promote continuity of care and to ensure that the identified needs of the service users are met by the appropriate services.

Box 10.6   Gavin's story (continued)

On initial contact the Assertive Outreach workers enquired how Gavin felt physically. He responded positively to an approach that did not launch into an inquisition about his mental health. However, he has not made any contact with his GP for many years. Gavin was concerned about having to wait in the surgery to be seen, and tentatively agreed to the Assertive Outreach team arranging for the doctor to meet on Gavin's doorstep.

The GP was pleasantly surprised to hear that the mental health services had managed to make some contact with Gavin. Despite not having seen Gavin at the surgery, the doctor appeared to be quite aware of his existence on the estate and was prepared to negotiate a time for a joint visit to his flat. At the appointed time, Gavin refused to open the front door but did talk with the doctor briefly through the closed door. The subsequent agreement was that the Assertive Outreach team would remain in occasional contact with the GP to update the continuing negotiations with Gavin about having direct contact to review his physical condition.

Gavin is quite intelligent, despite the impression most people seem to make of him from a brief encounter or a description. He has managed, with some help from his mother, to work out his finances and order and pay for the necessary goods he requires by mail order or home delivery. The Assertive Outreach team reflect back to him his skills and resourcefulness, while offering to make any connections with other agencies that he wishes. They are careful not to make any presumptions and to act in his knowledge as they appreciate that he only maintains contact with them because he trusts they are not going to misuse that trust.

Integrating the psychosocial interventions into practice

We are of the view that there is a synergy between the psychosocial interventions and Assertive Outreach. There are, we think, some underlying commonalities of approach across the psychosocial interventions, which make them highly congruent and compatible with Assertive Outreach – see Table 10.3 and Mills (2000) for a fuller discussion. The challenge, as is made clear in the application to practice sections that follow, is to implement the psychosocial interventions effectively, in the context of how Assertive Outreach teams actually work. It is, moreover, not a simple matter of training clinicians to use them. The numerous barriers to effective implementation of the psychosocial interventions need more sophisticated strategies than training alone. These are explored in depth and detail in Chapter 12. We would say that the following principles are firmly embedded within Assertive Outreach (see Chapter 3), and that in that important respect Assertive Outreach provides a natural 'home' for the psychosocial interventions.

Engaging the service user collaboratively

All the main proponents of the psychosocial interventions discussed here emphasize the huge importance of working collaboratively with the service user. Both the service user and the practitioner are engaged in generating shared goals and understandings and in achieving important outcomes and aspirations, which the user has owned. Many if not all service users wish at a minimum to avoid going back to hospital if at all possible – relapse prevention clearly has a key part to play here. Whilst medication adherence is rarely if ever a major goal in and of itself, it often serves as a means to help the user achieve goals which are important, such as staying out of hospital. The experience of voices and a raft of negative self-appraisals is often a difficult, sometimes frightening, experience – working with CBT approaches to address these issues is clearly an enormous advantage. Finally, for service users, as for the rest of us, having at least a manageable relationship with the family is an important arena, in which it is possible through family intervention to make improvements.

Emphasizing self-management

All the psychosocial interventions emphasize in different ways the importance of self-management. The more users feel that they do have a measure of control over the debilitating effects of their illness, the better. The more the various self-management strategies developed through the psychosocial interventions can be put into effect, then the more the service user can begin to feel that they are genuinely beginning to exercise control and hence engender a genuine sense of meaning and significance in their lives. A strengths approach to Assertive Outreach has precisely the same objective.

Understanding and addressing the impact of symptoms on the relationship between the service user and practitioner

One of the major realities of working with people with severe longterm mental illness is that their experience may, from time to time at least, be grounded in the existence of voices, which they hear and we do not. Sooner or later, it is highly likely that these voices will be present when we are meeting up with them. There may be occasions when our contact with the service user may turn out to be in itself a stress factor, when, for example, they are not taking medication and they fear that we may instigate readmission. An important part of the engagement process both with Assertive Outreach and with the psychosocial interventions is that it becomes possible for both the service user and the practitioner to acknowledge the existence of the voices, and the impact they may be having on our relationship with them.

Thorough assessment

It is already clear how central a part strengths assessment plays in this approach to Assertive Outreach. Careful, comprehensive assessment is also a central part of any of the psychosocial interventions. Each particular psychosocial intervention brings with it its own specialist assessment requirements, but strengths assessment in the context of Assertive Outreach will give a general orientation and an indication of where more specialist assessment needs to be undertaken.

Developing a shared understanding

The process both in strengths assessment and in the psychosocial interventions is to develop a shared understanding – of the user's own aspirations, the direction they wish to go in and the particular issues they need to address.

Developing coping strategies through the care plan

The strengths care plan is a very flexible tool. It can be used to develop care plans in any of the 'domains' of the strengths assessment from health, to housing, daily living or social support, etc. Within these categories, care plans can be developed relating specifically to a coping strategy linked to one of the psychosocial interventions. The criteria for using a psychosocial intervention is the same as with any other

Table 10.3 The integration of core skills and the psychosocial interventions

Core functions of strengths Assertive Outreach
• Engagement and non-office-based community outreach
• Strengths assessment
• Care planning
• Direct work with the service user
• Care co-ordination
• Monitoring and review

Core integrating principles (adapted with permission from Mills 2000)
• Engaging the service user collaboratively
• Emphasizing self-management
• Understanding and addressing the impact of symptoms on the relationship between the service user and practitioner
• Thorough assessment
• Developing a shared understanding
• Developing coping strategies through the care plan

Psychosocial interventions
• Relapse prevention
• Medication adherence
• Cognitive behavioural interventions – working with service user cognitive appraisals
• Behavioural family intervention

intervention that may be under consideration: does it assist the user in attaining their own goals and aspirations? If, for example, a user is committed to staying in the community and out of hospital, then a care plan linked to relapse prevention and medication adherence may well be indicated.

CONCLUSIONS

In Assertive Outreach, a focus on monitoring mental health, medication compliance, early warning signs of relapse, the need for family interventions and providing appropriate responses to crisis and risk, becomes less formalized and more interwoven in an informal conversational approach to the ongoing working relationship. The context for this complex fluid approach to engagement, assessment and service delivery

---

Box 10.7   Concluding Gavin's story

Five years after the first visit by the Assertive Outreach team Gavin remains in regular contact, and has had no further hospital admissions. He remains off medication and in regular discussion about the diagnoses of schizophrenia and personality disorder, and how they relate to his experiences. On one occasion, he called out the crisis intervention team at 9.30 pm on a false alarm, just to see if they would respond the way he had been informed they would. They did, and took it in good humour, because of the relationship they also had with the Assertive Outreach team.

Gavin knows all the members of the Assertive Outreach team. Three people have left the team since his first connection, and he has got used to new people without disruption to the overall working relationship. The psychiatrist and GP have both visited his maisonette accompanied by members of the Assertive Outreach team, which Gavin recognizes as progress – the first occasions he has met medical staff without the need for compulsory hospital admissions.

The environment of his home is largely clear of the original collections of bags and papers. He has invited his mother into his home on frequent occasions during the last few years, and ventured out to a local small specialist music shop with members of the Assertive Outreach team on a number of occasions. Gradual clearance of Gavin's home unearthed a large collection of music, which has proved to be a specialist interest of his. He enjoys discussing musical tastes with a couple of the team's workers, and with one particular sales assistant in the local shop. He has also revived an interest in pencil drawing – one of the team who shares a similar interest has helped Gavin to get one of his drawings framed and hung on his living-room wall.

He continues to be suspicious of other people on the estate but has not had the urge to carry a weapon about the home for some time. His appearance has changed very little but he is beginning to understand how it may affect the way other people think of him.

is set within recognized essential components of effective Assertive Outreach, particularly taking the service to where the service user feels more comfortable, taking a longterm view of service contact and variations on a team approach.

The messages arising from the research literature rarely offer sufficient guidance on how to accommodate the eccentricities of individual service user circumstances. Assertive Outreach is primarily about gaining the trust of people who choose either not to become actively involved with, or to actively resist, mental health services. Unlike other parts of the traditional delivery of services, Assertive Outreach workers are challenged not to adopt a blaming stance towards people who seem unmotivated by the mental health system in general. It requires an attitudinal shift that demonstrates a suspension of most judgemental faculties and personal standards, in order to be open to connect with the experiences of others. These are not easy conditions within which to replicate research findings. This requires adaptability and chameleon-like qualities of the outreach workers, and a constant desire to bring a feel-good factor into the working relationships whenever possible, e.g. sharing a sense of humour. 'Persistence', 'flexibility' and 'creativity' are essential elements of the approach to working with the service users and, above all else, the approach needs to be led by the service user's own pace.

The messages from 'evidence-based practice' are vitally important, and Assertive Outreach services will greatly benefit from accessing high-quality training, supervision and practice development initiatives in order to offer the highest quality services to their service users. However, the nature of circumstances frequently dictates that more basic and practical needs take priority, particularly in relation to accommodation needs, welfare benefits entitlements, essential activities of daily living and social networks. It is quite possibly a failure to acknowledge these priorities in the working relationship that causes some people to disengage from services.

References

Barrowclough C, Tarrier N 1992 Families of Schizophrenic Patients: Cognitive Behavioural Intervention. Chapman & Hall, London

Beck A 1976 Cognitive Therapy and the Emotional Disorder. International Universities, New York

Birchwood M 1996 Early intervention in psychotic relapse. In: Haddock G, Slade P (eds) Cognitive-Behavioural Interventions with Psychotic Disorders. Routledge, London

Birchwood M, Smith J, Macmillan F et al 1989 Predicting relapse in schizophrenia: the development and implementation of an early signs monitoring system using patients and families as observers. Psychological Medicine 19: 649–656

Birchwood M, Smith J, Macmillan F et al 1998 Early intervention in psychotic relapse. In: Brooker C, Repper J (eds) Serious Mental Health Problems in the Community: Policy, Practice and Research. Baillière Tindall, London

Brooker C 2001 A decade of evidence-based training for work with people with serious mental health problems: progress in the development of the psychosocial interventions. Journal of Mental Health 10 (1): 17–31

Brooker C, Falloon I, Butterworth A et al 1994 The outcome of training community psychiatric nurses to deliver psychosocial intervention. British Journal of Psychiatry 165: 222–230

Burns T, Firn M 2002 Assertive Outreach in Mental Health: A Manual for Practitioners. Oxford University Press, Oxford

Bustillo J, Lauriello W, Horan W et al 2001 The psychosocial treatment of schizophrenia: an update. American Journal of Psychiatry 15 (2): 163–175

Caplan G 1964 Principles of Preventative Psychiatry. Tavistock, London

Cardin V, McGill C, Falloon I 1986 An economic analysis: costs, benefits, and effectiveness. In: Falloon I (ed) Family Management of Schizophrenia. Johns Hopkins Press, New York

Cramer J, Rosenheck R 1999 Enhancing medication compliance for people with serious mental illness. Journal of Nervous Mental Disease 187: 53–55

Crow T, MacMillan J, Johnson A 1986 A randomised controlled trial of prophylactic neuroleptic treatment. British Journal of Psychiatry 148: 120–127

Curson D, Barnes T, Bamber R et al 1985 Long-term depot maintenance of chronic schizophrenic out-patients: the seven year follow-up of the Medical Research Council fluphenazine/placebo trial. III. Relapse postponement or relapse prevention? The implications for long-term outcome. British Journal of Psychiatry 146: 474–480

Department of Health 1999 National Service Framework for Mental Health: Modern Standards and Service Models. HMSO, London

Department of Health 2000 NHS National Plan. HMSO, London

Diamond R J 1998 Instant Psychopharmacology. Norton, New York

Dixon L B, Lehman A E 1995 Family interventions for schizophrenia. Schizophrenia Bulletin 21: 631–643

Drury V, Birchwood M, Cochrane R et al 1996 Cognitive therapy and recovery from acute psychosis: a controlled trial. I. Impact on psychotic symptoms. British Journal of Psychiatry 169: 593–601

Fadden G 1997 Implementation of family interventions in routine clinical practice following staff training programmes: a major cause for concern. Journal of Mental Health 6: 599–612

Fadden G 1998 Family intervention. In: Brooker C, Repper J (eds) Serious Mental Health Problems in the Community: Policy, Practice and Research. Baillière Tindall, London

French P, Walford L 2001 Psychological approaches to early intervention for psychosis: what it is and what it can achieve. Mental Health Care 4 (5): 158–161

Gamble C, Brennan G 2000 Working with Serious Mental Illness: A Manual for Clinical Practice. Baillière Tindall, London

Goldstein M, Rodnick E, Evans J et al 1978 Drug and family therapy in the aftercare of acute schizophrenics. Archives of General Psychiatry 35: 1169–1177

Hirsch S, Gaind R, Rohde P et al 1973 Outpatient maintenance of chronic schizophrenic patients with long-acting fluphenazine: double-blind placebo trial. Report to the Medical Research Council Committee on Clinical Trials in Psychiatry. British Medical Journal 1 (5854): 633–637

Hogarty G, Kornblith S, Greenwald D et al 1997 Three-year trials of personal therapy amongst patients living with or independent of family. II. Description of study and effects on relapse rates. American Journal of Psychiatry 154: 1504–1513

Johnstone L 1989 Users and Abusers of Psychiatry. Routledge, London

Kemp R, Hayward P, David A 1997 Compliance Therapy Manual. Maudesley Hospital, London

Kemp R, Kirov G, Everitt B et al 1998 Randomised controlled trial of compliance therapy. 18-month follow-up. British Journal of Psychiatry 172: 413–419

Kuipers E, Garety P, Fowler D et al 1997 London–East Anglia random controlled trial of cognitive behaviour therapy for psychosis. I. Effects of treatment phase. British Journal of Psychiatry 171: 319–327

Linszen D, Dingemans P, van der Does J et al 1996 Treatment, expressed emotion and relapse in recent onset schizophrenia. Psychological Medicine 26: 333–342

McFarlane W, Link B, Dushay R et al 1995 Psychoeducational multiple family groups: four-year relapse outcome in schizophrenia. Family Process 34: 127–144

McGlashan T, Miller T, Woods S 2001 Pre-onset detection and intervention research in schizophrenia psychoses: current estimates of benefit and risk. Schizophrenia Bulletin 27 (4): 563–570

McGorry P, Jackson H 1999 The Recognition and Management of Early Psychosis. Cambridge University Press, Cambridge

McGorry P, Edwards J, Mihalopoulos C et al 1996 EPPIC: an evolving system of early detection and optimal management. Schizophrenia Bulletin 22 (2): 305–326

Mills J 2000 Dealing with voices and strange thoughts. In: Gamble C, Brennan G (eds) Working with Serious Mental Illness: A Manual for Clinical Practice. Baillière Tindall, London

Minghella E, Richard R, Freeman T et al 1998 Open All Hours: 24-hour response for people with mental health emergencies. Sainsbury Centre for Mental Health, London

Morgan S 1993 Community Mental Health: Practical Approaches to Long-term Problems. Chapman & Hall, London

Mueser K, Bond G, Drake R 2001 Community-based treatment of schizophrenia and other severe mental disorders: treatment outcomes. Medscape Mental Health 6 (1): 1–26

Nuechterlein K H, Dawson M E 1984 A heuristic vulnerability – stress model of schizophrenic episodes. Schizophrenia Bulletin 10: 300–312

Onyett S 1992 Case Management in Mental Health. Chapman & Hall, London

Plaistow J, Birchwood M 1996 Back in the Saddle – A Guide to Relapse Prevention. North Birmingham Early Intervention Service, Birmingham

Rollnick S, Heather N, Bell A 1992 Negotiating behaviour change in medical settings: the development of brief motivational interviewing. Journal of Mental Health 1: 25–37

Shepherd G 1991 Foreword. In: Watts F N, Bennett D H (eds) Theory and Practice of Psychiatric Rehabilitation, 3rd edn. Churchill Livingstone, Edinburgh

South Camden Crisis Response and Resolution Team 2001 Operational Policy. Camden & Islington Mental Health and Social Care Trust, London

Tarrier N, Barrowclough C, Vaughan K et al 1988 The community management of schizophrenia: a controlled trial of behavioural intervention with families to reduce relapse. British Journal of Psychiatry 153: 532–542

Tarrier N, Lowson K, Barrowclough C 1991 Some aspects of family intervention in schizophrenia: financial considerations. British Journal of Psychiatry 167: 473–479

Tarrier N, Barrowclough C, Porceddu K et al 1994 The Salford intervention project: relapse rates of schizophrenia at five and eight years. British Journal of Psychiatry 165: 829–832

Tarrier N, Yussupoff L, Kinney C et al 1998 Randomised controlled trial of intensive cognitive behaviour therapy for patients with chronic schizophrenia. British Medical Journal 317: 303–307

Warner R 2001 The prevention of schizophrenia: what interventions are safe and effective? Schizophrenia Bulletin 27 (4): 551–562

Watkins P 2001 Mental Health Nursing: The Art of Compassionate Care. Butterworth-Heinemann, Oxford

Chapter 11

Risk taking

Steve Morgan

"If you don't risk anything, you may risk everything!"

(Anon)

INTRODUCTION

Definition

"Risk is the likelihood of an identified behaviour occurring in response to changing [*situations, events or*] personal circumstances. The outcomes are more frequently harmful to self or others, though occasionally they may have a beneficial aim in pursuit of a positive change" (Morgan 1998, p 8). [Italics added]

This type of definition reflects the importance of the 'context' of behavioural changes for the individual, the awareness of which contributes immensely to our overall understanding of a very complex issue. Considerations of risk are not just about defensive practices in the pursuit of restricting potentially negative outcomes, though this will be the primary focus on occasions. It is also about the potential for pursuing 'positive' risk taking (Morgan 2000a).

The assessment of risk involves complex considerations of many broad categories of behaviour. The predominant literature largely responds to the preoccupation with aggression and violence (Mason and Chandley 1999). However, considerations of suicidal ideas and actions, self-harm and self-injury, neglect, exploitation, harassment, abuse, loss and bereavement are some of the many categories that demand attention. A strengths approach recognizes that service users' experiences of risk are more likely to be in the role of victims than as perpetrators (Bingley 1997).

Risk assessment is primarily concerned with gathering information and analysing the potential outcomes of behaviour patterns. It involves a degree of predictive ability, though these abilities are hampered because we are being asked to make predictions on limited experience, the incidents of risk being rare (Hawton 1994, Reed 1997). Identifying specific risk factors of relevance to an individual, and the context in which they may occur, is a process fraught with uncertainty but it requires the linking of historical information to current circumstances, in order to anticipate possible future change. Ongoing risk research aims to refine the identification of risk factors (Borum 1996, Department of Health 2001). However, it is more frequently concerned with the negative factors, with little or no attention being paid in the literature to the factors that help us to identify and take risks in a positive framework.

Risk is the art of living with uncertainty; and positive risk taking will necessarily be characterized by degrees of uncertainty. However, it forms an essential component of effective risk management if the service users are to be genuinely included in the process, requiring a clear statement of plans and an allocation of individual responsibilities – translating collective decisions into real actions.

A number of important principles need to be borne in mind when considering risk assessment and risk management in practice:

1. Risk is dynamic, constantly changing in response to changing circumstances.
2. Risk can be minimized, but not eliminated.
3. Assessment is enhanced by multiple sources of information, but frequently you will be working with incomplete and possibly inaccurate information.
4. Identification of risk carries a duty to do something about it, i.e. risk management.
5. Assessment information and clinical decision making can be improved by engaging multidisciplinary, multi-agency collaboration, through discussions and joint care planning (including involvement of the service user and carers themselves, as much as possible).
6. 'Defensible' decisions are those based on clear reasoning.
7. Risk taking can engage positive collaboration with beneficial outcomes.
8. Confidentiality is a right but may be breached in exceptional circumstances when people are deemed to be at serious risk of harm.

9. Organizations should adopt reasonable expectations of a 'no-blame' culture but not condone poor practice.

(Based with permission on O'Rourke and Bird 2000)

WHAT DO WE MEAN BY RISK TAKING?

To take a risk is to take a chance, a gamble, an opportunity to learn, something that can have tangible positive gains to be acquired or achieved. To actively take a risk is to chance feeling alive, heightening awareness of our feelings and emotional reactions, through an increased state of alertness.

To be a passive recipient of unplanned risk taking potentially results in missed opportunities to learn, through a more likely loss of awareness, creativity, understanding, even life.

Positively and proactively taking risks can result in achieving combinations of desired personal goals, to:

- be informed
- exercise choices
- make decisions
- hold some control over the direction of our own destiny
- experience degrees of power
- collaborate with others positively
- make constructive use of opportunity
- experience autonomy
- weigh up consequences
- learn from experience
- want to change and grow
- exercise an unwritten human right.

> **Proposed definition**
>
> 'Positive risk taking' in mental health is the weighing up of potential benefits and harms of exercising one choice of action over another. It involves developing plans and actions that reflect the positive potentials and stated priorities of the service user, and using all accessible resources and support to achieve the desired outcomes, and to minimize the potential harmful outcomes.

When was the last time you took a risk? Do we pay real attention to the role that risk plays in our personal and working lives? We all take risks as a part of our daily lives, to differing degrees and differing intent. Making and taking risks can add a spark to life. We take risks in many different ways – career choices… lifestyle choices… leisure pursuits… right through to how and where and when to travel… even down to crossing the road.

How do we take these risks? Generally through a careful consideration of what we want, what we need to do, what we have to do, what our 'strengths' are... and by accepting the ultimate consequences, to varying degrees (Box 11.1). Sometimes risks are taken impulsively and/or subconsciously. Then there are those of us who take a more flighty approach to the whole issue of decisions and their consequences, sometimes preferring to attribute blame elsewhere.

For example, when it comes to changing a job, the decision-making process can be very complex and fraught with risks: whether to accept an increase in pay as the determining factor, influenced by the multiple needs for additional money that may impinge on your thinking at the time. What of the potential additional responsibility that may go with the new job, and the different skills required? To give up the comfort of the known, and the working relationships established with a group of colleagues, can be a more difficult decision for some people. This is only the tip of the iceberg in some decisions, not yet taking account of personal challenges and goals, issues of prestige, desires to travel, or simply the need to move on to something more stimulating. The potential list of factors is endless and highly individual but always involves degrees of risk taking, some of which may not become apparent until sometime beyond acting on a decision.

Conversely, not changing your job can also be a risk. Remaining with the status quo holds the possibility of stagnation of knowledge and ideas, a lack of challenges in order to stretch abilities or test the limits,

---

Box 11.1   Case vignette: Mike's story

Mike was diagnosed with multiple sclerosis and epilepsy, and inappropriately placed in a nursing home for the elderly at the age of 47 because there was no other facility suited to his needs in the local area. The initial care plan required him to bathe under close supervision or to be bathed by staff, because of the risk of a fit whilst in the bath. He frequently reacted in a verbally aggressive manner, had always preferred a shower and felt a strong need for greater personal dignity.

The care home had one fully adapted shower cubicle, with an alarm cord fitted in the event of a fall. The care home team, and staff from the wider local services, discussed a detailed risk assessment and a management plan that included Mike's need to inform staff of when he was using the shower, how he felt physically at the time, and regular checks by staff from outside the shower room when he was using the facility.

Mike greatly appreciated the sense of independence and dignity that the plan offered him. There were no significant problems for three years but one day he had a fit whilst lowering himself onto the shower seat, causing a serious head injury as he fell against one of the fixed rails. The local inquiry into the incident attached no blame to the care home or wider supporting team of people, fully supporting the plan and the way it had been enacted to Mike's benefit for the three years until the accident.

and a guarantee of continuing the same relationships and circumstances currently established. Such a situation also ensures the potential opportunities offered by other options remain unfulfilled.

Do the same rules and opportunities apply to people who experience severe and enduring mental health problems? In the field of mental health, the perceptions of the public, legislators and practitioners alike, all mitigate against the taking of risks:

- by promoting an epidemic fear of risk, seen only as the potential or real enactment of threats; failing to accept that it is a reality of many aspects of life, often needing to be seen as a challenge to be worked with
- by focusing the spotlight of attention on rare tragedies, with a consequence of painting them as the more usual picture of what is happening in mental health services
- by service providers focusing exclusively on the service user's history of failures and mistakes, rather than the often more challenging tasks of helping people to identify their strengths and celebrate their past achievements
- by fearing the consequences of getting something wrong, serving to paralyse the urge to take a chance and try something new
- by promoting a culture of blame, fuelling society's need to find a scapegoat when something goes wrong.

Harrison (1997) suggests we should be more explicit about the risks involved in defensive practice, particularly the failure to effectively involve and empower service users. Risk taking should be seen as a healthy part of community care, rather than as negligence or gambling with high stakes. It is the mechanism that resists an ongoing tightening of procedures in the false expectation of the elimination of risk. The kind of society that needs to perpetuate a culture of blame only serves to destroy the seeds of confidence before they have an opportunity to flourish; and the quashing of personal aspirations can only serve to contribute to the potential for serious risks, with damaging consequences taking place (Morgan 2000a).

Through the focus of media reporting (Philo et al 1993) and mental health risk research (Sheppard 1996), we are very good at generating the statistics of failure. Conversely, we are not good at generating or even interpreting potential statistics of success. We cannot be sure of the numbers of homicides or suicides that our interventions may have avoided.

However, the evidence from Taylor and Gunn (1999) strongly suggests that the number of homicides committed by people with a mental health problem has not increased in the way that the figures for the general population have, across the period from the mid-1950s to the mid-1990s. In fact, with a relatively stable total across this period for people experiencing mental health problems, the statistical proportion of total homicides is decreasing. The time-span broadly coincides with the implementation of the occasionally criticized policy of community care. Surely, it cannot all be attributed to luck; maybe more than a little good practice and clinical judgement has aided this statistical anomaly! Szmukler (2000) poses the pertinent question of whether it is reasonable to expect mental health services to prevent the unpredictable, yet goes on to highlight an important paradox "…if homicides are preventable by a service, and are rare, the service must be good."

The risk business

A criticism of the increased focus and attention on risk during the last decade, particularly by many practitioners working in the field, is a sense that the business of mental health has become the 'risk business'. Invariably, this is seen in a negative light, as somehow being detrimental to their work. Rose (1998) offers a discussion that challenges us to look more critically at the way risk has come to dominate the debate on mental health clinical practice. The term 'risk thinking' is used to describe a shift in the central obligation on mental health professions, developing a stronger emphasis on the function of administrative decision making. He suggests that the policy of community care is characterized by a complex institutional topography of clinics, centres, residential units and office bases, primarily shaped by an imperative to manage risk and defined by their ability to offer levels of security and containment.

A risk-thinking paradigm is characterized by a further shift, from the prominence of the clinical language of diagnosis, treatment, care and support, to the probabilistic language of risk. The latter attempts to bring the future into the present and make it a quantifiable entity. In this new scenario risk assessment seems to be less concerned with formulating good clinical judgement and more focused on providing 'defensible' decisions. Clinical issues become increasingly influenced by nonclinical agendas, and by expectations generated external to the helping relationship. Practitioners are having to make an additional assessment, i.e. the risk to themselves of litigation, through getting things wrong (Rose 1998).

Roy (1997) outlines the mechanisms of the inquiries and organizational procedures, and warns of the dangers of these taking a lead in shaping the demands on practitioner priorities. Within these emerging changes he suggests: "The individual clinician is well advised to consider the personal risks of clinical practice in the same way as one would ensure adequate insurance and pension arrangements for one's home and family."

Any new service models have to struggle to establish themselves within the context of the prevailing political climate, and undoubtedly UK mental health services are strongly affected by the media portrayal of risk, and its influence on public thinking and government responses. It appears on the surface that society is less tolerant of inabilities to manage the rare and the unpredictable. As unrealistic as it is, risk elimination remains the perceived benchmark of mental health service success; the whole service will continue to be tarred by each individual incident that occurs. If this situation is to change, all people involved in mental health services need to promote the real evidence, as portrayed by Taylor and Gunn (1999) and Szmukler (2000).

Just as cost-effectiveness in services is usually measured against hospital bed use, so there is the danger that new service models will become measured against their ability to resolve the narrowly focused public safety agenda. Morgan (2000a) warns against Assertive Outreach potentially being set up to become the new face of the risk business, with impossibly unrealistic expectations of risk elimination. The policy agenda for Assertive Outreach is becoming more closely aligned to that of providing legislative responses to the series of homicide inquiries of the last decade (Department of Health 1999, 2000). Talk of tracking resistant individuals, and using mechanisms of coercion and enforcement, to ensure more compliance with treatment and hence greater safety are ill founded, not least because it promotes service users' fears of 'aggressive outreach' and completely misses the underpinning philosophy and foundations of its effectiveness, i.e. engagement through creative and flexible collaboration.

What is so wrong about being in the risk business? Just as risk applies to the lives of everyone everyday, so risk has always been an integral part of daily working practice in mental health services. Perhaps the problem is not so much about seeing the work as risk oriented but more about the exclusively negative attention attributed to the risk element during recent years, and the perception that much of the increased bureaucratic workload can be attributed as a response to a risk-driven agenda.

A strengths approach to the issue would emphasize the more constructive view of risk, as a uniquely challenging aspect of the work, to positively engage service users' viewpoints and experiences, in a collaborative approach to identifying and managing the impact and consequences of different courses of action. In this scenario, risk taking is a reasonable activity to be expected of service providers, not a negligent failing of responsibility and duty. Nobody benefits by simply allowing risky situations to develop into serious incidents, least of all the service users or the practitioners.

Why 'positive risk taking'?

The case for not taking risks is largely based on the aforementioned fear of failure, leading to blame and scapegoating. A logical extension of the unrealistic expectations of risk elimination would be the creation of a risk-free world. If such an entity could exist, what would it look like? It fortunately defies the imagination, as it would probably resemble an extremely sterile existence. To give a glimpse of what this existence may resemble we need to look into the world of fiction: Aldous Huxley (1932) wrote an account of the 'ideal' society in *Brave New World*, which ultimately reads as a rather unsettling, loveless and even sinister world.

Rose (1998) concludes: "This culture of blame is intrinsic to and perpetuates the fantasy to which we are all prey: that there can be a life without risk; a life of unlimited self-enjoyment. Ultimately, it is this fantasy, the ethics which it embodies, the fears and anxieties which it produces and feeds off, and the hostility towards difference which it engenders, which must be challenged."

In reality, we all take risks, personally and professionally. Denying it does not mean they go away or go unnoticed. Quite the contrary, denial is more likely to serve the situation where risks occur in an unsupported and unthinking way with outcomes determined more by luck or chance – less of the positive, more of a recipe for disaster. By not pursuing a risk-taking approach we risk depriving people of opportunities for growth and change, giving good reasons for people to mistrust the so-called motives of helping and to consider disengaging from services.

Within mental health services, frequent risks confronted include:

- 'Discharge' from inpatient units, where the pressure on beds dictates that the person needing to be admitted is a higher priority of risk than the person being discharged; frequently the discharge decision will be commuted to 'extended leave', resulting in more than 100% bed use.
- Pressures on community caseloads; requiring members of staff to take a higher workload than they feel comfortable with or to take referrals that they do not feel particularly skilled to work with, or to make visits/ appointments based on limited information and without the safety and good working practice of appropriate joint working.

Such clinical decisions are made on a daily basis but perhaps not always sufficiently discussed, planned or thought through. However, even decisions that seem to be left more to luck and chance will be seen to have a basis in clinical judgement when put under closer scrutiny. Pressure of work may result in some decisions being made through intuition or gut reaction but these are generally skilled areas of functioning based on life and work experiences. Such processes are seldom random decisions with no basis to them, even though it may not be possible to pinpoint specific influencing factors. Morgan (2000b) suggests "…they are extremely valuable warning bells that may register a need for caution. Conversely, they are the messages that can quite often suggest a potential for taking a positive risk where other objective factors indicate or suggest otherwise… Where documented, they should be clearly referenced as gut reaction/intuition, to avoid being confused with objective fact-based evidence."

In the case of Assertive Outreach services, the constructive approach to taking risks is likely to yield a number of potential benefits:

- Helping to facilitate the function of engagement, which is a central responsibility charged to such services. The evidence for risk taking aiding engagement is largely anecdotal as this has not been an area attracting any research attention (Box 11.2).
- Promoting collaboration and user involvement, most specifically through the requirement to be more transparent in order to identify potential risks to be taken and the support mechanisms for facilitating them.
- Recognizing the reality of service users' experiences.
- To be more 'normalizing' in approach.
- To be real – everyone else takes risks.

Graley-Wetherell and Morgan (2001) document specific service user views on what they appreciate most from contact with an Active Outreach service. The examples of creative engagement, and involvement in the planning and delivery of care, are identified as going beyond the user's previously narrower experiences of what mental health services usually do. This can be interpreted as a significant risk in its own right but one that is unanimously met with positive reactions from the recipients of such an approach.

Risk taking in practice

Only an extremely small proportion of service users actively resist services at all costs. In these instances, an assessment of risk will occasionally require more restrictive measures and interventions in response. The majority of so-called resistant individuals do engage, to various degrees, where services are offered in a more flexible way that reflects their perception of needs. This approach often presents a challenge to the role of professional judgement but does not necessarily have to result in negative risks! The challenge to practitioners is one of becoming more flexible and creative in their active attempts to gain the trust of disaffected people.

Box 11.2   Assertive Outreach and engagement

Assertive Outreach workers recognize that engagement with their services is not something that happens automatically; it has to be earned and always monitored and worked at. It is frequently of a very tenuous quality, based on delicate negotiations, as follows:

- A reluctance to accept a mental illness diagnosis, or to discuss the need for medication, does not mean a person will not engage in conversations of other needs, e.g. housing, money and work. Strengths Assertive Outreach prioritizes the need to maintain contact through these conversations, thus developing trust, which may be subsequently used to negotiate on more delicate mental health issues, as well as providing the level of contact that enables ongoing assessment.
- For the suicidal person a hospital admission does not always offer a guarantee of safety or the best environment for addressing the causes and symptoms. Intensive support at home, particularly through active and empathic listening, may communicate the necessary messages that the intense distress is being understood and appropriately managed.
- Agitation and verbal aggression that is quickly medicated may lead to further volatility and resentment with services. Appropriate supervision may be offered in some instances through respectful and non-judgemental support. Not all aggression results in escalation to violence, and sometimes it is relevant for a person to express levels of aggression as a means to dissipate anger and frustration.
- Expectations of increased skills development for the self-management of neglectful behaviour is not always the most appropriate response for chronically institutionalized individuals. Continued tenure of independent accommodation may occasionally be supported by a plan of regular short respite placements out of the home, in order for cleaning services to restore the standard of the environment.

Risk taking requires a balanced understanding of the seriousness of possible outcomes with the probabilities of their occurrence based on specific risk factors (Carson 1994), i.e. good risk assessment. However, this approach still implies a focus on the negative elements of risk. In reality, it is more about comparing and balancing what we consider the likely benefits and harms of a situation to be. Linking this information to the individual's personal motivations for change can increase the likelihood of positive gains.

Decision-making processes

"Risk-taking has at least four levels of analysis and responsibility:

1) the assessment and control of specific risk factors;
2) taking account of situational or contextual risk factors;
3) acknowledging and controlling the problems and calling in aid the potential of the decision-making process;
4) managing the total decision-making process."

(Carson 1996)

Risk decisions are often extremely complex, fraught with uncertainties and dependent on subjective factors. However, it is always possible to make reasonable decisions through being more explicit about the process undertaken. Risk decisions need to be clearly justifiable, not based on flippant notions of hoping for the best advice from someone else, and avoiding the use of identifiable risk decision-making processes. It is about thinking through issues rigorously, most frequently as a collective venture, to discover what decisions can be genuinely justified.

If you have reason to believe that an event is possible but unlikely then you should declare and record that likelihood in an explicit form. Unless it can be shown that your estimate was inappropriate it will prove powerful in discouraging any court, or other form of inquiry, from utilizing hindsight in order to conclude that harm, which has now occurred, was more likely than it then seemed. Helping others to see how you arrived at a decision offers you some control over their ability to use hindsight against you.

In relation to service users' involvement in the processes, Carson (1994) points out that the legal position is one of the individual's 'capacity, competence and consent'. They are presumed capable and the tests are of understanding not wisdom, i.e. the person must be able to understand the nature and consequences of a particular question.

Maltsberger (1994) suggests that practitioners take calculated risks only through having steps in place to protect themselves legally. Most commonly, these would involve demonstrating that the decisions are not neglectful or open to claims of malpractice. This is achieved through thorough documentation of the decision-making processes and a full risk assessment, demonstrating how risk taking is an important step in the treatment and care plan of the individual's return to recovery.

In the case of suicide risk, the timing of when to take calculated risks is generally when an informed considered opinion has been reached that continued close monitoring of a person will be more likely to lead to negative outcomes (Maltsberger 1994). At this stage practitioners would be calling on their own practice-generated evidence that it is appropriate to hand back a large degree of responsibility for decisions and actions to the service user. This is one of the broad aims of the strengths approach, alluded to but not often practised by service providers, i.e. to create a healthy interdependence rather than an unhealthy dependence on mental health services.

ASSERTIVE OUTREACH TEAMS AND RISK TAKING

Risk taking naturally pervades most functions of effective Assertive Outreach teams:

- The primary focus on 'engagement' demands a risk-taking approach, with the team often having to be open in their negotiations of the priorities to be worked on, with the service user taking more control in directing the helping relationship.
- By definition of the client group, risk is central to the considerations of how to work with people. Most service users accepted as appropriate for Assertive Outreach services will have some history and/or currently identified issues of risk, specifically the potential risks associated with their reasons for disengaging from services.
- Staff will take some risks in the way they offer the service, i.e. outreach necessitating the great majority of the work to be away from service settings, largely on the service user's territory, raising issues of safety and the need for reasonable safeguards and mechanisms of support.
- In order to change service user perceptions of the more usual service responses to them, the Assertive Outreach team will need to establish a real difference in the way it works with and relates to the service user. As such, they will frequently be required to challenge the more conventional methods of service delivery (Box 11.3). Thinking differently means occasionally flying in the face of the 'usual' way of thinking and working, with the potential consequence of having to manage the resistance to innovation from other parts of the system, or even degrees of hostility and attempts to undermine such challenges.
- The strengths approach to Assertive Outreach promotes more inclusive risk management thinking by encouraging staff to develop the crucial links with other people and agencies important and/or relevant to the needs of the individual service user. This often involves more creative connections with a much broader range of service providers than a narrow focus on 'mental health' would usually prioritize, e.g. utilities companies (gas; water; electricity), housing organizations, the benefits agency and a diverse voluntary sector.

The more usual process of working within a context of Assertive Outreach involves mechanisms that will support effective risk taking:

- identifying the risks with the service user, including the potential gains and losses of choices and decisions made
- identifying real strengths from an appreciation of past successes and achievement, current resources and positive future potential

- working on the service user's own terms and pace, without imposing any judgement or standards on them
- developing recognition of 'early warning signs' through relapse signatures at an earlier behavioural stage before psychiatric symptoms become more evident
- developing crisis and contingency plans that respond to the early signs of difficulty or potential negative outcomes
- constant information sharing and discussion with the service user, to aid informed choice, and to check out the level of understanding of behaviours and consequences of action
- agreed team decisions, monitored through daily handover meetings. Such a team approach provides conditions that enable safer risk taking, through a sense of continuity of service delivery and the intensity of contact.

The overall context is one of achieving truly integrated teams working in a multiskilled, multidisciplinary (and multi-agency) network. As such, effective communication and co-ordination within the team and with the relevant external agencies are essential, not simply desired options. Dvoskin and Steadman (1994) offer an example of how many of the above elements of effective team functioning, combined with elements of an advocacy role, provide an example of effective risk management where issues of aggression and violence may be the predominant risk.

Box 11.3   Case study: beyond conventional thinking

Ritchie is 24 years old, with a diagnosis of paranoid schizophrenia derived over four hospital admissions during the last five years. He has an established pattern of using cannabis and crack cocaine, with each admission resulting from police intervention following threatening behaviour with acts of violence causing actual bodily harm. Ritchie is usually detained for periods under Section 3 of the Mental Health Act 1983, and on periods of probation. He complies grudgingly with medical treatment whilst under probation orders but disengages from services when the orders cease, feeling that services only see him as the 'illness' rather than attempting to understand his experiences and needs.

Aim

To promote Ritchie's understanding of the links between his drug use, mental state and acts of aggression. To help Ritchie better manage his pattern of living to minimize relapses of mental state, causing him to respond to paranoid phenomena through violent acts.

Failed conventional wisdom

The established service responses have been documented as repeated focused attempts to persuade Ritchie to cease taking illegal drugs, to attend regular outpatient appointments and to remain compliant with prescribed depot medication through fortnightly visits to the psychiatric clinic.

Risk-taking thinking

Ritchie is young and frustrated by the lack of opportunities life is offering him. Drug taking offers him an identity and social connections that he would not give up without something very positive to put in its place. A more productive starting point would be to explore a strengths assessment with Ritchie, to discover potential interests and abilities. The next step would be to acknowledge his drug-taking behaviours are based on 'skills' (which just happen to be deployed in a negative direction at present). Rather than focusing on the negative outcomes of drug taking, the short-term plan should be to recognize the skills (time management; negotiation; budgeting; social interactions; risk-taking decisions) and help Ritchie to employ the same skills in more productive directions.

Risks

The approach is a longterm process of promoting positive change, where the gains of engagement need to be earned rather than just assumed. In the short term, the more immediate anxiety-provoking concerns of drug taking versus medication compliance need to take a lesser prominence, with the fear that potentially aggressive behaviours may repeat themselves.

Challenges

Where the traditional service responses have proved repeatedly to fail, new thinking is justified. Reasonable safeguards need to be incorporated into risk-taking thinking but elimination of the potential for aggressive and violent behaviours can never be guaranteed. Wide-ranging anxieties and the propensity to blame need to be carefully managed.

Applying a strengths approach

Is the strengths approach a natural process for practitioners to perform in their daily work? In its simplest form, the approach is one of identifying the:

- strengths of the service user, informal and formal support networks
- nature and detail of the risk to be taken
- timing of when it is appropriate to take risks
- mechanisms to be in place to support its successful outcome, and minimize potential for damage or loss.

Applying a strengths approach to the assessment of risk is more likely to underpin the potential for taking risks. Common sense would suggest that if our assessment focused entirely on the deficits and potential for negative outcomes it would be extremely difficult to identify the conditions for risk taking. The confidence to take risks is much more likely to arise from investigating previous successes, current positive potentials and resources, and the future desires and aspirations of the individual. In this way, both the strengths assessment and risk assessment become inextricably entwined in the pursuit of plans that enable rather than restrict service user recovery and growth. Such an approach is also likely to be a greater motivator for the service user to engage in realistic discussions of risks, encouraged by the possibility that others may see beyond just labelling them as a negative risk potential.

The concept of risk taking is closely aligned to the strengths principle regarding the service user's desire to learn, grow and change (see Chapter 3). We all learn more from trying out something new and being allowed to draw our own lessons from the occasional failures. For many practitioners the need to demonstrate a pseudoscientific credibility and a 'professional' approach conflicts with their ability to truly implement a strengths-based risk-taking approach. The commonsense simplicity of a strengths approach feels very close to the way we wish to work, or even dare to hope that we do work. However, most people are prevented from doing so by the burden of unrealistic demands and expectations linked to the more restrictive public safety agenda.

What is needed to enable risk taking to happen in reality?

1. Service user and carer perspectives of risk having a prominent place in the whole assessment and management process, counterbalancing the current predominance of flawed media–public–government misrepresentations and unrealistic expectations.
2. A focus on strengths, giving a more positive base on which to build potential plans that will support beneficial risk taking. Considering the strengths and abilities of the service user, of their wider network and social systems, and of the wide-ranging services potentially available (statutory and voluntary sectors, and most importantly non-mental health resources).
3. A willingness on behalf of all people associated with the Assertive Outreach team to think and work in this way. It presents significant challenges to the more traditional ways of working and requires people with a mindset that relishes such challenges and the pursuit of new ideas. People who pay lip-service to innovation never push the limits of what is routine and comfortably known.
4. The whole team signed up to the approach and to the identified risks to be supported; not only the members of the Assertive Outreach team but hopefully the service user, carers and the wider span of services that may be involved in the specific care plan. If parts of the wider network are not signed up then confidence in being able to sustain positive risk taking becomes undermined as the fears associated with a blame culture are more likely to permeate the thinking and threaten the implementation of creative ideas.
5. High-quality supervision and support are essential for discussing and refining ideas, as well as providing a 'reality check' to prevent idealism overwhelming realism.

6. The development of appropriate crisis and contingency plans for the 'fears' and possibilities of failure. These will aid prevention of some harmful outcomes, and minimization of others. Risk taking should be pursued in a context of promoting safety not negligence.

7. It should become part of the culture of ideas and team training. Risk taking should not be seen as a one-off experiment. Assertive Outreach teams should see this approach as their natural first line of thinking. Whole team training will be essential if the approach is to be fully understood and practised by all team members, as a routine part of its culture.

8. Managerial support from the organizational hierarchy, preferably up to senior management and board levels. Understanding of the rationale behind positive risk taking needs to be vertical throughout the organization if it is to instil the necessary confidence in practitioners to take calculated risks. Nobody will be expected to take positive risks if they are fearful that failure will only introduce blaming processes from higher up in the organization. Such understanding needs to start with its articulation in the organization's statement of beliefs and to be further detailed in all aspects of policymaking and organizational procedures.

9. Adequate resources to enable creative work to take precedence over 'what usually just happens.' Resources are never open-ended, but the Assertive Outreach team needs organizational support to sustain the components of effective practice outlined in the research literature. Beyond this, the team needs to use its collective imagination to access real community resources creatively, not just to be limited by consideration of mental health services resources.

10. Shifting the organizational and team 'culture' to 'no blame' and to a 'can-do' attitude respectively. There is no good reason for not doing what is happening by default anyway! The team needs to feel confident that mechanisms are in place to support it to cope with the extra degrees of uncertainty, beyond that which is only to be expected with human behaviour and unpredictable mental health factors.

11. Risk taking is further enhanced by limiting the duration of the decision, i.e. working to shorter timescales and with smaller goals broken down. This has a strong analogy with weather forecasting, whereby the predictions are more accurate for the next few hours than they would be for the next few days (Monahan and Steadman 1996). It is also enhanced by having mechanisms in place to check on progress, and an ability to change previous decisions quickly when needed, including intervening in a more restrictive way.

12. Accountability and responsibility – Morgan (1998) indicates that individual practitioners can reasonably be expected to accept responsibility for the professional standards of conduct set out by their professional body and for the care co-ordination/keyworker role within the local implementation of the guidance and legislation. However, there are also collective responsibilities for information sharing, decision making and care planning, belonging more with

the team than the individual in isolation. The organization also holds responsibilities, as outlined above.

ORGANIZATIONS AND RISK TAKING

Most mental health organizations react conventionally towards the constant bombardment of negative messages from the media misrepresentation and government rhetoric, by targeting limited resources on those deemed potentially violent. Munro and Rumgay (2000) suggest that this may lead to serious injustices to people who are seriously ill but pose no danger. Organizational priorities need to acquire a degree of risk taking – they could do much more to support the risk-taking decisions of their own staff, and reverse the more usual current practitioner perceptions of feeling 'guilty until proven innocent'. They could take a significant beneficial risk on behalf of their staff by promoting the message of realistic expectations and risk taking outside of the service, by flying in the face of the more usual media–government–public expectations, using the available evidence they could tell it as it is, rather than the way others falsely would like to see it.

What does a 'no-blame' culture organization look like? Ideally, it would adopt all of the following responsibilities:

- providing a clear policy on risk taking with service users
- clearly articulating its support for properly taken risk decisions, even when they ultimately result in some form of harm
- providing appropriate training and support in risk decision making for multidisciplinary practitioners
- helping everyone to learn from decision-making experiences
- enabling practitioners to obtain quality information and data, and to interpret service philosophies before making risk decisions.

Most importantly, it would develop more supportive arrangements for investigating incidents of harm within its own structure. With very rare exceptions, the point at which a risk has become an incident is a traumatic time for practitioners as well as everyone else involved. No gain arises out of reacting in ways that make the practitioner feel more anxious and unnecessarily guilty about the outcome. The opposite effect is more usual, in that where practitioners are left feeling unsupported at times of highest need it has a major negative impact on perceptions and morale much more widely across the organization. The first messages to those involved in an incident should be that:

- the organization believes you did everything you could within the circumstances in which you were required to work
- you will be offered any support or supervision that you feel is appropriate to your needs at this time
- we have to determine the sequence of events that led up to the unfortunate incident, but you should feel involved and informed throughout the process.

Where the rare cases of negligent or bad practice are subsequently identified, they can then be dealt with appropriately. There is no merit in giving the impression that everyone behaved negligently until the majority are proved otherwise – the final sense of relief at being exonerated is little compensation for the period of time kept in the dark and feeling inadequate at your job. However, such an approach may not sit comfortably with other people who hold the loss and trauma associated with serious incidents – victims and/or carers, for example. The organization adopting a 'no-blame' culture should offer appropriate comfort, support and information to meet their needs, without succumbing to the witch-hunt.

TOOLS AND GUIDELINES FOR PRACTICE

The practice of risk assessment and management in recent mental health practice is rife with research and paper-based assessment tools, largely in response to the repeated recommendations from the homicide inquiries. In this reactive role, they generally focus on the identification of negative risk factors (Worthing Priority Care 1995, O'Rourke and Hammond 2000), with little or no attention to the strengths, resources and potential for positive risk taking. Indeed, they rarely pay any significant attention to the concept of risk management, preferring to focus almost entirely on risk assessment. Morgan (2000b) partially redresses the balance, with a few references to 'positive potentials' accompanied by small spaces for documenting this type of information but with a greater than usual structuring of the risk management guidance.

For the element of risk-taking practice to become incorporated into the routine work of practitioners requires something that offers a tangible reminder. However, is it another assessment 'tool' or is it something more in the way of guidelines for practice? The concept of risk taking has been discussed as a way of supporting clinical practice, not the changing of practice just to fit another paperwork tool. The following case study (Box 11.4) is offered as an example to illustrate risk taking in practice. It provides the necessary background information, which is then used in the structure provided (Box 11.5). This offers a guide to individual and collective thinking and discussion, as well as a subsequent format for documenting the information.

Box 11.4   Case study: Sandra

Personal history

Sandra is 43 years old. Both parents are deceased; little is known about her father but her mother was a known local prostitute. She has two sisters and two brothers, all living locally. Her younger brother is in residential care for people with learning disabilities, and Sandra visits him approximately monthly. Her elder brother is generally aggressive and abusive towards all the family members and towards services that attempt

box continued

contact with him through Sandra. There is sufficient cause to assume that Sandra has been sexually abused at various stages of her life, including within the family when she was younger, and by other men coming to her brother's house when she has had to live there temporarily. She has no children but has alluded to having two abortions.

She has been married twice: her first husband died in a traffic accident when Sandra was 22, and the second marriage was an abusive relationship towards her, ending in divorce after only two years at the age of 26. Sandra has been in a relationship for most of the last 10 years but this man also has another female partner, causing regular arguments and anxiety. Despite this situation, he remains the person she feels closest to.

Psychiatric history

Sandra has experienced a history of contact with mental health services over more than 24 years; the whole family appear to have been known to social services for a much longer time. She has had three hospital admissions during this time and spent much of the last 15 years in and out of temporary and supported accommodation. She has a diagnosis of psychotic depression and is generally compliant with monthly depot medication, which she prefers to receive from her GP practice.

Community support

Sandra has tended to resist contact with community mental health workers, feeling that they try to interfere with her own sense of independence. She is clear that she wants to have her own flat, located close to her boyfriend, and to live life by her own choices. Community services have frequently placed her in supported accommodation, and set targets for achieving standards of daily living skills before she could consider living independently in her own accommodation. This has caused Sandra to occasionally rebel against the institution or to leave and make herself homeless ending up either temporarily with her elder brother or in temporary accommodation.

She chooses to eat takeaway food or to make sandwiches and snacks. She becomes quite frustrated by programmes that set her up to shop for and cook elaborate meals. Sandra is a very gregarious person out on the street but feels that services are setting her up with social skills training as a way of saying she cannot cope with life without running the risk of being exploited by others. She also sporadically attends a local drop-in centre, where she is well known, meets people she has come to know, and occasionally has a light meal.

At times when supported accommodation staff have set boundaries that she cannot tolerate Sandra has retreated to her room for days, presenting as depressed. The residential unit and community mental health team staff have attributed this and potential suicidal ideas to her inability to manage on her own, further strengthening the need for her to prove to them that she can achieve the necessary standards to live independently.

Assertive Outreach

On the latest self-imposed leaving of the supported accommodation, the CMHT referred Sandra to the Assertive Outreach team, as a vulnerable person who had repeatedly disengaged from services. After a protracted period of engaging and assessing needs and wants with Sandra, it was determined that a different risk-taking approach was warranted with her. This is set out as an example using the guiding format in Box 11.5.

Box 11.5   GUIDELINES FOR CONSIDERING AND DOCUMENTING 'POSITIVE RISK TAKING'

What are the service user's experiences and understanding of risk?

Sandra feels that she has been treated poorly at various times of her life, by family members, friends of her brother, and by the community services. She feels she has been exploited for sex and her benefits money.

What are the carers' experiences and understanding of risk?

Her brother is very abusive and aggressive towards every one in hospital and community services. He states that they should not interfere with the family, and all the problems are caused by workers who are 'snooping around where they do not belong'.

What risks does the person wish to take?

Sandra is clear that she wants her own flat close to her boyfriend's, and to be allowed to get on with her own life. She does not see this as a risk but states that she would keep contact with the Assertive Outreach team if they could help her have her own place to live.

What are the desired outcomes?

That she could sustain a lifestyle of her own choosing whilst still sustaining regular contact with the Assertive Outreach team.

What strengths can be identified?

Sandra is very consistent and clear about her wishes. She has sustained positive relationships with people who do not impose judgements and standards on her, e.g. staff and other users of the drop-in. Her relationship with her boyfriend is unconventional, occasionally turbulent, but longstanding and generally warm and supportive. The Assertive Outreach team has established working relationships with all people close to Sandra, except her elder brother.

What are the planned stages (for risk taking)?

- Establish Sandra as a high priority for re-housing in the locality where her boyfriend lives.

box continued

- The Assertive Outreach team to work closely with Sandra to understand her daily living choices, and how she enacts them.
- To develop with Sandra a detailed package of intensive support that reflects her choices of where and how she wishes to live.
- Regular monitoring of how the support package is working, and the potential for Sandra to be exploited in the same ways as previously.
- Regular informal meetings with the people who Sandra sees the most.

What may be the pitfalls (including estimates of likelihood)?

Once she has her own accommodation there is a slight chance Sandra may disengage from the support of the Assertive Outreach team. It is felt to be slight because Sandra and much of her support network have developed a trust and liking for the Assertive Outreach workers' style and approach. Despite regular monitoring Sandra may still fall prey to local men who have used and exploited her previously.

Other parts of the statutory sector services retain their view that this is not the appropriate way forward, and that Sandra would be safer if she remained in supported accommodation for the longer term.

What safety nets (including crisis and contingency plans) can be identified?

- Sandra's closest supports do not wish her to be exploited as before, and will report any suspicions to the Assertive Outreach team.
- Sandra will have a mobile phone provided by the Assertive Outreach team, and a range of contact numbers to call in emergencies.
- She will be known by the whole team (not just one worker).
- An emergency bed can be arranged with a local voluntary sector agency who operate the drop-in, at reasonably short notice if the independent accommodation placement is breaking down or in need of respite for cleaning.

Early warning signs

- Experiencing an increasingly disturbed sleep pattern for three nights in succession. Sometimes linked to abusive contacts from her elder brother.
- Loss of appetite.
- Not answering the door, or the calls on the mobile phone during the next three days.
- Concerns expressed by Sandra's boyfriend that she is not her usual self.
- Remaining in bed for most of the day, feeling depressed.
- Hearing derogatory voices in her head.

What happened the last time this course of action was followed?

The last occasion that Sandra had her own independent accommodation was about 15 years ago, with no support that she felt was appropriate to her needs. Her self-neglect and neglect of the flat led to hospital admission and subsequent loss of the tenancy.

> **How was it managed?**
> The situation deteriorated with no support or help.
>
> **What needs to change and what can change?**
> The Assertive Outreach team can offer and co-ordinate a much more intensive and responsive package of support.
>
> **How will progress be monitored?**
> Daily visits by Assertive Outreach staff, with monitoring and communication through daily handover team meetings.
>
> **Who agrees to this approach?**
> Sandra, her boyfriend, one of her sisters, the Assertive Outreach team, consultant psychiatrist, and the voluntary sector drop-in service.
>
> **Date 1/7/02**
>
> **How and when reviewed**
> Daily handover meetings and six-monthly wider review.

CONCLUSIONS

We operate within the context of government legislation and a research agenda that remains more in tune with theoretical possibility, rather than practical reality and the experiences of service users who are served by flexible and creative teams (Graley-Wetherell and Morgan 2001). Within this scenario, Assertive Outreach faces the danger of becoming more narrowly associated with enforced restriction and compliance to medication regimes. Short-sighted expectations imply that if hard-to-engage people are closely policed and made to take their medication, risks to the public will be reduced. Assertive Outreach is potentially being set up to become the new face of the 'risk business', entrusted with the role of tracking resistant individuals and equipped with the mechanisms of coercion and enforcement. No consideration will be given to the reasons why people disengage, and service users' worst fears of 'aggressive outreach' will be fulfilled. The potential benefits of collaborative Assertive Outreach will be shattered as more people feel driven to greater extremes of service avoidance.

The challenge to service providers is to be more flexible and creative in their attempts to engage trusting relationships. It is not about reducing complicated social, cultural and environmental factors down to narrow identification of symptoms, risk factors and strategies for restrictive management. Assertive Outreach has a positive record of effectively linking the function of engagement to practical tasks and evidence-based clinical interventions. Flexible and creative services hold benefits for both service users and providers who engage within them. They also offer a constructive approach to managing risks (Box 11.6).

> **Box 11.6   Risk taking**
>
> To laugh is to risk appearing a fool.
> To weep is to risk appearing sentimental.
> To reach out for another is to risk involvement.
> To expose feelings is to risk exposing one's true self.
> To place your ideas, your dreams before the crowd is to risk their loss.
> To love is to risk not being loved in return.
> To live is to risk dying.
> To hope is to risk despair.
> To try is to risk failure.
> But all risks must be taken because the greatest hazard in life is to risk nothing.
> The person who risks nothing, does nothing, has nothing... is nothing.
> He may avoid suffering and sorrow but he simply cannot learn, feel, change, grow, love, live.
> Claimed by his certitude he is a slave.
> He has forfeited his freedom.
> Only a person who risks is free.
>
> (Anon)

References

Bingley W 1997 Assessing dangerousness: protecting the interests of patients. British Journal of Psychiatry 170 (Suppl 32): 28–29

Borum R 1996 Improving the clinical practice of violence risk assessment: technology, guidelines and training. American Psychologist 51 (9): 945–956

Carson D 1994 Risk-taking and Risk Assessment in Mental Disorder Services. Paper presented to Division of Psychiatry, Guy's and St Thomas' Medical School, 13th April

Carson D 1996 Risking legal repercussions. In: Kemshall H, Pritchard J (eds) Good Practice in Risk Assessment and Risk Management. Jessica Kingsley, London p 3–12

Department of Health 1999 A National Service Framework for Mental Health. The Stationery Office, London

Department of Health 2000 NHS Plan. HMSO, London

Department of Health 2001 Safety First. Five-Year Report of the National Confidential Inquiry into Suicide and Homicide by People with Mental Illness. HMSO, London

Dvoskin J A, Steadman H J 1994 Using intensive case management to reduce violence by mentally ill persons in the community. Hospital and Community Psychiatry 45 (7): 679–684

Graley-Wetherell R, Morgan S 2001 Active Outreach: An independent service user evaluation of a model of assertive outreach practice. Sainsbury Centre for Mental Health, London

Harrison G 1997 Risk assessment in a climate of litigation. British Journal of Psychiatry 170 (Suppl 32): 37–39

Hawton K 1994 The assessment of suicide risk. In: Barnes T R E, Nelson H E (eds) The Assessment of Psychoses: A Practical Handbook. Chapman & Hall, London, p 125–134

Huxley A 1932 Brave New World. Penguin, London

Maltsberger J T 1994 Calculated risks in the treatment of intractably suicidal patients. Psychiatry 57 (8): 199–212

Mason T, Chandley M 1999 Managing Violence and Aggression: A Manual for Nurses and Health Care Workers. Churchill Livingstone, Edinburgh

Monahan J, Steadman H J 1996 Violent storms and violent people. American Psychologist 51 (9): 931–938

Morgan S 1998 Assessing and Managing Risk: Practitioner's Handbook. Pavilion, Brighton

Morgan S 2000a Risk-making or risk-taking. Openmind 101: 16–17.

Morgan S 2000b Clinical Risk Management: A Clinical Tool and Practitioner Manual. Sainsbury Centre for Mental Health, London

Munro E, Rumgay J 2000 Role of risk assessment in reducing homicides by people with mental illness. British Journal of Psychiatry 176: 116–120

O'Rourke M, Bird L 2000 Risk Management in Mental Health. Mental Health Foundation, London

O'Rourke M, Hammond S 2000 Risk Management: Towards Safe, Sound and Supportive Services. Surrey and Hampshire Borders NHS Trust and South Thames Research and Development Fund

Philo G, Henderson L, McLaughlin G 1993 Mass Media
Representation of Mental Health/Illness. Report for the
Education Board of Scotland. Glasgow University Media
Group, Glasgow

Reed J 1997 Risk assessment and clinical risk management:
the lessons from recent inquiries. British Journal of
Psychiatry 170 (Suppl 32): 4–7

Rose N 1998 Living dangerously: risk-thinking and risk
management in mental health care. Mental Health Care
1 (8): 263–266

Roy D 1997 Clinical risk management: an emerging agenda
for psychiatry. Psychiatric Bulletin 21: 162–164

Sheppard D 1996 Learning the Lessons, 2nd edn. The Zito
Trust, London

Szmukler G 2000 Homicide inquiries. Psychiatric Bulletin
24: 6–10

Taylor P J, Gunn J 1999 Homicides by people with mental
illness: myth and reality. British Journal of Psychiatry
174: 9–14

Worthing Priority Care (1995) The Worthing Weighted Risk
Indicator. Worthing, Sussex

Chapter **12**

Practice–based evidence

Steve Morgan

From where you stand look back for the clues to a better future

INTRODUCTION

Throughout this book, we have endeavoured to offer glimpses of what strengths-based Assertive Outreach can look like in practice. The challenge that faces contemporary mental health services, in Assertive Outreach and all other service developments, is to consider how good ideas can be realistically translated into routine practice. "Mental health care has struggled with the notion of translating research into practice ever since it began to focus on treatment rather than segregation" (Dodd 2001). A potential strength for Assertive Outreach is its claim to be one of the most researched components of mental health service delivery (Mueser et al 1998, Stein and Santos 1998). The problem in the context of its research base arises from the diversity of evidence available, with a complex array of potential outcome measures. This can frequently result in service commissioners, managers, practitioners and service users describing their requirements of the service from different perspectives – focusing on service costs, medical outcomes, social outcomes or service satisfaction.

Warner et al (2001) provide valuable commentary on an expert panel report (Sainsbury Centre for Mental Health 2001), identifying a complex range of obstacles that challenge the potential for the workforce to accept the current radical agenda for change. "The discrepancy between the capabilities needed by the mental health workforce and their current capabilities needs to be urgently addressed in terms of training. But ensuring the right organisational culture, which enables staff to use their knowledge and practise their skills effectively, is equally important." Beyond the wealth of research underpinning the current trend to 'evidence-based practice', they rightly identify that effective implementation of ideas will be further influenced by local cultural factors, including local management structures, and even strong individual personalities.

Kitson et al (1998) reinforce the context of environmental culture and strength of leadership but raise further issues of staff attitudes influencing the way evidence is assimilated into a system, and a hierarchy of research methods which places emphasis on the academically driven sources of evidence above the experiences of service users and everyday practice. There is little doubt that a gulf exists between the worlds of research and practice, with many practitioners feeling unable or unwilling to access the messages of research, and in some cases feeling that their practice is or will be threatened by the need to change in order to deliver evidence-based practice. Training is seen as the key to implementing the evidence into practice. However, Morgan and Juriansz (2002a,b) argue that training alone will have only a minor impact, particularly because of its inability to address the complexity of issues outlined above, with its greater attention to academic credentials in the *workshop* than individual practice and team functioning in the *workplace*.

Presenting a more effective approach to the development and implementation of good practice requires all of the following ingredients (Box 12.1). Notably, research and training have a key role to play but not in the relative isolation of workshop and conference settings. The pivotal components to developing effective services are 'practice development' and 'practitioner/team reflection'. These are the mechanisms specifically focused on the realities of implementation, providing the foundations for *'practice-based evidence'*.

Box 12.1   Components of effective service implementation

- Understanding the messages from the 'research.'
- 'Training' initiatives linking research to specific service need.
- 'Practice development' initiatives to support the application of training.
- Adherence scales designed to monitor effective implementation.
- 'Supervision' and practitioner/team 'reflection.'
- Strengths-based 'tools.'
- The 'enabling' managerial context.

EVIDENCE–BASED PRACTICE

Dodd (2001) reminds us that "Practitioners need to be reassured that the interventions they give actually make a difference." The focus of evidence-based practice is driven by the ideals of identifying and examining what specific components of clinical practice and social functioning can be proved effective, and in what ways they should be delivered in order to maximize the benefits of interventions for service users. Mueser et al (1998) offer an extensive synthesis of worldwide (but predominantly US) research into models of intensive case management and assertive community treatment (ACT), offering significant evidence for a range of service and service user outcomes. More specifically focused on the strengths model, Marty et al (2001) report a remarkable level of agreement of 28 'expert' opinions on what constitutes the critical ingredients for effective delivery of the model of case management, with evidence for consistent positive outcomes through several studies.

With all the existing quantity of evidence available, and a strong message that 'fidelity to the model' is what ensures effective practice (Teague et al 1998), there should be little problem in replicating good services into the emerging picture of UK mental health practice. This is not the case for two specific reasons: firstly, Clement et al (2002) advise: "Some caution must be observed however in applying findings from the US to the European context, given that standard mental health care in Europe is very different to that available in the USA." Galvin (2000) offers a thorough critique of the evidence from the USA and subsequent debates in the UK mental health press, and identifies that many of the critical ingredients are non-culture specific, therefore applicable to UK settings, but that further enquiry is needed into the reasons why some UK attempts at implementation have proved less effective. Secondly, the detailed messages from the research are difficult for practitioners to access and implement without support beyond just hearing the message.

The need for this continuing examination through research methods is unquestionable. We have less need for replicating the types of research that already inform us of the broad range of critical ingredients. Burns and Firn (2002) remind us of a need to use research more specifically to determine the efficacy of individual elements and influences on clinical practice in the UK setting. However, Galvin (2000) also outlines the most recent debate where UK studies have challenged the efficacy of Assertive Outreach, and have been challenged in reply for failing to implement the model correctly in their research protocols. For the majority of busy practitioners this level of debate and disagreement is seen as being 'a spat between academics fighting for their own theoretical high ground', and of little significance to the realities of everyday practice. However, simplistic dismissal ignores the real impact that such research debates do have in influencing government and organizational agendas, and hence practice.

The message is important. However, what we do with the message determines the effectiveness of subsequent service development. Understanding the messages from the research offers a significant foundation for developing good practice. For evidence-based practice to be implemented more effectively will require a more enlightened appreciation that practitioners do not just need to be told the message through the medium of training, they also need more direct and practical help in the workplace to negotiate changes of practice that adopt and adapt the messages as appropriate. This is *'practice-based evidence'*, which contributes to enriching our knowledge of what works by combining the experience of daily practice with the experience of the research message.

TRAINING: COMMUNICATING THE MESSAGE

The issue about training needs to be seen from a strengths perspective: the question is not whether it is an effective instrument in service development but one of how to make it a *more* effective instrument. All too often training workshops will be based around the notion of the 'expert stance,' most usually with a presenter giving information to a passive audience. Models of practice and research outcomes are delivered to a diverse audience of people from different parts of a service or system, with different levels of prior knowledge. Discussion encouraged will be of a superficial nature, predominantly to support the importance of the 'message' that the research holds the key to practice. The result often leaves some people new to the subject area feeling enlightened as to the possibilities of change but with no confidence in how to initiate desired changes in services or to practice. For others who already held a degree of prior knowledge, the experience often leaves them further frustrated in that they have had no opportunity to take their level of knowledge beyond what it was, and still feel disabled in terms of implementing meaningful change.

The outline programme of a one-day workshop (Box 12.2) was presented by Steve Morgan in April 2001, and monitored (feedback notes) by David Juriansz. The participants were all from one local service in the UK. Whilst it is an attempt to make the experience more interactive through the predominant use of discussion and case studies, it is still unable to address the important next step of real implementation into practice, because the presenters would have no further contact with participants beyond the one-day workshop discussion (and a possible tutorial to support academic study). Frustration lies on both sides: from the participants' point of view it was expressed that it would have been useful to have a knowledgeable presenter working briefly in their service alongside them, to help implement the ideas raised. For the presenters, they would feel their job was more complete if they could follow the information through to confronting the realities of local implementation.

The workshop in Box 12.2 is structured to present an overview of the main issues for a mixed group of community-based and inpatient-based practitioners. The orientation of the lead presenter ensured that a strengths perspective informed the structure, content and subsequent discussions (he had also facilitated a workshop on the strengths approach for the same audience before this day and would be focusing more specifically on strengths assessment subsequently). The focus of sessions and main discussion points are listed in Box 12.3.

Box 12.2 Assertive Outreach (one-day workshop)

Learning outcomes

Participants will be given the opportunity to:

1. Describe the meaning and functions of Assertive Outreach.
2. Determine the target audience for Assertive Outreach services.
3. Develop strategies for engagement through a team approach.
4. Consider local needs for developing an Assertive Outreach function.

Session 1   Assertive Outreach exercise
09.30–10.50   (using exercise sheet)

- Introduction to the day.
- Begin with group's 'issues and expectations' on flipchart.
- Handout sheet with 10 questions for discussion.
- Gain feedback and pick up on specific questions.

Session 2   Defining client groups exercise
11.10–12.30   (using exercise sheet)

- Who should be prioritized to receive an Assertive Outreach approach?
- Use small groups exercise with case studies and flipchart analysis of '4 levels' (severe – complex – high risk – disengaged).
- Feedback and discussion in large group.

Session 3   Implementing a team approach exercise
13.30–14.50   (using exercise sheet)

- Exercise designed to help practitioners appreciate the challenges involved in working as a truly effective team.
- Using case studies plus exercise sheet and small group work.
- Feedback and discussion in large group.

Session 4   Local service development exercise
15.10–16.30   (using exercise sheet)

- Exercise to help practitioners appreciate the challenges involved in developing an Assertive Outreach team/function in the local area.
- Use exercise sheet and small group work.
- Feedback and discussion in large group.

Questions to ask (session 4):

1. Is the 'local development' a team or a function?
2. How does it measure against essential components of the research literature?
3. What impact does the rural setting have on Assertive Outreach?

Box 12.3 Trainer's notes on the delivery of the day (David Juriansz)

Session 1

1. Policy overview – why assertive outreach is effective; cost factors; cornerstone of mental health policy.
2. Research overview, including PRiSM and UK700, both concluding that Assertive Outreach is no more effective than standard care.
3. Opportunity for issues and expectations raised by the audience.
4. Small groups – 'What is Assertive Outreach?'

Some relevant issues raised:

- Implications of Assertive Outreach for Community Mental Health Teams 'picking up the dregs'!
- Need to tap into activity – practical and functional help. Suited to occupational therapists – other team members needing to work in this way.
- Care and control issues.
- Assertive Outreach teams don't get rid of hospital beds. About helping disengaged clients.

Session 2

- Who is Assertive Outreach for?
- Flipchart analysis – use of priority groups targeting – 4 levels (severe and enduring mental health, complex needs, high risk, disengaged people).
- Discussion of case studies in small groups (Wesley – appropriate for Assertive Outreach; Colin – excluded because of 'personality disorder').
- Lively feedback from groups. Discussion about dual diagnosis – inclusion in Assertive Outreach?

Session 3

1. Team approach.
2. Introduction.
3. Exercise 2, and explain task for small groups (30 minutes).
4. Case study: Shirley (and Brian).

Issues raised:

- Group came back with practical things for Shirley – better childcare, etc., interventions to manage stress.
- Good large group discussion about personalities, attitudes in teams and the abilities to deliver practical interventions.
- Anecdotal evidence about doctors mucking in to clean up mess (Steve's 'marigolds').

Session 4
Small groups – local service development issues (30 minutes).

General issues raised:

- No close policy – how to deal with full Assertive Outreach caseloads.
- Waiting for people to fit into our criteria – are we failing them?
- Evidence-based randomized controlled trials versus user perspectives.
- Need for practice-based evidence.

Specific local issues:

- Separate Manager of CMHT and Assertive Outreach teams (less than ideal).
- On CMHTs – intensive support for more care co-ordination clients – feels like Assertive Outreach!
- Intranet available but how do staff find out all this information? 'You have to seek it yourself.' 'Evidence-based practice' group being set up but difficult to disseminate information.

This programme (see Box 12.3) illustrates the dilemma training faces: a good deal of 'expert knowledge' was communicated, discussed and explored, but what next? How did it help the participants to go away and actually put into practice what they had heard and discussed?

One possible solution that has been extensively attempted would be to develop a more detailed programme, tailored for a specific Assertive Outreach team. Such a programme may well spread across five or ten days and would enjoy the benefit of being able to tailor its content to meet the more detailed evidence of specific processes and interventions related to Assertive Outreach, e.g. an Assertive Outreach training content of engagement and assessment, relapse prevention, crisis intervention, dual diagnosis, medication management and family interventions. Each of these would last one day, totalling six days in all.

However, the same issues arise regarding implementation of evidence into practice. Workshops can be packed with useful information and discussion but they still do not usually involve the presenters or facilitators 'outreaching' into the workplace to examine and support the difficulties of real implementation. Reliance is still left entirely on the practitioners (including team managers) to grapple with the issues of implementation by themselves, often whilst having to maintain some kind of existing service.

The argument from trainers may well be that issues of implementation are local to the service, and as such should be managed by the local service itself. However, this cuts little ice where the people delivering the message also portray 'fidelity to the model' as some kind of inflexible mantra – and failure to comply implies some level of service failure to be shouldered by practitioners. Maybe if presenters spent just a little more time experiencing the realities of the service they are preaching about they may realize the importance of bending the message to accommodate local factors, without losing the value of the message. They might just have to alter their own views on the message itself, in the light of the evidence generated by the interface of ordinary service users and ordinary practitioners. This is practice-based evidence.

PRACTICE DEVELOPMENT AND PRACTICE–BASED EVIDENCE

The term 'practice development' is widely used in mental health practice with very little clarity about what it really means. Garbett and McCormack (2002) applied a concept analysis approach to existing published literature, and individual and group interviews. As a result, they identified practice development to be a systematic and rigorous activity underpinned by facilitation processes, with intended outcomes of changes in the behaviours, values and beliefs of the staff involved. Their definition will be adopted here: "…a continuous process of improvement towards increased effectiveness in patient-centred care. This is brought about by helping healthcare teams to develop their knowledge and skills and to transform the culture and context of care. It is enabled and supported by facilitators committed to systematic, rigorous continuous processes of emancipatory change that reflects the perspectives of service users."

In considering the conditions that would most likely support effective implementation of evidence-based practice, Kitson et al (1998) suggested that the context or culture of the service, and the nature of skilled facilitation, will be as important as the research evidence itself. In close harmony with these ideas, Dodd (2001) reminds us that "The development of assertive outreach is based on sound evidence, but the process of implementation of 'evidence based practice' is extremely complex, and needs a strategic approach to ensure practitioners can deliver effective models." Such a strategic process is unlikely to be established in a workshop alone, and service managers are frequently as ill informed as the practitioners regarding the details of contemporary advances in services such as Assertive Outreach.

The answer lies in the skilled workshop facilitators following through their role into the workplace. The experience of Morgan and Juriansz (2002b) with CMHTs was initially developed from work in the field of Assertive Outreach. The approach to facilitation, applied to a rigorously constructed process of practice development, has been found to promote an environment where practitioners feel more valued for their ideas, and where development reflects individual needs and those of the team. Greater initiative, self-reliance and motivation were reported from these approaches. Garbett and McCormack (2002) suggest this approach not only promotes the optimal conditions for evidence-based practice to be assimilated but that it also fits well with the government agenda for improved quality of services through clinical governance (Department of Health 1998).

Examples of implementing Assertive Outreach in the recent UK literature emphasize the importance of the messages from research, and the need for good-quality training (Ford and McClelland 2002, Greatley and Ford 2002), but there is no mention of practice development and skilled facilitation in the workplace. A gap remains between delivering the message to the practitioners and the practitioners delivering the most effective service to the service users. Practice development offers the hitherto elusive answers to the 'application to implementation' conundrum, through flexible adaptation of good ideas (Morgan and Juriansz 2002a,b).

Much evidence-based practice flows in one direction: communication about the research services presented in various ways to other services. A further essential element that contributes to practice-based evidence is the lessons to be learned from the service users themselves. Dodd (2001) suggests that "Qualitative data can highlight some of the richest and most thought-provoking experiences that can affect practice, but is often undervalued by practitioners, who may assume the myth that academia is uninterested in people's stories." The emphasis within this statement should shift more from the practitioners to the academics. It is not just an assumption as academics do show an interest in people's stories but only as a lower level of evidence than the 'gold standard' of randomized controlled trials and other forms of academic interest.

Ryan et al (1999) report on an earlier study, one of the first to incorporate an independent service user evaluation of its emerging model of practice. The overall outcomes of the service were variable, with very positive responses to engagement and service linkages, and less consistent outcomes in hospital bed reductions and cost-effectiveness. However, the service user views reported by Beeforth et al (1994) were found to be valuable. The study by Graley-Wetherell and Morgan (2001) of the Active Outreach team in Julian Housing, Norwich, amplifies the importance of hearing the service user's voice when we consider the effectiveness of models of practice. The richness of their messages is not picked up in the more usual satisfaction measures of research reports. Hopkins (2002), in reference to this latter study, suggests "…if users are to be truly at the centre of services, their views should be central to any evaluation of those services."

THE ROLE OF ADHERENCE SCALES

The two approaches that have been most refined in terms of developing model adherence scales, and which have received most dissemination, are those of McGrew and Bond (1995) and Teague et al (1998). Both approaches have used the same 'expert panel' approach for their development: a listing of all the critical features of Assertive Outreach is generated; an expert panel of 20 or so 'experts in the field' is convened, and asked to rate the relative importance of the contribution of each 'critical feature' to the ACT model; the responses of the 'expert panel' are analysed, critical features of the model where there are high levels of agreement are retained, and those with lower levels of agreement rejected.

Both these approaches have been generated in the USA, and therefore reflect US assumptions concerning service structures and systems, and staff groupings and categories, which are current in the USA but not necessarily in the UK.

Both McGrew and Bond and Teague et al organize their ACT model around three major factors:

- staffing/human resources
- organizational systems and structures
- specific service components including intensity and location of delivery.

In transferring their model to a UK policy and practice environment, it needs to be recognized that there are major staffing and service system differences between the two countries, which render a literal transfer of every element of the US model difficult if not impossible. Firstly, the configuration of the mental health workforce is different in the two countries. As an example, a role has to be found in the UK for occupational therapy, a profession for which there is no direct equivalent in the USA. Equally, Teague's requirement to have one full-time equivalent vocational rehabilitation specialist on every ACT is difficult to implement in the UK, as such specialists are very thin on the ground.

So far as organizational systems and structures are concerned, in the UK it is difficult to directly implement the 'team approach' with shared team caseload responsibility, since the National Service Framework clearly endorses the principle of individual accountability through the CPA care co-ordinator system.

In terms of the third component of the model, concerned with specific service elements, there is probably more transferability here. However, even in this area, there are likely to be difficulties in achieving high levels of adherence with respect to the intensity and duration of delivery. Evidence from a number of recent UK research studies would suggest that many UK Assertive Outreach teams might struggle to achieve the recommended contact levels of three or four home visits per week, with about two hours per week of direct contact time.

For all these reasons, serious thought needs to be given as to what adjustments to the US model need to be made in order for it to be applicable in the UK policy and practice environment. The Department of Health's Policy Implementation Guide (Department of Health 2001) has done precisely this, and has articulated a model of Assertive Outreach for UK policy and practice conditions; see also Ryan (2001) for a practice development approach to adherence. Viewed from this perspective, applying an adherence scale can be useful. It can give detailed information about what specific organizational and service intervention ingredients are seen as necessary. These can then be used to critically examine and reflect upon how best they can be translated into practice. By using an adherence scale as a guide to critical and reflective practice (see below), they can serve a useful function in translating theory into practice.

SUPERVISION AND REFLECTION

It is the philosophy of practice-based evidence that truly effective changes to clinical practice, in line with the messages from the research, can only be achieved through the sharper focus offered by a presence alongside practitioners and teams in their daily routines. This requires a facilitative style of supervision, prompting practitioners to reflect on and change identified aspects of individual and team practice. It requires much the same approach as would be expected in the work with individual service users:

- engaging a trusting relationship with practitioners and teams
- establishing a baseline of current knowledge, skills and attitudes
- reflecting existing strengths and good practice
- suggesting, modelling and supporting ideas for change
- monitoring and measuring changes.

The challenges for successful implementation require the manager of the process to perform many of the following functions (though this is not an exhaustive list):

- being a regular presence, working alongside people, as time and consistency are essential elements in the change process
- supporting all functions of the team and all team members, managerial and clinical (supporting the team leader, not taking over), and providing a trusting impartial conscience and inquisitor within the team
- chairing meetings, to propose changes through constructive discussion, e.g. implementing a strengths approach within a broadly problems-oriented culture (Box 12.4)
- shadowing and co-working a range of planned and unplanned interventions (assuming the roles of guide and mentor, as required) – What are the aims of a specific contact? What if it doesn't go to plan? What contingency plans do you have in place? What have you learned after the event?
- encouraging active personal reflection through a process of in vivo supervision
- reviewing the administrative process of care, e.g. note-keeping and other forms of required documentation
- reviewing existing policies and procedures, e.g. CPA and risk management, defined client groups and caseload management
- identifying and working with resistance
- providing copies of relevant educational materials, e.g. articles, references and clinical tools
- providing in vivo training that responds to the immediate needs of the individuals or teams in a client-centred way, rather than planning a series of training workshops to fulfil a predetermined programme in a service-centred way
- promoting service user involvement and evaluation, as well as practice development manager reports of progress and evaluation.

Box 12.4   Case example: team meetings

Baseline issue for change

A team identifies that it is not using its regular multidisciplinary meeting very effectively. It generally starts late, people often avoid it by double-booking other work, and the atmosphere is one of poor motivation and passive resistance from the majority, and dominance of discussion and decisions by a small minority of people. A decision is made that the meeting is vitally important to the team but needs to be reviewed with the intention of improving its effectiveness.

The options considered are to access 'training' around team meetings or to introduce a 'practice development' change process.

Training option

The team leader investigates options for a training solution. Very little opportunity arises to access a conference or external course that will focus specifically on the need to review team meetings. Contact with the organization's own training department indicates that a half-day workshop is run once every three months centrally within the organization, with spaces available for staff in the team to be nominated to attend.

The team leader asks for the workshop to be run within the team, for the whole team. This is not seen as a priority for the finite resources of the training department but the compromise solution is for the team to nominate four of its 12 staff to attend the next session.

The half-day workshop covers a range of different types of meeting that occur in teams, broadly discusses the roles and functions of team meetings, and finishes with a one-hour discussion between all participants about their experiences from their own parts of the service. The participants attending were from all parts of the organization's clinical and administrative/managerial sections; consequently, the content remained very general.

The four team members reported their experience at the next team meeting. No specific solutions to the team's needs were identified and the outcome was little change to the structure and atmosphere of the meetings.

Practice development option

An external practice development consultancy was invited to sit in and observe/review the working of the team meeting. All team members were briefly interviewed about their views and ideas for the meeting. The practice development worker put together proposals for change, which were discussed with the team leader initially, then the whole team. The practice development worker agreed to chair the meetings for a period of a couple of months, to support the implementation of changes. At the point of subsequent review of the changes, three existing team members volunteered to take on the chairing role, with support and supervision from the practice development worker.

> At the collective review, all staff agreed that the team meeting could always be improved in different ways. The response to the practice development initiative has been a major internal review of the meeting in relation to other team functions. Attendance and participation are both greatly increased.
>
> NB The above scenario is based on a real example of the author's work with a CMHT in north London. The ideas of 'group supervision' (see Chapter 5) can be introduced to this process, in order to promote more creative responses to the needs and functions of the team meeting, where appropriate.

STRENGTHS 'TOOLS'

As a starting point for identifying practitioner strengths in relation to Assertive Outreach work, one of the authors has recrafted a strengths assessment tool to meet the needs of interviewing individual practitioners. The tool (Fig. 12.1) is also accompanied by written guidelines (Box 12.5) for use within team workplace and/or workshop settings. Further tools have been adapted to Assertive Outreach, for identifying individual responses to team development needs – Creative Capability Interview Parts 1 and 2 (these have been developed through Practice Based Evidence by Steve Morgan, based on work with David Juriansz in community mental health teams: Morgan and Juriansz 2002b).

Figure 12.1 Active/Assertive Outreach

'Staff' strengths assessment

Area 1: Applying 'values' and 'principles' of strengths-based practice

Past achievement:

Current skills & knowledge:

Future aspiration:

Area 2: Imaginative 'collaborations' with service users and agencies

Past achievement:

figure continues

Current skills & knowledge:

Future aspiration:

Area 3: Implementing 'creative' and 'flexible' ideas in practice

Past achievement:

Current skills & knowledge:

Future aspiration:

Area 4: Experiencing and/or managing 'team approaches' in practice

Past achievement:

Current skills & knowledge:

Future aspiration:

Area 5: A relevant knowledge base drawing on 'theory' and 'practice'

Past achievement:

Current skills & knowledge:

Future aspiration:

Personal priorities for development
(from 'aspirations' above)

Outline desired outcomes, timescales for achievement and potential 'resources'/'allocation of responsibilities' needed for success

1
2

Staff member: _____   Period of assessment: _____

© Steve Morgan – Practice-based evidence

Box 12.5   Active/Assertive Outreach

Guide to using 'Staff strengths assessment'

General guidance

- The exercise is usually to be performed through the medium of a one-to-one interview but can be something built up through personal reflection.
- The task does not have to be completed under the time pressure of a one-off interview but may be comfortably completed in a short time in some circumstances.
- The process is not one of attempting to document long lists. It will benefit from reflection on several experiences and ideas but needs to arrive at one preferred option in each section of each area. Do not feel pressured into having to document the first idea that arises in each section. The process of interviewing is intended to enable deeper reflection.
- Read and understand the requirements of all five areas and the final priorities before launching into the first area of discussion.
- Reflect on and discuss the five areas in any order you, the interviewee, wish.
- All 'Future aspiration' sections should be completed as far as possible. However, other sections across each area may occasionally be left blank, where appropriate (note in these sections that careful consideration has been made even though nothing specifically has been currently identified).
- A strengths assessment is about identifying and noting positive statements and ideas. Problems/difficulties may be discussed in interview but only if they help to clarify a positive point or strength.

box continues

- Future aspirations and priorities can be related to you personally and/or the wider 'team.' However, team actions need to include you in any identified changes or actions.
- When the five future aspirations have been identified, the interviewee (with help from the interviewer) should review all five with the intention of identifying two priorities for developing detailed actions.
- Documented action on the priorities should result from careful and detailed analysis, not on noting down the first ideas to arise. Actions should be imaginative and achievable (first ideas and simple solutions can often be the best).

Specific areas

1. 'Values' and 'principles':

- Focus on the uniqueness of the Active Outreach approach, as you know or believe it to be.
- Think about how values and principles really influence routine practice not just their intellectual currency in academic or theoretical discussion.

2. 'Collaborations':

- Focus on imaginative ways of 'engaging' the service user in the working relationship. Include consideration of ways that may provide real service user involvement.
- Consider the need for addressing the engagement of other parts of the 'system' (health and broader social considerations).
- Consider the imaginative potential for longterm disengagement of service users from Active Outreach into resources that are real for their needs (i.e. not always back to CMHTs).

3. 'Creative' and 'flexible' ideas:

- Focus on the service user's personal needs and wishes and how the services respond to meet these.
- Considerations should not rely on mental health resources unless the service user has specified the wish for them.
- Consider 'how' ideas have been enabled to develop uniquely to individual circumstances and not so widely to several people or teams.

4. 'Team approaches':

- Focus on examples or ideas of good team working. There is no specific blueprint to restrict your consideration of what a team approach is or should be.
- Consider what qualities you identify as representing good teams.

5. 'Knowledge base':

- Consider what people need to do their job to the fullest potential as individuals and as teams.

> • Appreciate the importance of theoretical knowledge/applied research, and equally the importance of everyday practice for informing us of what works, and how.
>
> © Steve Morgan – Practice-based evidence

The 'Creative Capability Interview Part 1' tool (Fig. 12.2) is designed as a confidential individual interview, with practitioners being offered choices of one option from each category to discuss (or all categories, depending on time), reflecting personally on the current state and needs for change across the team. It is not meant to be a tool for interrogation of individual practice.

Figure 12.2   Creative capability interviews

Creative Capability Interview: Part 1
(Active/Assertive Outreach)

Ethical practice

1. Working with 'service users' should be primarily about respecting individual difference, and promoting their right to make choices about individual needs and care.

2. Workers in teams need to possess values that promote 'acceptance,' 'patience,' 'commitment' to the individual, and challenge some of the more rigid orthodoxies of mental health service delivery.

Care process

3. 'Engagement' and 'assessment' of the service user's strengths and personal motivations is the most important foundation of collaborative working.

4. 'Creativity' and 'flexibility' should be the most essential considerations underpinning all aspects of working relationships.

Team working

5. The 'capabilities' of a team will be maximized through developing robust mechanisms of collaborative working across the whole team.

6. Good 'service' and 'team' leadership requires a strong commitment to a clear and unified purpose.

Knowledge in practice

7. Practical experience with service users is equally as valid for informing good practice as the messages from research.

8. Knowledge and experience should be openly shared within local teams, and across wider services.

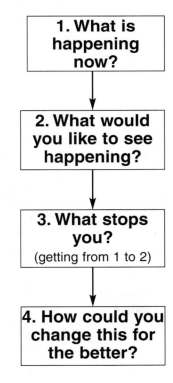

1. What is happening now?

2. What would you like to see happening?

3. What stops you? (getting from 1 to 2)

4. How could you change this for the better?

© Steve Morgan – Practice-based evidence

figure continues

Creative Capability Interview: Part 2
(Active/Assertive Outreach)

Ethical practice	1. Service users determine the 'priorities' for the working relationship	DISAGREE 1 2 3 4 AGREE 5
	2. As a team, we regularly examine and review the impact of our values and principles on practice	DISAGREE 1 2 3 4 AGREE 5

Care process	3. Time for creative approaches to engagement is a priority	DISAGREE 1 2 3 4 AGREE 5
	4. Our assessment of needs includes the identification of service user strengths	DISAGREE 1 2 3 4 AGREE 5
	5. We identify and manage the broad range of risks effectively and positively	DISAGREE 1 2 3 4 AGREE 5
	6. Our working practice draws on a broad range of practical and research-based approaches	DISAGREE 1 2 3 4 AGREE 5

Team working	7. The 'management team' are clear about the 'purpose' of AO	DISAGREE 1 2 3 4 AGREE 5
	8. We are clear about our 'purpose' in the local AO team	DISAGREE 1 2 3 4 AGREE 5
	9. The local AO team has a clear model of team working	DISAGREE 1 2 3 4 AGREE 5
	10. We link effectively with other parts of the mental health system (including primary care)	DISAGREE 1 2 3 4 AGREE 5
	11. We have good systems of support and supervision	DISAGREE 1 2 3 4 AGREE 5

Knowledge in practice	12. We access and use practical as well as theoretical knowledge and experience within the local AO team	DISAGREE 1 2 3 4 AGREE 5
	13. We share skills, knowledge and expertise across the AO service	DISAGREE 1 2 3 4 AGREE 5

[Circle the three numbers that correspond to the priorities you feel need addressing]

© Steve Morgan – Practice-based evidence

The 'Creative Capability Interview Part 2' tool (see Fig. 12.2) is designed as a measurement of change across time. Each individual rates the team currently against 13 positive statements of practice, using a Likert Scale of 1–5 Disagree–Agree. The whole team responses can be amalgamated for one point in time, and compared at subsequent intervals, to identify whether targeted training and practice development have achieved any positive changes in the perceptions of team functioning.

MANAGEMENT BY ENABLING

Buckingham and Clifton (2002) suggest that "The great organisation must not only accommodate the fact that each employee is different, it must capitalise on these differences. It must watch for clues to each employee's natural talents and then position and develop each employee so that his or her talents are transformed into bona fide strengths." We spend too much time defining a role and then appointing people into the roles with a subsequent need for training in order to meet the requirements. We are not identifying and making sufficient use of individual personal strengths in relation to the roles we define. A more radical proposal would be to identify personal strengths first, and then build the functional roles around the individuals. In this way we might begin to receive positive answers to the following question of our staff members: "At work do you have the opportunity to do what you do best everyday?" The Gallup Organization has devoted 30 years to asking this question of 1.7 million people worldwide, in all types of business activity, and only approximately 20% of people interviewed could answer Yes (Buckingham and Clifton 2002).

Buckingham and Clifton (2002) suggest that most organizations appear to be operating by two flawed assumptions:

1. Each person can learn to be competent in almost anything.
2. Each person's greatest room for growth is in his or her areas of greatest weakness.

At best, these assumptions lead to individuals raising their poorer standards of performance to levels of acceptance or mediocrity but rarely any further. If we wish to set our sights on achieving excellence, we need to accept the challenge of focusing our efforts on the following assumptions:

1. Each person's talents are enduring and unique.
2. Each person's greatest room for growth is in the areas of his or her greatest strength.

These assumptions should be equally applied by practitioners to service users, and by organizations to their practitioners. In this way the previous strengths assessment tool can be applied for practitioners in much the same way as we would expect practitioners to apply strengths assessment for service users (see Chapter 8).

Another aspect of an enabling management culture is described by Rapp (1998) as the 'inverted hierarchy'. In this scenario, the human resources organizational map takes the opposite appearance to what you would traditionally expect. In this instance, the service users are at the top of the tree, with Assertive Outreach workers, team managers and service management on successive steps downward. We would usually expect to see the service manager at the top with service users at the bottom of such a diagram. What this represents in practice is the need to see practitioners as servants of the service users. Similarly, the function of service management is to act as servants to the practitioners. The new function of management becomes that of serving practitioners through creating the right environment and resources for them to do their jobs to the maximum effectiveness, through:

- providing direction
- providing tools
- removing obstacles and constraints
- establishing a reward-based environment.

(Rapp 1998)

It is not the role of leadership, as identified through the constant stream of administrative directives that more frequently hinder effectiveness. A leadership function can be accommodated in the instance where an individual, team or service requires external direction. The skilled manager is one who understands that good management is about giving guidance but then standing back in a permissive role, only intervening where their skill and knowledge is needed. The skill is to be aware of the need for flexibility of response to different practitioner needs and in different situations. In its fully evolved form, it would take on more of the role of the facilitator outlined earlier in 'Practice development'.

CONCLUSIONS

The dominant stance of research and training in recent decades has led to one of the great paradoxes in mental health practice: it has successfully challenged practitioners to examine the quality and efficacy of what they do, whilst simultaneously letting them down when it comes to the all-important support for implementing good practice. The academically oriented minds that populate the world of research and training have largely opted to stay physically removed from the inconsistencies and challenges of gritty reality. They occupy a comfortable place where models and theories can be developed with clean edges and symmetry, and tools can be developed to help replicate so-called reality in 'experimental' conditions. The results are often important messages for practitioners to hear but the lack of any support following the delivery of 'the message' through training initiatives does very little to promote the high-class services that service users are entitled to (Morgan and Juriansz 2002a).

The primary source of failure lies in the disconnection between the artificially created world of research and training, and the real world of practice. Conferences and workshops have the occasional ability to energize staff through the messages of 'what could be', raising their personal expectations and those of others (service users, carers, managers, commissioners and politicians). However, they are left to interpret these messages for themselves, within the reality of the complexity of their own service resources and configurations. Messages about 'fidelity to the model' (Teague et al 1998, Hemming et al 1999) are well intentioned but often serve only to further frustrate practitioners who cannot replicate the research picture rigidly prescribed.

The true failure lies not so much with the practitioners who could not meet the 'requirements of fidelity' but with the researchers and trainers who do not follow the message through into the complexities of implementation. The requirement for practitioners to attend the workshop or forum needs to be matched by the requirement for those delivering the message to attend the workplace, i.e. practice-based evidence (Morgan and Juriansz 2002b). By working alongside practitioners in the workplace, the important factors that contribute to good practice can be better tailored to the situations that arise.

References

Beeforth M, Conlan E, Graley R 1994 Have We Got Views For You: User Evaluation of Case Management. Sainsbury Centre for Mental Health, London

Buckingham M, Clifton D O 2002 Now, Discover your Strengths: How to Develop Your Talents and Those of the People You Manage. Simon & Schuster, London

Burns T, Firn M 2002 Assertive Outreach in Mental Health: A manual for practitioners. Oxford University Press, Oxford

Clement S, Freeman J, Ford K et al 2002 Assertive Outreach in the North East, Yorkshire and Humberside. Northern Centre for Mental Health, Durham, UK

Department of Health 1998 Clinical Governance: Quality in the New NHS. HMSO, London

Department of Health 2001 The Mental Health Policy Implementation Guide. HMSO, London

Dodd T 2001 Clues about evidence for mental health care in community settings: Assertive Outreach. Mental Health Practice 4 (7): 10–14

Ford K, McClelland N 2002 Assertive Outreach: development of a working model. Nursing Standard 16 (23): 41–44

Galvin S 2000 Justifying the use of a model for assertive community treatment: a critical appraisal of the effectiveness literature. Unpublished working paper, Local Health Partnerships NHS Trust. (Copies available from Ipswich Outreach Team, 72 Foundation Street, Ipswich, Suffolk IP4 1BN)

Garbett R, McCormack B 2002 A concept analysis of practice development. Nursing Times 7 (2): 87–100

Graley-Wetherell R, Morgan S 2001 Active Outreach: An independent service user evaluation of a model of assertive outreach practice. Sainsbury Centre for Mental Health, London

Greatley A, Ford R 2002 Out of the Maze: Reaching and Supporting Londoners with Severe Mental Health Problems. King's Fund and Sainsbury Centre for Mental Health, London

Hemming M, Morgan S, O'Halloran P 1999 Assertive Outreach: implications for the development of the model in the United Kingdom. Journal of Mental Health 8 (2): 141–147

Hopkins G 2002 Research into practice. Community Care, 5–11 December: 45

Kitson A, Harvey G, McCormack B 1998 Enabling the implementation of evidence based practice: a conceptual framework. Quality in Health Care 7: 149–158

Marty D, Rapp C A, Carlson L 2001 The experts speak: the critical ingredients of strengths model case management. Psychiatric Rehabilitation Journal 24 (3): 214–221

McGrew J, Bond G 1995 Critical ingredients of assertive community treatment: judgements of the experts. Journal of Mental Health Administration 22 (2): 113–125

Morgan S, Juriansz D 2002a Practice based evidence. Openmind 114: 12–13

Morgan S, Juriansz D 2002b Uncovering creative capability. Mental Health Today, July: 25–28

Mueser K T, Bond G R, Drake R E et al 1998 Models of community care for severe mental illness: a review of research on case management. Schizophrenia Bulletin 24 (1): 37–73

Rapp C A 1998 The Strengths Model: Case Management with People Suffering from Severe and Persistent Mental Illness. Oxford University Press, New York

Ryan P 2001 Project 2 in Doctoral Submission. Middlesex University, London

Ryan P, Ford R, Beadsmoore A et al 1999 The enduring relevance of case management. British Journal of Social Work 29: 97–125

Sainsbury Centre for Mental Health 2001 Comparing the Capabilities of the Mental Health Workforce with the Capable Practitioner Framework. The capable practitioner expert panel's report. Sainsbury Centre for Mental Health, London

Stein L, Santos A 1998 Assertive Community Treatment of Persons with Severe Mental Illness. Norton, New York

Teague G B, Bond G R, Drake M D 1998 Program fidelity in assertive community treatment: development and use of a measure. American Journal of Orthopsychiatry 68 (2): 216–232

Warner L, Hoadley A, Ford R 2001 Obstacle course. Health Service Journal, 4 October: 28–29

Index